Pharmacy Law and Practice

Third Edition

Jonathan Merrills
BPharm, BA, BA (Law), FRPharmS,
Barrister (Middle Temple)

and

Jonathan Fisher
BA, LLB (Cantab),
Barrister (Gray's Inn)

A complimentary reference book from the
Pharmacy Mutual Insurance Company

PMI – First for Pharmacists and Pharmacy Students

b

Blackwell
Science

© 1995, 1997, 2001 by J. Merrills and J. Fisher

Blackwell Science Ltd
Editorial Offices:
Osney Mead, Oxford OX2 0EL
25 John Street, London WC1N 2BS
23 Ainslie Place, Edinburgh EH3 6AJ
350 Main Street, Malden
    MA 02148 5018, USA
54 University Street, Carlton
    Victoria 3053, Australia
10, rue Casimir Delavigne
    75006 Paris, France

Other Editorial Offices:

Blackwell Wissenschafts-Verlag GmbH
Kurfürstendamm 57
10707 Berlin, Germany

Blackwell Science KK
MG Kodenmacho Building
7-10 Kodenmacho Nihombashi
Chuo-ku, Tokyo 104, Japan

Iowa State University Press
A Blackwell Science Company
2121 S. State Avenue
Ames, Iowa 50014-8300, USA

First edition published 1995
Reprinted 1996
Second edition published 1997
Reprinted 1998, 1999
Third edition published 2001
Transferred to digital print 2003

Set in 9.5/11.5pt Palatino
by DP Photosetting, Aylesbury, Bucks

Printed and bound in Great Britain by
Marston Lindsay Ross International,
Oxfordshire

DISTRIBUTORS
Marston Book Services Ltd
PO Box 269
Abingdon
Oxon OX14 4YN
(*Orders:* Tel: 01235 465500
        Fax: 01235 465555)
USA
Blackwell Science, Inc.
Commerce Place
350 Main Street
Malden, MA 02148 5018
(*Orders:* Tel: 800 759 6102
                781 388 8250
        Fax: 781 388 8255)
Canada
Login Brothers Book Company
324 Saulteaux Crescent
Winnipeg, Manitoba R3J 3T2
(*Orders:* Tel: 204 837-2987
        Fax: 204 837-3116)

Australia
Blackwell Science Pty Ltd
54 University Street
Carlton, Victoria 3053
(*Orders:* Tel: 03 9347 0300
        Fax: 03 9347 5001)

A catalogue record for this title
is available from the British Library

ISBN 0-632-05932-X

Library of Congress
Cataloging-in-Publication Data

Merrills, Jonathan.
    Pharmacy law and practice/J. Merrills,
J. Fisher. — 3rd ed.
        p. cm.
    Includes bibliographical references and
index.
    ISBN 0-632-05932-X
    1. Pharmacy — Law and legislation —
Great Britain.   2. Drugs — Law and
legislation — Great Britain.   3. Pharmacists
— Legal status, laws, etc. — Great Britain.
I. Fisher, Jonathan.   II. Title.

KD2968.P4 M47 2001
344.41'0416 — dc21

                                2001037520

For further information on
Blackwell Science, visit our website:
www.blackwell-science.com

Contents

Preface to the Third Edition

When we wrote the first edition, our object was to describe the law rather than just list the Acts, regulations and cases which make up the law applying to community pharmacy.

That is still our object, but to achieve it in the face of the volume of new laws affecting pharmacy has meant a complete rewrite of the book for the third edition. As always there had to be a compromise between including everything we would have liked, and producing a readable text.

Once again we have concentrated on the laws which apply to community pharmacy and we have extended into other areas only where we consider it relevant to the community pharmacist. Although community pharmacists sometimes deal with agricultural products and veterinary medicines, we have generally left out the detailed laws in these areas. Instead we have included sections on the law which affects day to day practice as a pharmacist.

We have sought to produce an accessible text for both the community pharmacist and the pharmacy student. Any errors are ours – we hope there are none.

New challenges continue to confront the community pharmacist and we hope that this book will be a useful companion in meeting those challenges.

The law is stated as at 1 June 2001.

Jon Merrills
Jonathan Fisher

Table of Cases

The following abbreviations of law reports are used:

AC   Law Reports Appeal Cases Series
All ER   All England Law Reports
App Cas   Law Reports, Appeal Cases
Ch   Law Reports, Chancery Division
COD   Crown Office Digest
CMLR   Common Market Law Reports
ECJ   European Court of Justice
EG   Estates Gazette
Ex D   Law Reports, Exchequer Division
ICR   Industrial Cases Reports
IRLR   Industrial Relations Law Reports
LS Gaz   Law Society Gazette
KB   Law Reports, King's Bench Division
QB   Law Reports, Queen's Bench Division
SJ   Solicitors' Journal
WLR   Weekly Law Reports

Table of Statutes

*Asterisked Acts have been totally repealed.

Table of Statutory Instruments

List of Abbreviations

ABPI	Association of the British Pharmaceutical Industry
ABRHP	Advisory Board on the Registration of Homeopathic Products
ACBS	Advisory Committee on Borderline Substances
ACD	Advisory Committee on Drugs
ACMD	Advisory Council on the Misuse of Drugs
AHA	Area Health Authority
AHA(T)	Area Health Authority (Teaching)
ANPN	Appropriate Non-proprietary Name
BAN	British Approved Name
BMA	British Medical Association
BNF	British National Formulary
BP	British Pharmacopoeia
BPC	British Pharmaceutical Codex
CD	Controlled Drug
CDSM	Committee on Dental and Surgical Materials
CHC	Community Health Council
CHImp	Commission for Health Improvement
CPMP	Committee for Proprietary Medicinal Products
COSHH	Control of Substances Hazardous to Health (Regs)
CRC	Child Resistant Container
CRM	Committee on Review of Medicines
CSA	Central Services Authority
CSAG	Central Standards Advisory Group
CSM	Committee on Safety of Medicines
DGM	District General Manager
DoH	Department of Health
DHA	District Health Authority
DHSS	Department of Health and Social Services
DMU	Directly Managed Unit
DPB	Dental Practice Board
DPF	Dental Practitioners' Formulary
DT	Drug Tariff
EC	European Community
ECJ	European Court of Justice
EEC	European Economic Community
EMEA	European Medicines Evaluation Agency

EP	European Pharmacopeia
EU	European Union
FHSA	Family Health Services Authority
FPC	Family Practitioner Committee
FP10	Form used by GPs for NHS prescriptions
FSMPs	Food(s) for Special Medical Purposes
GDS	General Dental Services
GM	General Manager
GMP	General Medical Practitioner
GMS	General Medical Services
GP	General Practitioner
GSL	General Sale List
HA	Health Authority
HEA	Health Education Authority
HO	Home Office
HPC	Health Professions Council
HPSS	Health and Personal Social Services (Northern Ireland)
HSC	Health Services Circular
HSPG	Health and Social Policy Group (Northern Ireland)
HSSE	Health and Social Services Executive (Northern Ireland)
INN	International Non-proprietary Name
IPA	Indicative Prescribing Amount
LAC	Local Advisory Committee
LHCC	Local Health Care Co-operatives (Scotland)
LHG	Local Health Group (Wales)
LLP	Limited Liability Partnership
LMC	Local Medical Committee
LPC	Local Pharmaceutical Committee
MA	Medicines Acts
MAFF	Ministry of Agriculture, Fisheries and Food
MC	Medicines Commission
MCA	Medicines Control Agency
MDA	Misuse of Drugs Act; Medical Devices Agency
M(H)	Minister of Health
MHAC	Mental Health Advisory Committee
ML	Manufacturers Licence
MS	Manufacturer 'specials'
NHS	National Health Service
NHSE	National Health Service Executive
NHS & CC Act 1990	National Health Service and Community Care Act 1990
NHS MB	National Health Service Management Board
NHS SA	National Health Service Supplies Authority
NHS TA	National Health Service Training Authority
NMC	Nursing and Midwifery Council
OGL	Open General Licence
OTC	Over the Counter Medicine
OP	Original Pack
OPD	Original Pack Dispensing

P	Pharmacy Only Medicine
PAC	Public Accounts Committee
PACT	Prescribing Analysis & Cost
PCG	Primary Care Group
PCT	Primary Care Trust
PDC	Pharmaceutical Disciplinary Committee
PGD	Patient Group Direction
PHLS	Public Health Laboratory Service
PIL	Product Import Licence; Patient Information Leaflet
PL	Product Licence
PL(PI)	Product Licence (Parallel Import)
PMR	Patient Medication Record
POM	Prescription Only Medicine
PPA	Prescription Pricing Authority
PPRS	Pharmaceutical Price Regulation Scheme
PRP	Pharmacy Review Panel
PS	Pharmaceutical Services
PSC	Pharmaceutical Service Committee
PSNC	Pharmaceutical Services Negotiating Committee
PSNI	Pharmaceutical Society of Northern Ireland
RDC	Rural Dispensing Committee
RGM	Regional General Manager
RHA	Regional Health Authority
RP	Responsible Person
RPB	Retail Pharmacy Business
RPM	Resale Price Maintenance
RPSGB	Royal Pharmaceutical Society of Great Britain
SHA	Special Health Authority
SHHA	Special Hospitals Health Authority
SHHD	Scottish Home and Health Department
SMAC	Standing Medical Advisory Committee
SNMAC	Standing Nursing & Midwifery Advisory Committee
S of S	Secretary of State
SPAC	Standing Pharmaceutical Advisory Committee
SPC	Summary of Product Characteristics
TOS	Terms of Service
VPC	Veterinary Products Committee
WDL	Wholesale Dealers Licence
WO	Welsh Office
ZD	Zero Discount

The National Health Service

The National Health Service (NHS) has been described as the most magnificent feature of the UK's post-World War II landscape. The National Health Service Act 1946, which created the NHS as we know it, was extensive in scope. It covered the funding of the service, and created a national network of hospitals operating in a tiered management structure. Benefits were extended to the whole of the population, which was provided free of charge with medicine and the services of hospitals, doctors, dentists and opticians.

The National Insurance Act 1911

Before 1911 the provision of medical care was haphazard. There were some voluntary health insurance schemes, often based on a particular industry. By 1900 about 7 million people in the country were covered. In return for flat rate payments they had the services of a doctor and were provided with free medicine.

In 1911 the Prime Minister, Lloyd George introduced a compulsory health insurance scheme. It was based on a German scheme which had been introduced in 1883 by Bismarck.

The National Health Insurance Act 1911 covered all employees below a certain income level. The worker paid into a scheme run by a trade union, a friendly society or a commercial insurance company. In return, when he was ill he received cash, the free services of a doctor, and the necessary medicines.

Dispensing by pharmacists

The 1911 Act gave statutory recognition to the principle, long advocated by pharmacists, that the dispensing of prescriptions should be carried out under normal conditions only by or under the supervision of pharmacists. It applied this principle to the large class of the community which received its medicines under the provisions of the Act.

The National Health Service statutes

There remained a number of problems with the provision of health services. The hospitals were very variable in quality of buildings and quality of care. Many were run by charities. Only those persons who actually paid the insurance were covered for treatment. There was no provision for dependants. The problems, especially those of the hospitals, were highlighted during World War II. The new Socialist government of 1946 immediately implemented the National Health Service Act 1946, which brought the NHS into being on 5 July 1948.

The NHS Act 1946

Section 1 states:

(1)   'It shall be the duty of the Minister of Health to promote the establishment in England and Wales of a comprehensive health service designed to secure improvement in the physical and mental health of the people of England and Wales and the prevention, diagnosis and treatment of illness, and for that purpose to provide or secure the effective provision of services in accordance with the following provisions of this Act.

(2) The services so provided shall be free of charge, except where any provision of this Act expressly provides for the making and recovery of charges.'

The Minister was to provide throughout England and Wales, hospital and other medical and nursing services 'to such extent as he considers necessary to meet all reasonable requirements'.

The Act vested in the Minister a range of facilities and services which had previously been owned or provided by local health authorities, voluntary hospital authorities and other voluntary organizations, by the government under the 1911 scheme, and by doctors practising privately.

The Act recognized the right of doctors to continue to practise privately, either wholetime or in combination with certain types of NHS contract. They could admit patients to private beds in NHS hospitals.

The Act embodied the principle of the 1911 Act, that medicines were normally to be dispensed at pharmacies, and that normally doctors were not to dispense for their patients. Regulations could lay down the conditions for departing from this.

The 1946 Act set up a tripartite structure to administer the new arrangements. Different authorities controlled the hospitals, the primary care service and the mental hospitals.

The NHS took over control of 2688 hospitals from local authorities, charities and commercial bodies. The new structure consisted of 14 regional boards. Below them were 388 hospital management committees. The special position of teaching hospitals was recognized by the creation of 36 teaching hospital groups. Within each hospital the management was in the hands of an administrator, a matron and the senior doctor.

Local health authorities (HAs) were to administer ambulance services, midwifery, home nursing, and provision of care for the mentally ill.

The primary health care services were to be run by 134 executive councils. The health professionals, i.e. general practitioner, dentist, optician and pharmacist were (and remain) independent contractors. By contrast staff in the hospital services were employees.

This original structure has been changed over the years as the amending legislation reflected changes in both government and management theory.

The National Health Service Act 1977

This repealed the whole of the 1946 Act and consolidated a number of previous measures into one Act. It is now the principal Act dealing with the NHS. Since its introduction the structure of the NHS has again been altered by both primary and secondary legislation. The 1977 Act, as amended, sets out the duties of government in the NHS, while the later Acts deal with the current structures of accountability and command, and with the more detailed arrangements for service delivery.

General principles, scope and nature of the current NHS

Section 1 of the 1977 Act re-enacts the provisions of the original 1946 Act by placing a duty on the Secretary of State (S of S) to:

'continue the promotion in England and Wales of a comprehensive health service designed to secure improvement:

(a) in the physical and mental health of the people of those countries, and
(b) in the prevention, diagnosis and treatment of illness, and for that purpose to provide or secure the effective provision of services in accordance with this Act.'

Free services

Section 1(2) of the 1977 Act states 'the services so provided shall be free of charge except in so far as the making and recovery of charges is expressly provided for by or under any enactment, whenever passed.' In other words, the NHS is to be free except where a charge may lawfully be made.

Other duties

Besides the primary duty imposed by section 1 of the 1977 Act, sections 3, 4 and 5 impose further duties.

To the extent that he considers it necessary, the S of S must provide:

- hospital accommodation
- accommodation for other services
- medical, dental, nursing and ambulance services
- parenatal services and services for nursing mothers and young children
- services for the prevention of illness, care of the ill, and convalescence
- other services for diagnosis and treatment
- contraceptive services.

'Special hospitals' must also be provided for persons subject to detention under the Mental Health Act 1983 and who require treatment in high security institutions.

Section 2 of the 1977 Act gives power to the S of S to:

'provide such services as he considers appropriate for the purpose of discharging his duties, and

do anything else which is calculated to facilitate or be conducive or incidental to the discharge of his duties.'

The S of S also has power to provide:

- invalid carriages
- treatment outside the UK for tuberculosis sufferers
- a microbiological service
- assistance for relevant research.

Health and Medicines Act 1988

Section 7 of the Health and Medicines Act 1988 gives specific powers to the NHS to engage in income generation schemes. The schemes as such are not defined in the Act, which merely provides a framework for activities to take place. The DoH has issued guidance.

Income generation schemes

An income generation scheme is defined as one which seeks to provide a level of income which exceeds total costs, or at least provides an income contribution over and above the direct unit cost involved. HAs are still subject to legal and administrative constraints in this area. NHS services must still be provided free of charge. Non-NHS services should be charged for on a commercial basis. This includes the provision of private beds, and the treatment of overseas visitors in hospital.

The S of S's power may only be exercised by bodies set up under the 1977 Act. The powers conferred by section 7 were delegated by the S of S to HAs by a Direction issued in 1989.

The 1977 Act does not permit HAs to provide FHS pharmaceutical services. HAs cannot themselves be granted an NHS dispensing contract. The effect of sections 4 and 5 of the Health and Social Care Act 2001 on this remains to be seen.

National Health Service and Community Care Act 1990

The majority of NHS services are provided by NHS Trusts, which assumed responsibility for the ownership and management of hospitals or other establishments which were previously managed or provided by Regional, District or Special HAs. Trusts may be either physical units such as an acute hospital, or more nebulous institutions such as an ambulance service.

The Health Act 1999

- Abolished fund-holding practices
- established Primary Care Trusts (PCTs)
- allows the making of Regulations to ensure practitioners (including pharmacists) are insured
- sets out that the remuneration for providing Part II services shall be determined by the S of S
- provides for a price regulation scheme (PPRS) which may be voluntary or compulsory, and provides powers to set prices charged to the NHS for medicines
- makes it a criminal offence to evade paying NHS patient charges
- extends the powers of the NHS Tribunal to disqualify persons guilty of fraud
- allows for the pharmacy profession to be regulated by Orders
- sets up the Commission for Health Improvement (ChImp).

The Act also repeals the Professions Supplementary to Medicine Act 1960, the Health Service Joint Consultative Committees (Access to Information) Act 1986 and the Nurses, Midwives and Health Visitors Act 1979.

Health and Social Care Act 2001

This Act implements the NHS Plan 2000. The Act is in five parts:

- Part 1 changes the way the NHS, including family health services, is run and funded in England and Wales.
- Part 2 deals with pharmaceutical services in England and Wales and some aspects of such services in Scotland.
- Part 3 provides for the establishment of Care Trusts and for the transfer of staff in connection with partnership arrangements.
- Part 4 changes the way long-term care is funded and provided in England and Wales.
- Part 5 deals with the control of patient information and the extension of prescribing rights as well as various miscellaneous and supplementary provisions.

Part 1 – changes the way the NHS is run

The following are of particular relevance to pharmacy.

Public private partnerships
Section 4 inserts a new section 96C into the 1977 Act. The Secretary of State and the National Assembly for Wales, as well as Health Authorities, Special Health Authorities, Trusts and Primary Care Trusts may participate in public private partnerships with companies that provide facilities or services to persons or bodies carrying out NHS functions.

The S of S may form or participate in forming companies to provide facilities, services, loans, guarantees or other financial provisions to the NHS.

Section 5 allows NHS bodies to form or invest in companies for income generation. Such activities must not interfere with any duties under the 1977 Act or operate to the disadvantage of patients. They are subject to any directions given by the S of S.

New arrangements for patient involvement
Sections 7–12 establish new arrangements for public and patient involvement in the NHS to run alongside the existing CHCS. See later.

- Local Authority overview and scrutiny committees (OSCs) will scrutinize the NHS and represent local views on the development of local health services.
- NHS organizations have a duty to involve patients and the public in decision making about the operation of the NHS.

Abolition of Medical Practices Committee
Sections 14 and 15 transfer arrangements for managing the numbers and distribution of GPs to HAs.

Regulation of Health Service Practitioners
Sections 17–22 introduce new arrangements covering the regulation of family health service practitioners.

- Only practitioners, including deputies and locums, who are included in lists maintained by HAs will be able to deliver family health services.
- Criteria to be admitted to (and to remain on) a list include probity and positive evidence of good professional behaviour and practice. This will involve a system of declarations, annual appraisal and participation in clinical audit.
- HAs may refuse to include a practitioner on the relevant medical, dental, ophthalmic or pharmaceutical list on the grounds of unsuitability.

Section 21 provides powers to make regulations providing for a persons inclusion in a HA list to be subject to conditions.

Section 24 provides for HAs to keep supplementary lists of deputies and assistants who provide the various family health services (including GPs, dentists and people who provide pharmaceutical and optical services).

Financial interests and gifts
Section 23 requires practitioners to declare financial interests and the acceptance of gifts or other benefits.

Discipline arrangements
Section 25 provides for new arrangements for HAs to suspend and remove practitioners from the relevant lists on the grounds of inefficiency, fraud or unsuitability.

Section 27 creates the Family Health Services Appeals Authority as an independent body whose functions will include dealing with appeals by these practitioners against HA decisions.

Abolition of NHS tribunal
Consequently Section 16 provides for the abolition of the NHS Tribunal.

Part 2 – concerns pharmaceutical services

Chapter 1 provides for new arrangements under which community pharmacy and related services may be provided, initially on a pilot basis.

- These services will be known as local pharmaceutical services (LPS).
- HAs may designate neighbourhoods or premises in connection with pilot schemes, and must conduct at least one review of each pilot scheme.
- Health authorities have power to vary or terminate pilot schemes.

New health service bodies
Section 33 allows potential providers of local pharmaceutical services to apply to the relevant authority to become health service bodies. One result will be that certain arrangements they make with other health service bodies will become NHS contracts.

Patient charges
Section 35 enables charges corresponding to those for pharmaceutical services under Part II of the 1977 Act to be levied for local pharmaceutical services, subject to exemptions.

Pilot schemes
Section 37 permits regulations to be made preventing the provision of pilot scheme services from the same premises as pharmaceutical services under Part II of the NHS Act 1977, except as provided in the regulations. It also permits regulations to make provision about the inclusion, re-inclusion, removal and modification of entries in pharmaceutical lists held under Part II of that Act.

Section 38 permits regulations to prescribe the extent to which pilot schemes are to be taken into account when considering applications for inclusion in those lists.

Section 40 deals with the provision of full scale permanent Local Pharmaceutical Services (rather than under pilot schemes). The Secretary of State or the NAW may only bring this section into effect if the results of pilot schemes show that the continued provision of Local Pharmaceutical Services would be in the interests of the NHS.

Chapter 2 introduces changes to the existing arrangements for the provision of pharmaceutical services.

Section 42 inserts a revised section 41 into the 1977 Act on the arrangements for pharmaceutical services. See Chapter 5.

Remote dispensing
Section 43 authorizes arrangements made by Health Authorities to include arrangements for the provision of these pharmaceutical services by remote means.

The intention is to facilitate, and provide a means to control, the development of Internet, mail order, home delivery and other arrangements which may involve dispensing across HA boundaries.

Part 3 – establishes Care Trusts

New powers establish Care Trusts to provide integrated care.

Part 4 – changes the way long term care is funded and provided

Nursing care is excluded from community care services. Local authorities are responsible for meeting the care needs of people whose long term care is funded through preserved rights to income support and jobseekers allowance.

Part 5 – Patient information

Part 5 deals with the control of patient information and the extension of prescribing rights as well as various miscellaneous and supplementary provisions.

Use of NHS information
See Chapter 19.

Section 60 permits regulations to control the use of patient information. The Secretary of State may require or permit patient information to be shared for medical purposes where he considers that this is in the interests of improving patient care or in the public interest.

Section 61 establishes a Patient Information Advisory Group.

Extension of prescribing rights
Section 63 makes provision for the extension of prescribing rights to health professionals other than doctors, dentists and certain specified nurses, health visitors and midwives who already have prescribing rights. This part also includes a number of supplementary provisions.

The interests of the public

Access to meetings

HAs are subject to the Public Bodies (Admission to Meetings) Act 1960. This states that generally the public have access to any formal meeting of the authority. An exception may be made where the authority resolves to exclude the public because of the confidential nature of the business to be discussed.

The DH has issued guidance indicating that authorities are expected to conduct their business in as open a manner as possible.

Non-executive members are appointed for their personal skills and experience, and not as representatives of any particular professional group. They are expected to have links with the local community. The DH advise that those working in provider units managed by the authority, or in units which have a contract with the authority should not be appointed. This is to avoid a conflict of interest.

The Health Service Commissioner

The National Health Service Reorganisation Act 1973 provided for the creation of the post of Health Service Commissioner. His function is to investigate and report and make recommendations on complaints about the activities of HAs and those for whom they are responsible.

Separate Commissioners were created for England and for Wales. The NHS (Scotland) Act 1972 created a similar post for Scotland. The provisions of the 1973 Act were repeated in the consolidating Act of 1977. The current provision is the Health Service Commissioner Act 1993.

How to complain

The Commissioner acts only on a written complaint, received within a year of the event. The complaint must be made by the person who has suffered the injustice (unless he is unable to act for himself).

Jurisdiction

The Commissioner investigates complaints that a person has suffered injustice or hardship because of a failure by an HA to provide services properly, or as a result of maladministration.

From 1 April 1996 the jurisdiction of the Commissioner was extended by the Health Service Commissioner (Amendment) Act 1996.

- Section 1 adds family health service providers and independent providers to the list of those about whom the commissioner may investigate complaints.
- Section 6 removes a statutory bar on the Commissioner investigating matters of clinical judgement.
- Section 7 allows the Commissioner to investigate complaints about family health services.

Community Health Councils

CHCs were established for each district by the 1973 Act to represent the public interest in the local provision of the NHS, and to be a channel for consumer views.

They are now governed by the Community Health Councils Regulations 1996, SI No.640 which became effective on 1 April 1996, and which are amended by the CHC (Amendment) Regulations 2000 SI No. 657.

The councils consist of between 18 and 24 members. Members are nominated as follows:

- one third by local authorities
- one third by voluntary organisations
- one third by themselves and appointed by the S of S.

There are certain exclusions from membership, e.g. NHS employees.

The Secretary is a paid employee of the RHA. The operating budget is provided by the NHS Executive. An annual report must be published, which is discussed by the Health Authority.

CHCs have the following statutory rights:

- access to relevant information from the NHS
- access to certain NHS premises
- the right to be consulted on substantial changes in provision
- the right to have observers at meetings.

They have a duty:

- to keep under review the operation of the health service in their district
- to make recommendations to improve the service
- to advise health authorities and PCTs.

Strengthened involvement of patient and public

The Health and Social Care Act 2001 set out a number of provisions designed to strengthen the arrangements for public and patient involvement in the NHS.

Local Authority overview
Overview and scrutiny committees (OSCs) are sub-committees of Local Authorities, set up under the Local Government Act 2000. Section 7 of the HSC Act allows those committees to exercise new functions in relation to the NHS, in those LAs which hold responsibility for social services. The OSC can review and scrutinize health service matters, and make reports and recommendations.

Duty to involve patients
Section 11 of the HSC Act 2001 confers on each Health Authority, Primary Care Trust and NHS trust a new statutory duty to involve patients and the public in the planning and decision making processes of that body. In relation to HAs, this covers both the hospital and community health services for which they are responsible and the family health services provided by practitioners in their area.

Independent Patient Advocacy Services
Section 12 of the HSC Act 2001 imposes a new duty on the S of S to arrange independent advocacy services (IAS) for people who wish to complain about the servicve they or someone they care for has received from the NHS. The ISA may be provided by the local authority or by other persons or bodies.

Patient Advocacy and Liaison Services (PALS)
The new arrangements are to be complemented by a new non-statutory arrangement, Patient Advocacy and Liaison Services (PALS). PALs will be new trust-based services able to assist and support patients. They will be able to provide information and resolve problems and difficulties. It is intended that they will be situated in or near main reception areas of hospitals and act as a welcoming point for patients and carers. The PALS will also advise patients on how to access independent advocacy to support their complaints.

NHS Executive's Code of Practice on Openness in the NHS

This Code of Practice sets out the basic principles underlying public access to information about the NHS. It came into effect in 1995. The basic principle of this Code is that the NHS should respond positively to requests for information, except in certain circumstances identified in the Code. For example, patients' records must be kept safe and confidential.

The Code of Practice covers the following NHS organizations in England: Regional Health Authorities, Family Health Services Authorities, District Health Authorities, Special Health Authorities. NHS Trusts, the Mental Health Act Commission and Community Health Councils. It also covers family doctors, dentists, optometrists (opticians) and community pharmacists.

Specific requirements are detailed in separate annexes. Annex C describes the information which General Medical Practitioners, General Dental Practitioners, Community Pharmacists and Optometrists must publish or make available. For pharmacists the Code refers only to practice leaflets. It also describes the information Family Health Services Authorities must provide.

Advice from the health professions

Professional advisory committees

The 1973 Act set up both local and national advisory committees for the professions. At the national level the 1973 Act set up the Central Health Services Council as the main advisory body. This was abolished by the Health Services Act 1980. However, the 1973 Act also continued the Standing Advisory Committees, for medicine, dentistry, nursing, ophthalmology and pharmacy. These committees were originally constituted under the 1946 Act. Their operation is now governed by the NHS (Standing Advisory Committees) Order 1981, SI No. 597, made under section 6(3) of the 1977 Act. The committee on ophthalmology has since been abolished.

The Order states the function, which for pharmacy is:

'to advise the Secretary of State for Health and the Secretary of State for Wales on the pharmaceutical services including the hospital pharmaceutical services.'

The Standing Pharmaceutical Advisory Committee (SPAC) has 12 members appointed by the S of S for Health with the agreement of the S of S for Wales. The President of the Royal Pharmaceutical Society of Great Britain (RPSGB) is an ex-officio member. Each appointed member serves for a four year term, with half the members being appointed every two years. Members are chosen for their knowledge and experience in pharmacy.

Local advisory committees

At local level a system of committees was set up to advise in both the primary and secondary care sectors.

For pharmacy the primary care committees are the Local Pharmaceutical

Committees (LPCs). These consist of either nine or 15 members who provide pharmaceutical services as either contractors or employees. The HA is obliged to consult them on certain matters, e.g. on applications for dispensing contracts. They must be consulted before local agreements for allocation of pharmacy monies are implemented. Health Circular FHSC(96)9 – 'Local pharmacy budgets 1996/7' makes this clear. They may offer advice at any time.

The LPCs are constituted under section 44 of the 1977 Act. This now states that where the Health Authority is satisfied that a committee formed for its area is representative of the persons providing pharmaceutical services in that area, the HA may recognize that committee.

Section 43 (6) of the Health and Social Care Act 2001 amends section 44 to clarify that notwithstanding that people in the HA's area may receive pharmaceutical services from people whose premises are outside that area, the LPC need only be representative of persons who are included in a HA's own pharmaceutical list, in order to be recognized by it.

LPCs are elected by the contractors in the area. They adhere to the constitution adopted by the Pharmaceutical Services Negotiating Committee (PSNC), which represents contractor interests at national level.

The functions are set out in section 45 of the Act. LPCs are to be consulted about certain matters by the HA, and may exercise any other functions which are given to them.

The expenses of an LPC may be met by a levy on local contractors. Section 45(2) allows HAs to deduct sums from moneys due to contractors. This is paid to the LPC. The S of S must approve the amounts.

Professional advice to Health Authorities

The Health Authorities Act 1995 amends the 1977 NHS Act at Section 12(1) to provide for professional advice to the authority.

Section 12(1) states:

'Every HA shall make arrangements for seeing that they receive from
a) medical practitioners, registered nurses and midwives
b) other persons with professional expertise and experience of health care advice appropriate for enabling the HA effectively to exercise the functions conferred or imposed on them under or by virtue of this or any other Act'.

The Health Act 1999 inserts a new provision into 1977 Act:

'Advice for Health Authorities and Primary Care Trusts. 16C. – (1) Every Health Authority shall make arrangements with a view to securing that they receive advice appropriate for enabling them effectively to exercise the functions exercisable by them from persons with professional expertise relating to the physical or mental health of individuals.
(2) This section applies to Primary Care Trusts as it applies to Health Authorities.'

Pharmaceutical Services Negotiating Committee

At a national level the S of S has recognized the PSNC as a body 'representative of the general body of chemists'. Negotiations over pay for pharmaceutical services take place between the PSNC and the DoH. The PSNC is formally consulted on changes in the relevant Regulations and in Terms of Service.

Acts of Parliament mainly concerned with the NHS

The National Health Service Act 1946*
The National Health Service (Scotland) Act 1947
The National Health Service (Amendment) Act 1949
The National Health Service Act 1951*
The National Health Service Act 1952*
The National Health Service (Amendment) Act 1957*
The National Health Service Act 1961*
The National Health Service (Hospital Boards) Act 1964*
The National Health Service Act 1966
The National Health Service (Family Planning) Act 1967*
The Health Services and Public Health Act 1968
The National Health Service (Scotland) Act 1972
The National Health Service (Family Planning) Amendment Act 1972*
The National Health Service Reorganisation Act 1973
The Health Services Act 1976*
The National Health Service Act 1977
The National Health Service (Scotland) Act 1978
The Health Services Act 1980
The Health and Social Security Act 1984
The National Health Service (Amendment) Act 1986
The Health and Medicines Act 1988
The National Health Service and Community Care Act 1990
The Health Authorities Act 1995
The NHS Amendment Act 1995
Health Service Commissioners (Amendment) Act 1996
National Health Service (Private Finance) Act 1997
National Health Service (Primary Care) Act 1997
Audit Commission Act 1998
Health Act 1999
Health and Social Care Act 2001

*Asterisked Acts have been totally repealed.

Chapter 2

Administration of the NHS

The Secretary of State for Health is the political head of the Department of Health (DoH). He is responsible to Parliament for the operation of the NHS. The Secretary of State is assisted by a Minister of Health and a number of junior ministers.

The Department of Health

The DoH is organized into four main 'businesses':

- social care
- public health
- NHS Executive
- resources and services.

In relation to the NHS, the main functions of the DoH are to negotiate with the Treasury for funding, to set the policy framework and to monitor the performance of Trusts and Health Authorities.

NHS Executive

The NHS Executive (NHSE) manages the NHS directly through Health Authorities (HAs). It is organised in two parts – a central unit (mainly located in the Department's Leeds office), and eight regionally located offices. All offices are staffed by civil servants. The Chief Executive of the NHS is responsible to the Secretary of State.

The NHS Executive sets a strategic framework for the NHS in accordance with the policy of the government. It manages the NHS to ensure that policy is implemented through the health authorities and trusts. It gives out advice and information on good practice.

Health Authorities

In England and Wales, locally based HAs are responsible for assessing the health needs of local people and making arrangements for services to be provided by NHS Trusts and other agencies. There are 100 health authorities whose activities focus on three main areas: strategy, support and administration.

HAs were created by the Health Authorities Act 1995, which substituted new sections 8 and 10 in the 1977 Act. The new authorities merge two previous classes of authority – the Family Health Services Authority which was responsible for primary care and the District Health Authority which was responsible for hospital and community health services. Individual Health authorities in England were established by the Health Authorities (Establishment) Order 1996, SI No.624 which became effective on 1 April 1996. It established authorities to act for the areas of England specified in the Order.

Their responsibilities are:

- Planning the health needs of the population.
- Developing new patterns of service and effecting health improvements.
- Contracting for the provision of primary and secondary care.

The Health Act 1999 placed a statutory duty on HAs, with other NHS bodies and local authorities, to produce Health Improvement Programmes (HlmPs). These are plans for tackling local health issues, involving all local organizations with a part to play.

HAs are given power to delegate certain functions to PCTs. This power does not extend to community pharmacy contracts, which remain with HAs.

Health Authority boards

These comprise:

- a non-executive chairman
- five non-executive members
- five executive members, including the chief executive and director of finance.

Non-executive members are appointed for their personal skills and experience, and not as representatives of any particular professional group. They are expected to have links with the local community. The DoH advise that those working in provider units managed by the authority, or in units which have a contract with the authority should not be appointed. This is to avoid a conflict of interest.

Committees

HAs have considerable discretion as to how they arrange committees which advise the HA or carry out its functions. A Schedule to the 1990 Regulations contains the rules for the conduct of meetings.

Management

The day-to-day operation of an HA is in the hands of the Chief Executive. This title has changed over the years from Clerk, to Administrator to General Manager, and now Chief Executive.

Accountability

The route of accountability is through the chairman, who is appointed by the Secretary of State, and can be removed from office.

Funding

HAs are each allocated budgets by the NHS Executive.

NHS contracts

The DoH has described the contractual funding system for hospital services as central to the reforms. The aim is to provide a mechanism whereby hospitals and other units are funded more directly for the work which they do.

Although section 4 of the National Health Service and Community Care Act 1990 (NHS & CC Act) defines an 'NHS contract' in terms of an arrangement between two health service bodies, purchasers are not limited to buying within the NHS hospital organization. They can buy from commercial organizations, e.g. private hospitals, and from other parts of the NHS such as community pharmacists. Contracts between health service bodies are not legal ones, but are service agreements between the HAs or general practitioner (GP) fund-holders (as purchasers of health services) and hospitals or other units (as providers of health services). Any disputes about such NHS contracts are to be resolved by a disputes procedure. These measures avoid recourse to the courts. There is a conciliation procedure at regional level. If this does not resolve the issue the Secretary of State has power to appoint an arbiter who will take the final decision.

Section 4 defines the expression 'NHS contract' as:

'the arrangement under which one health service body (the acquirer) arranges for the provision to it by another health service body (the provider) of goods or services which it reasonably requires for the purpose of its functions.'

A health service body is any of the following:

(a) a health authority
(b) a health board
(c) the Common Services Agency for the Scottish Health service
(d) an NHS Trust
(e) a recognized fund-holding practice
(f) the Dental Practice Board or the Scottish Dental Practice Board
(g) the Public Health Laboratory Service Board
(h) the Secretary of State.

NHS Trusts

The majority of NHS services are provided by NHS Trusts.

Sections 5 to 11 of the NHS & CC Act deal with NHS Trusts, which according to section 5 are bodies established by the Secretary of State to:

(a) Assume responsibility for the ownership and management of hospitals or other establishments which were previously managed or provided by Regional, District or Special HAs; or

(b) provide and manage hospitals or other establishments or facilities.

From 1 April 1991 hospitals were gradually established as NHS Hospital Trusts. The Act allows that hospital trusts may be either physical units such as an acute hospital, or more nebulous institutions such as an ambulance service. The Act provides for statutory public consultation of the establishment of Trusts.

Establishment as a Trust gives considerable freedom to manage affairs. The Trust is run by a Board, which is able to employ its own staff, set rates of pay, borrow capital and dispose of assets. Such activities are severely restricted within the main NHS structure. Staff employed by Trusts are still considered as NHS staff. The property remains NHS property, although vested in the Trust.

The Secretary of State retains certain powers over the Trusts. In particular he is able to direct them as to the services which they must provide, and in this way he is able to ensure that essential services such as Accident and Emergency remain available locally. Each HA has a responsibility to ensure that certain core services are available locally.

The powers of a Trust

The Secretary of State may make an order to confer on a Trust specific powers in addition to those contained in paragraphs 10–15 of Schedule 2 of the NHS & CC Act.

The specific powers are:

(a) To enter into NHS contracts as a provider.
(b) To undertake research.
(c) To train Trust staff and those likely to become employed by the Trust.
(d) To make facilities for training available to a university.
(e) To join with another body or individual to carry out its functions.
(f) To make charges for its services to private patients.
(g) To generate additional income using the powers in section 7(2) of the Health and Medicines Act 1988.

There are some general powers:

(h) To deal in land.
(i) To enter into legal contracts.
(j) To accept gifts of money, land or property.
(k) To employ staff.
(l) To do anything necessary or expedient to carry out its functions.

Status

According to Schedule 2, paragraph 18, a Trust shall not be regarded as the servant or agent of the Crown or except as provided by this Act, or as enjoying any status, immunity or privilege of the Crown. An NHS Trust's property shall not be regarded as the property of or property held on behalf of the Crown.

Financial objectives of Trusts

Section 10 requires the NHS Trusts to break even, taking one year with another, and to achieve any financial objectives which they are set.

Primary Care Groups

Since 1999 Primary Care Groups (PCGs) have replaced the previous internal market and GP fundholding arrangements as commissioning bodies. There are 481 PCGs in England, and each is responsible for around 100,000 patients.

Primary Care Groups were initially set up as sub-committees of HAs, but are intended to evolve into Primary Care Trusts (PCT).

Four levels of PCG are found, with levels 1 and 2 remaining as sub-committees of the HA. Level 3 groups act as free-standing bodies but remain accountable to the HA. Level 4 groups are able to become Trusts after a consultation process. This process must include canvassing public opinion, and that of local representative bodies including the Local Pharmaceutical Committee.

The NHS Executive has stated that it expects all PCGs to become Trusts by 2004.

Primary Care Trusts

PCTs were established by section 2 of the Health Act 1999, which inserted new provisions in the National Health Service Act 1977 – section 16A. – (1) The Secretary of State may establish bodies to be known as PCTs with a view, in particular, to their:

(a) providing or arranging for the provision of services under this Part of this Act

(b) exercising functions in relation to the provision of general medical services under Part II of this Act, and

(c) providing services in accordance with section 28C arrangements.

Each PCT shall be established by an order made by the S of S (referred to in this Act as a PCT order). A PCT shall be established for the area specified in its PCT order and shall exercise its functions in accordance with any prohibitions or restrictions in the order.

The creation of trusts began in April 2000.

The legislation allows Level 4 Trusts to merge with community trusts. Level 4 Trusts are direct providers and managers of community services. They are responsible directly to the S of S.

PCTs are allowed to commission and provide services, to employ staff and to own property. They are not prevented from setting up community pharmacies, although the S of S could give directions prohibiting this, as is done in the case of HAs.

Boards of PCT

The board consists of five lay members, plus the CE, FD and three professional members of the executive.

Funding

PCTs are funded by the HAs which make allocations to them. They receive a unified budget covering hospital and community services, GP prescribing and the general practice infrastructure.

Each financial year is complete in itself, so funds (or arrears) cannot be carried over to subsequent years. HAs are required to provide services within the set budgets.

PCTs are accountable to HA for outcomes.

HAs are required by the HA 1999 to pay to PCTs their share of Part II primary care expenditure.

Special Health Authorities

Special HAs have been created to administer specialised areas of service provision. They are directly accountable to the Secretary of State. A number of specialist postgraduate teaching and research hospitals in London, e.g. the Hammersmith, have SHA status. The Special Hospitals (those dealing with the care of seriously disturbed offenders, e.g. Rampton) also have SHA status. Other SHAs have support roles, e.g. the Prescription Pricing Authority.

The following have been designated SHAs:

- UK Transport (UKT)
- NHS Litigation Authority
- Centre for Applied Microbiology and Research (CAMR)
- Mental Health Act Commission
- National Clinical Assessment Authority
- Prescription Pricing Authority
- Retained Organs Commission
- Health Development Agency
- National Blood Authority (England)
- Ashworth Hospital Authority
- Broadmoor Hospital Authority
- Rampton Hospital Authority
- NHS Logistics Authority
- NHS Information Authority
- National Institute for Clinical Excellence.

Prescription Pricing Authority

The Prescription Pricing Authority (PPA) was created in 1978 as a Special Health Authority under provisions in the 1977 Act. It was reconstituted in 1990 by the Prescription Pricing Authority Consititution Order 1990, SI No. 1718.

The Authority consists of eight members:

- the chairman
- a general medical practitioner
- a pharmacist providing pharmaceutical services
- a chief officer of an HA
- the chief officer of the PPA
- three lay members, i.e. persons who are not and have never been a doctor, dentist, pharmacist, optician or nurse.

The appointment and tenure of office of the members is governed by the Prescription Pricing Authority Regulations 1990, SI No. 1719.

Members are appointed, by the Secretary of State, for a period not exceeding three years. The Secretary of State also appoints the Chairman.

The functions of the PPA relate to the examining, checking and pricing of prescriptions for drugs, listed drugs, medicines and listed appliances supplied as part of pharmaceutical services. These functions are carried out on behalf of HAs. In addition the Secretary of State may direct the PPA to carry out other tasks.

Effects of devolution

The services are organized slightly differently in each of the countries of the UK. The regional tier is absent, and the functions are provided either by the local health authorities or at national level.

Wales

During 1999 the National Assembly for Wales took on responsibility for the management and performance of the NHS in Wales. The NHS Directorate in Wales has a similar role to the NHSE. The Directorate is accountable to the Assembly.

In Wales there are currently five health authorities, 16 Trusts, and 22 Local Health Groups (LHG) which are similar to the PCGs found in England. The health authorities' role includes quantifying the health care needs of their area and commissioning the necessary care accordingly, supporting the contractor professions, protecting public health, and responding to the views of people and organizations in their area. NHS Trusts are charged with providing services and operate hospitals, community health service, ambulance services and other health facilities in accordance with contracts they have with health authorities. In Wales the responsibility for producing health Improvement Programs lies with the LHGs. There are two special health authorities (the Welsh Common Services Authority and the Health Promotion Authority for Wales). Community health councils in Wales report to the Welsh Assembly.

The Health Promotion Authority for Wales and parts of the Welsh Health Common Services Authority will also become part of the Assembly.

Northern Ireland

In Northern Ireland the Department of Health and Social Services (DHSS) is required, under the provisions of the Health and Personal Social Services (Northern Ireland) Order 1972, to secure the provision of an integrated service designed to promote health and social welfare of the population.

Part of this provision is the Health Services in Northern Ireland which is managed by the Health and Social Services Executive (HSSE).

The Health and Social Policy Group (HSPG) of the DHSS is responsible for promoting wider health and social gain. It sets the overall strategy for health and personal social services; promotes voluntary activity and community development in Northern Ireland; takes the lead in targeting health and social need; and is responsible for health promotion and protection, developing social policy and social legislation. The strategy of the DHSS has three main aims:

- to promote health and social well-being
- to target health and social need
- to secure and improve the provision and delivery of health and social services.

Health and Social Services Executive

The Health and Social Services Executive is the Northern Ireland counterpart to the NHS Executive in England. Its primary purpose is to secure improvements to the health and social well-being of people in Northern Ireland. Its main functions are:

- To provide leadership, direction and support to the Health and Personal Social Services (HPSS) in Northern Ireland.
- To set and ensure the achievement of specific objectives and targets for the HPSS in accordance with national and regional policies and priorities.
- To monitor the performance of HPSS in assessing need and improving health and social well-being of the population.
- To allocate resources and ensure that they are used effectively, efficiently and economically, in accordance with the required standards of public accountability.
- To promote the managerial environment necessary to achieve these objectives.
- To provide advice, information and support to Ministers relating to the management and performance of the HPSS.

The HSSE is headed by a Chief Executive who is supported by six directors.

Health and Social Services Boards

There are four Health and Social Services Boards in Northern Ireland. They act as agents of the DHSS in planning, commissioning and purchasing health and social services for residents in their areas – functioning in a similar role to HAs in England.

Each Board has a non-executive chairman, six executive and six non-executive members. The chairman and non-executive members are appointed by the

Minister with the approval of the Secretary of State. By statute two of the executive members are the chief executive/general manager and director of finance.

As commissioners and purchasers, Boards are required to plan, secure and pay for the services needed to meet the health and social care needs of their population. In deciding which services are needed, the Boards assess the population's health and social care needs by collecting information about patterns of death, illness and community care needs and by consulting local people. They also liaise with GPs and statutory and voluntary agencies to build up a picture of the health and social care needs of their residents.

Health and Social Services Trusts

The HSS Trusts are the providers of health and social services. They are responsible for the management of staff and services at hospitals and other establishments previously managed or provided by Boards. The Trusts control their own budgets and, although managerially independent of Boards, they are accountable to the HSSE. There are 20 Trusts in Northern Ireland. It is the only part of the UK which, because of the integrated health and social services, has Trusts based solely on the delivery of community health and social services.

Each Trust is managed by a Board of Directors which contains up to five non-executive members and a non-executive chairman, who are appointed by the DHSS with the approval of the Secretary of State and five executive members who are employees of the Trust.

Scotland

The Scottish Health Service is responsible to the Scottish Parliament. The Management Executive within the Scottish Office Department of Health is responsible for health service policy and central management. The Management Executive sets national objectives and priorities, agrees corporate contracts with area Health Boards and monitors their performance.

Health Boards have a strategic management role and are responsible for planning and commissioning hospital and community health services for the people who live within their area. Health Boards are also responsible for the primary care services provided by GPs, dentists, community pharmacists and opticians, who are independent contractors. There are 15 Health Boards covering the whole of Scotland (12 mainland and three island Boards).

There are 46 NHS Trusts in Scotland responsible for providing hospital and/or community services in a particular area, under contract to Health Boards and others. Non-executive directors are referred to as trustees. All trust chairs are members of the appropriate health board. There is one national Trust responsible for the Scottish Ambulance Service. The Scottish Ambulance Service is a special Health Authority Board.

Health Boards, with the exception of the larger ones, have one acute and one Primary Care Trust (PCT). There are 28 acute hospital trusts and 13 primary care trusts. PCTs are responsible for primary care, mental health, learning disabilities and community hospitals. Each Trust is accountable to the Secretary of State via the Management Executive.

Each PCT operates through Local Health Care Co-operatives (LHCC) whose role is to plan and provide service delivery at a local level. There are 70 LHCCs. The PCT senior management team has representatives from each LHCC.

There are also a number of other national organisations responsible for associated services and include the Common Services Agency, the Health Education Board for Scotland, the State Hospitals Board for Scotland. The patients' and public's interests in the NHS are represented by 16 Local Health Councils (one for each Health Board area except for the Western Isles which has two).

New proposals for the National Health Service in Scotland were set out in the Government's White Paper: *Designed to Care*. This announced that the 15 Health Boards would remain but that there would be a smaller number of Trusts of two types: acute hospital Trusts and primary care Trusts.

Chapter 3

Applications to Dispense NHS Prescriptions

This chapter is concerned mainly with the provisions governing the opening of a pharmacy, and the application for an NHS contract in an urban area. The rural dispensing arrangements are dealt with in Chapter 4.

Neither this chapter nor the one on rural dispensing arrangements is intended to give a step-by-step set of instructions on how applications should be made or how they are processed. Instead we aim only to outline the procedures.

The opening of a new pharmacy is subject to a number of controls. One set of controls relates to professional matters. This set derives from the Medicines Act 1968 and from the law governing the profession of pharmacy. These are dealt with in Chapter 9. The other set of controls relates to the granting of an NHS contract. A pharmacy may open without an NHS contract although such pharmacies are few in number.

Applications for NHS contracts

Until 1983 an application to dispense NHS prescriptions in a pharmacy was automatically granted. Since 1983 there have been a number of restrictive measures.

In 1987 amending regulations introduced a system of control to link the number of persons included in a pharmaceutical list as closely as possible to the need of the local population for reasonable access to the full range of NHS pharmaceutical services. At the same time they were intended to take account of the cost to the taxpayer of providing pharmaceutical services. A new contract was only to be granted if it was 'necessary or desirable' to secure adequate provision in the neighbourhood.

The main law is now found in the National Health Service (Pharmaceutical Service) Regulations 1992. The Regulations have been amended several times. A guide to the part of these regulations dealing with applications to dispense has been issued by the DoH as Annexes to Health Service Guidance HSG(92)13/FPN560. Since 1992 there have been a number of court decisions which have attempted to clarify the Regulations.

The 'pharmaceutical list'

The HA has a duty to keep 'pharmaceutical lists' of persons who undertake to provide pharmaceutical services. The lists are of:

- those who provide drugs (pharmacies)
- those who provide appliances
- oxygen concentrator suppliers

Each list contains the names of the contractors, the addresses of premises where services are provided and the hours at which services are provided. The list of pharmacies must also indicate whether or not the pharmacy has undertaken to provide additional professional services.

Different types of application

Applications fall into a number of categories which are dealt with in different ways:

(1)   Applications for a new contract in an urban area.
(2)   Applications for a new contract in a rural area.
(3)   Applications for minor relocation of premises.
(4)   Applications for change of ownership of premises.
(5)   Applications to supply appliances only.
(6)   Applications for variation of an existing contract.

Who may apply for a contract?

Section 43 of the NHS Act 1977 limits the classes of persons who may provide pharmaceutical services.

'1)   No arrangements shall be made by an HA (except as may be provided by regulations) with a medical practitioner or dental practitioner under which he is required or agrees to provide pharmaceutical services to any person to whom he is rendering general medical services or general dental services.

2)   No arrangements for the dispensing of medicines shall be made (except as may be provided in regulations) with persons other than persons who are registered pharmacists, or are persons lawfully conducting a retail pharmacy business in accordance with section 69 of the Medicines Act 1968 and who undertake that all medicines supplied by them under the arrangements made under this part of this Act shall be dispensed either by or under the direct supervision of a registered pharmacist.'

HAs have been advised by the DoH to summarily reject applications to dispense medicines which are from persons who are not entitled to conduct a retail pharmacy business. The Health Service Guidance on Procedures HSG(92)13 states that all applications for inclusion in the pharmaceutical list must be rejected if they are not from pharmacists, partnerships of pharmacists or from companies.

Applications may be made by a chemist (Reg. 14(1)). In this context 'chemist' must mean a person who wishes to open a pharmacy and who would be able to lawfully operate a retail pharmacy business.

A full application

Full applications must be made in the form set out in Part I of Schedule 3 of the Regulations. 'In the form' means that the application must be in the style set out, not that a specific printed form must be used. For that a phrase such as 'on a form provided by the HA and as set out in . . .' would be necessary. Typed or photocopied applications comply. The services to be provided must be specified, as must the proposed opening hours. The applicants have to give reasons in support of the contention that it is necessary or desirable to grant the application. HSG(92)13 states that further written statements in support of the application may be made.

Effect of grant of application

Normally the grant is effective for a period of six months. The applicant will be put on the list when he starts to provide the specified services. He must give 14 days' notice of his intention to start providing services (Reg. 4(9)). The HA may grant the application in respect of all or only some of the services offered in it (Reg. 4(6)).

Crucial times are:

- 24 weeks after the grant of an application, the date by which notice to commence services must be given; and
- 26 weeks after the grant, the date by which services must have been provided.

The six month period may be extended by the HA for a further period of up to 24 months.

Change of address of premises

During the six month or 24 month period mentioned above, the applicant may notify a change of address to the HA.

Change of address of premises before opening

During the six month or 24 month period allowed after the grant of a full application, the applicant may notify a change of address to the HA.

An applicant granted preliminary consent in respect of premises may seek to change the location at which he proposes services, during the 12 month or 24 month period before he must apply for a full grant.

The grant will be amended to the new address provided:

- The same service is to be provided.
- The neighbourhood is the same.
- The HA is satisfied that the change is a minor relocation (Reg. 4(10)).

The procedure is the same as that for dealing with a request by an established contractor to change premises. That means the HA will have to decide if the change is minor or not (Reg. 4(3)).

An applicant granted preliminary consent who wishes to make a relocation which is considered not to be minor before being entered on the list shall be treated as though he has made a new full application (Reg. 4(2)). The applicant must pass the 'necessary or desirable' test in relation to the new address.

Since the precise address need not be stated on a preliminary application it is presumably possible for the applicant to make a change of address without changing the location at all.

The 'necessary or desirable' test

The HA has to consider whether the new pharmacy is necessary or desirable. Regulation 4(4) states:

'An application ... shall be granted by the HA only if it is satisfied that it is necessary or desirable to grant the application in order to secure, in the neighbourhood in which the premises from which the applicant intends to provide the services are located, the adequate provision, by persons included in the list of the services, or some of the services specified in the application'.

This test is applied to every application except those for:

- minor relocation of premises
- change of ownership of premises
- supply of appliances only
- supply of oxygen concentrators.

The test can be met in either of two possible ways. The application may be necessary or it may be desirable. The two words are not mutually exclusive, so presumably an application may also be necessary *and* desirable.

HSG(92)13 indicates that each application should be decided on its merits and there should be no fixed rules for example about distance between pharmacies. The test considers the adequacy of the services to patients, not the effect on existing pharmacies.

The Court of Appeal gave guidance on the 'necessary and desirable' test in *Ex parte Lowe No. 2*, 2001.

The Court said:

- an application can only be granted for the purpose of securing the adequate provision of pharmaceutical services by pharmacists
- adequacy is a question of degree. A spectrum of adequacy runs from 'wholly adequate' to 'wholly inadequate'
- the real issue is where on that spectrum of adequacy does a particular case belong
- that question has a variety of answers, which include:
  - wholly adequate: there is no doubt that the existing provision is sufficient and hence it would be neither necessary nor desirable to grant the application
  - wholly inadequate: there is no doubt that the existing provision is

insufficient and hence it would be both necessary and desirable to grant the application
- marginal: some point between the two answers above, where it is not necessary to grant the application, but it might be desirable to do so in order to secure the adequate provision of services
- decisions must be pragmatic because there are spaces on the spectrum between marginal and wholly adequate or wholly inadequate.

'Persons on the pharmaceutical list'

The test refers to persons on the pharmaceutical list. This formulation excludes dispensing doctors. Thus services provided by dispensing doctors are excluded when consideration is given to the need or desirability, in the locality, of services provided by pharmacists.

What is a neighbourhood?

In a Northern Ireland case (Re: An application by Boots, 1994), Lord Justice Murray in the NI High Court said people must 'live in some proximity' to be neighbours.

The High Court ruled in 1996 that absence of a resident population did not prevent a shopping centre from being a 'neighbourhood'. Mr Justice Tucker said:

'I have reached a clear finding that shopping centres can indeed constitute neighbourhoods.'

He also said that when assessing the adequacy of existing pharmacy provision the authority should pay regard to the needs of everyone who might be expected to be in, but not necessarily resident in, the neighbourhood at any time and for any purpose *(Ex parte Boots the Chemists Ltd* – the 'Cribbs Causeway' case.)

In another High Court case in 1996 the court suggested

'There must be some communality for a neighbourhood'. (*Ex parte Baker*)

In 1999 Mr Justice Kay, again in the High Court (*ex parte* Tesco) ruled that a superstore was not a neighbourhood in its own right, but was part of a neighbourhood which included local villages. He rejected an argument that it was irrelevant to consider whether or not an area had a resident population.

Preliminary consent

Applications for a new contract may be either 'full' applications or applications for 'preliminary consent'. The NHS (General Medical and Pharmaceutical Services) Amendment Regulations 1983, SI 1983 No. 313, introduced the notion of 'preliminary consent'. Prior to 1983 there was no control of entry to the pharmaceutical list, and an application to go on the list was automatically granted.

Preliminary consent allowed a likely contractor to 'test the water' without committing himself. It was not necessary to specify the exact location of premises in an application for preliminary consent, so the applicant was able to maintain some degree of commercial confidentiality. An applicant who was granted preliminary consent was automatically granted admission to the pharmaceutical list on subsequent application. This dual system caused some problems when the test of 'necessary or desirable' was introduced.

The 1992 Regulations now provide that an application for preliminary consent is to be subject to the same test as a full application.

An application for preliminary consent may be made regardless of whether the premises are situated in a rural area or in an urban area.

Making an application for preliminary consent

Applications for preliminary consent are dealt with in Regulations 14 and 15.

Applications must be in writing

The application must be in writing (Reg. 14(2)). No form is prescribed in the regulations. The application must state the location of the premises. 'Location' is not the same as address and is less specific, although it must in each case be sufficiently precise to enable the 'necessary or desirable' test to be applied.

Effect of the grant of preliminary consent

Once a person has been granted preliminary consent then the HA must grant any full application made during the preliminary consent period, provided the premises are in the same location.

The HA may grant the application in respect of all, or of some of the services specified in it. This full application must specify the address of the premises. HSG(92)13 states that the applicant is free to amend the services to be provided to the extent that it does not affect the basis on which preliminary consent was granted.

Preliminary consent is effective for 12 months. The HA has a power to extend that 12 month period for any further reasonable period. The decision to do so must be made before the expiry of the 12 months. The extension must be reasonable in the circumstances (Reg. 14(5)). If during that time the applicant makes a full application, then this must be granted provided the premises are in the same location.

Applications for a minor relocation

A person who is on the pharmaceutical list may apply to change the address from which he provides services. If the HA is satisfied that the change is a minor relocation, and other conditions are satisfied, then the application must be granted.

The other conditions are that:

- The same services are being provided.
- The provision of services has not been interrupted (unless the HA has allowed an interruption).

What is a minor relocation?

A minor relocation is not defined in the Regulations, but HSG(92)13 states that it is minor if the HA decides that there would be no significant change to the population served.

'Minor relocation' has been judicially considered in *R*. v. *Cumbria FPC, ex parte Boots the Chemists Ltd* and the relevant portion of the judgment reads:

'We have been asked to give guidance on the meaning of "minor relocation". We do so with hesitation; it is a matter of fact and degree. The primary consideration is geography, whether the move is over a short distance. But what is a short distance depends on the circumstances. In a densely populated town a move of a few hundred yards might not be minor. In the depths of the country a move of several miles might be.

   Second, the FHSA must consider if the population served in the new premises will be the same as the old. It might be that the distance is small, but a physical barrier – a river, a motorway – would mean that the new premises would be difficult to reach by the population served by the old premises. The FHSA is entitled to take account of this, and of the availability of public transport and whether the population is pedestrian or car-borne, bearing in mind that major users are elderly ...'

The Court of Appeal gave judgements in two cases in 1995 on the interpretation of various phrases relating to applications for minor relocation.

The facts in *R* v. *Yorkshire Regional Health Authority, ex parte Gompels* were as follows. The doctors' surgery in a small town decided to move from the High Street to purpose-built premises nearby. Two of the pharmacies in the town applied to relocate their premises from the High Street to near the new surgery. Another High Street pharmacy opposed the minor relocation applications on the grounds *inter alia* that the relocations could not be minor if the redistribution of prescriptions would threaten the viability of that pharmacy.

The Court of Appeal held that the continuing viability of adversely affected pharmacies was irrelevant. The application has to be granted if 'within the neighbourhood ... the Health Authority is satisfied that the change is a minor relocation'.

As to what constitutes a 'minor relocation' the Court of Appeal was divided. One judge said that the essential question was one of geography and topography. He said

'The words "minor relocation" are plain English words which mean no less and no more than they say'.

The other two judges disagreed. One said that the HA must also consider the significance and consequence of the move as they affect users of the service. He thought the word 'minor' was synonymous with 'unimportant'.

The other referred to the 1988 case above and suggested that it would be a minor relocation if the new location is substantially as convenient to the population served as the old location.

The facts in the second case were similar. (*R* v. *Yorkshire Regional Health Authority, ex parte Suri*) The two appeals were heard together.

Applications for change of ownership

A person taking over the ownership of an NHS pharmacy must apply to the HA to provide NHS pharmaceutical services. The application must be made in the form specified in Part I of Schedule 3 of the Regulations. The application must be granted by the HA provided that:

- When the application is made a person on the list is providing services from the premises specified.
- The same services will be provided from those premises.
- The provision of services will not be interrupted.
- The new owner does not fall into the 'European diploma' category.

European diplomas

The Regulations place certain restrictions on pharmacists who hold diplomas in pharmacy granted by universities in other EU countries. Such pharmacists are required to satisfy the HA as to their knowledge of English before an application can be granted (Reg. 4(5)).

Removal from pharmaceutical list

The HA must remove a name from the list where it determines that:

(1) The contractor has died (Reg. 17(1)(a)).
(2) The contractor is no longer a pharmacist or retail pharmacy business (RPB) (Reg. 17(1)(b)).
(3) The contractor has not provided services for six months (Reg. 17(3)).

There are provisions in the Medicines Act for a RPB to be carried on by representatives where a pharmacist has died or has been declared legally incompetent, e.g. because of mental illness. The representative 'stands in the shoes of' the pharmacist and the business remains on the list. The main requirement for the carrying on of the business by representatives is that a pharmacist be employed to handle professional matters (see Chapter 9 under the heading 'Representatives'.)

Regulation 17(2) enables the representatives to continue on the list.

Where the contractor has not provided services for six months the HA is required to follow the following procedure:

- the contractor must be given 28 days' notice of the intention to make a determination
- he must be given an opportunity to make representations
- the HA must consult the LPC.

The meaning of Regulation 17(9)(b) at first seems obscure, *viz*. 'nothing in this regulation shall affect a chemist who is performing a period of relevant service and no removal under paragraph (3) shall be effected in respect of any such chemist until six months after he has completed that service'. However the definition section of the Regulations clarifies matters. The 'relevant service' is service in the armed forces in a national emergency.

Applications from appliance contractors

Applications from appliance contractors, or from those who wish to provide only appliances, are dealt with in a broadly similar way. However, there is no requirement that the applicant be a pharmacist. The necessary or desirable test applies. The rules relating to controlled localities have no application for appliance contractors. The availability of appliances from pharmacies in the locality is a factor to be considered when determining whether the existing service is adequate.

Planning law

The planning regulations which affect pharmacies are found in the Town and Country Planning (Use Classes) Order 1987. This lists the various classes of activity for which planning permission may be granted.

An explanatory note attached to the order says that 'dispensaries' will fall into Class A1. This is the class for shops. If the 'dispensary' is ancilliary to a hospital then it may fall into Class C2 (residential institutions). Under a previous order it was possible for pharmacies which were 'dispensing-only' to fall into a category of professional use of residential premises, thereby avoiding planning restrictions applicable to shops.

It is not necessary for the relevant planning permission to have been granted prior to the granting of an application for minor relocation or for a new contract.

Chapter 4

Rural Dispensing

History

Doctors and pharmacists have argued over who should dispense for patients in rural areas since the advent of the NHS. In 1975 the two professions agreed a voluntary standstill on changes in dispensing arrangements while they engaged in discussions. Following these discussions a number of systems were put into place:

- 1977, 'Report of the National Joint Committee of the medical and pharmaceutical professions on the dispensing of NHS prescriptions in rural areas' – commonly known as the 'Clothier Report'
- 1983, the Rural Dispensing Committee (RDC) was to determine applications for dispensing in rural areas, and to determine the 'rurality' of an area
- 1990, RDC abolished and decisions made by FHSAs (now HA).

The current rules

The NHS Act 1977 made it clear that doctors would only be allowed to dispense drugs in exceptional circumstances and that the prime suppliers of medicines would be pharmacists. Exceptions were made in rural areas where there was no pharmacy and where patients would have extreme difficulty in getting to a pharmacy. (Lord Justice Schieman in *R. v. North Staffs HA, ex parte Worthington* 1996).

Controlled locality

The current rural dispensing rules apply to areas termed 'controlled localities'. A controlled locality is an area which has been determined by the HA to be 'rural in character'. The HA is required to delineate the boundaries of the controlled areas on a map. Where a previous determination of rurality has been made under the NHS (GMPS) Amendment Regulations 1983, then that area continues as a controlled locality.

An HA must determine rurality if requested in writing by the LPC or LMC (Regulation 9).

The 'five year rule'

Regulation 9(11) states that where a HA has decided whether or not an area is rural, the question may not generally be considered again in the next five years.

The exception is where the HA is satisfied that there has been a 'substantial change of circumstances' in relation to the area, or to a part of it, since the matter was last determined.

Meaning of 'substantial change'

No definition is given in the Regulations. The Guidance document states that each case should be considered on its merits. Examples are given such as changes in the size of the population, changes in transport facilities, changes in levels of services.

What does 'rural' mean?

The DoH issued guidance in HSG 92(13). This states that it is essentially a matter of common sense, but factors to be taken into account include:

- size of the community
- distance between settlements
- overall population density
- public transport arrangements
- level of local services.

The guidance document specifically states that an area is not rural simply because a doctor receives a rural practice allowance. Areas which have not been classed as 'controlled' are not necessarily urban.

Applications by pharmacists to dispense in rural areas

Applications to dispense in 'controlled localities' are subject to the procedures set down in Regulations.

Two tests are applied to the application.

Stage 1

The HA must first of all determine whether to grant the application would prejudice the proper provision of general medical services or pharmaceutical services in an area.

Regulation 12(13) states:

'The HA–
   (a) shall refuse an application to the extent that it is of the opinion that to grant it would prejudice the proper provision of general medical services, personal medical services, dispensing services or pharmaceutical services in any locality'.

The application may not be granted if there would be prejudice to *either* medical *or* pharmaceutical services. Thus an application from a pharmacy to dispense may not be granted if to do so would prejudice the proper provision of pharmaceutical services, for example those provided by the doctor.

The Regulations lay down a timetable, and indicate which other persons or bodies should be consulted before a decision is taken.

Location

At this stage an application is not required to give the exact address of the proposed pharmacy, but the location must be given sufficiently clearly for the test to be applied. In practice that seems to mean that it must be possible to look at the population within a one mile radius of the proposed site, so as to determine how those people are affected.

What is meant by 'proper provision'?

Proper provision means provision of the service to the standard which the contractor is obliged to provide in order to comply with the Terms of Service.

What is meant by 'prejudice'?

The services will be prejudiced if the contractor would be unable to comply with the Terms of Service. A reduction in the standard of service will not, in itself, constitute prejudice to the proper provision. This interpretation has been approved by the S of S in a number of decisions. It is also given in the Guidance document.

Stage 2

If the HA finds that there is no prejudice it must then determine, as a separate decision, whether the application is 'necessary or desirable'. The two stages are distinct and separate, and must be done in the correct order. The same people, at the same meeting, may make the decisions.

The 'necessary and desirable' stage for pharmacists is the same as that which governs the applications for dispensing in urban areas. See Chapter 3.

Applications by pharmacies already on the list

Applications made under Regulation 4(2)(b) are not mentioned in Regulation 11, and hence fall to be determined as if they were applications made for a non-controlled area. Applications covered by Regulation 4(2)(b) include those by persons already included on a list who wish to:

- open additional premises within the area
- change premises
- provide other pharmaceutical services from existing premises.

This apparent oversight in the Regulations has been the subject of several challenges in the courts. In 1996 Lord Justice Schiemann held in *ex parte Worthington* that the court had no power to strike out words (the 'loophole') that were perfectly clear.

Applications by doctors

Doctors may apply for 'outline consent' to dispense for those of their patients who live more than one mile from a pharmacy (Reg. 21). The same test is used, i.e. whether granting the application would prejudice the proper provision of general medical or pharmaceutical services.

The application must specify the area for which the grant of 'outline consent' is sought. The application must be in writing, but no particular form is specified.

The effect of a grant is that the doctor may then dispense to any of his patients residing in the specified area, who request him to dispense, and who live more than one mile from an NHS pharmacy.

In certain circumstances doctors are enabled to dispense for patients without making an application as outlined above.

Immediate treatment
Regulation 19(a) of the NHS(PS) Regulations 1992 states that a doctor shall provide to a patient any appliance or non-scheduled drug which is needed for immediate treatment.

Personal administration
Regulation 19(b) allows doctors to provide directly to their patient any medicine which is going to be administered to the patient by the doctor or the doctor's staff. This covers items such as vaccines.

The 'serious difficulty' rule
Regulation 20 of the NHS (PS) Regulations 1992 states:

> 'Where a patient satisfies a HA that he would have serious difficulty in obtaining any necessary drugs or appliances from a pharmacy by reason of distance or inadequacy of means of communication he may at any time request in writing the doctor on whose list he is included to provide him with pharmaceutical service.'

This provision applies to any patient, including those resident in urban areas.

Other paragraphs of this Regulation deal with the detail of the arrangements between the doctor and the HA.

In considering whether the patient has a serious difficulty, the HA is expected to consider:

- personal circumstances of the patient
- local arrangements for medical and pharmaceutical services
- transport
- any collection and delivery services
- availability of telephones
- any other relevant factors.

There is no appeal procedure from a decision of the HA that the patient does not have any serious difficulty.

Temporary residents
Doctors who provide pharmaceutical services to at least some of the patients on their list may also dispense to any temporary residents whom they accept.

Appeal procedure

An appeal may be made to the Health Services Appeals Authority. The Appeals Authority may, but is not required to, hold an oral hearing.

An appeal against a decision made under the Regulation 12 procedure may be summarily dismissed by the unit if it decides the appeal is frivolous, vexatious or discloses no reasonable grounds of appeal.

Chapter 5

Terms of Service

The Health Authority's duty

HAs are under a legal duty to arrange for the supply of pharmaceutical services to patients in their area.

According to section 41 of the NHS Act 1977 (as amended by the Health and Social Care Act 2001) they must arrange for the supply of 'proper and sufficient drugs and medicines and listed appliances' when they are ordered by a medical practitioner under the NHS.

They must also make similar arrangements for the supply of the limited range of drugs and medicines which may be ordered by a dental practitioner, nurse or other 'prescribed person' under the NHS.

The services which are so provided are known as 'pharmaceutical services'. The details of those arrangements are dealt with by Regulations.

Section 41 of the 1977 Act entitled 'Arrangements for pharmaceutical services' now reads:

'It is the duty of every Health Authority, in accordance with regulations which shall be made for the purpose, to arrange as respects their area for the provision to persons who are in that area of –

a) proper and sufficient drugs and medicines and listed appliances which are ordered for those persons by a medical practitioner in pursuance of his functions in the health service, the Scottish health service, the Northern Ireland health service or the armed forces of the Crown;

b) proper and sufficient drugs and medicines which are ordered for those persons by a dental practitioner in pursuance of –

    (i) his functions in the health service, the Scottish health service or the Northern Ireland health service (other than functions exercised in pursuance of the provision of services mentioned in paragraph (c)); or

    (ii) his functions in the armed forces of the Crown;

c) listed drugs and medicines which are ordered for those persons by a dental practitioner in pursuance of the provision of general dental services or equivalent services in the Scottish health services or the Northern Ireland health service;

d) such drugs and medicines and such listed appliances as may be determined by the Secretary of State for the purposes of this paragraph which are ordered for those persons by a prescribed description of person in accordance with such conditions, if any as may be prescribed, in pursuance of functions in the health service, the Scottish health service, the Northern Ireland health service or the armed forces of the Crown; and

e) such other services as may be prescribed.'

The persons referred to in (1)(d) may be PAMs, pharmacists, dental auxiliaries, ophthalmic opticians, osteopaths, chiropractors, nurses, midwives, health visitors, or any other health professionals the S of S specifies.

The current Regulations are the NHS (Pharmaceutical Services) Regulations 1992, SI 1992 No. 662. These Regulations consolidate some 30 previous Regulations into one document. A similar new consolidated set of Regulations deals with general medical services, *viz.* the NHS (General Medical Services) Regulations 1992, SI 1992 No. 635. Updated NHS (Service Committees and Tribunals) Regulations 1992, SI 1992 No. 664 have also been enacted, and amended.

The NHS (Pharmaceutical Services) Regulations 1992 have already been amended by nine sets of Amendment Regulations: SI 1993 No. 2451, SI 1994 No. 2402, SI 1995 No. 644, SI 1996 No. 698, SI 1998 No. 681, SI 1998 No. 2224, SI 1999 No. 696, SI 2000 No. 121 and SI 2000 No. 593.

Pharmaceutical services

Pharmaceutical services consist of:

(1) the supply of drugs and medicines as above
(2) the supply of appliances
(3) the provision of certain 'additional professional services'
(4) the supply of contraceptive substances and appliances.

Pharmaceutical services may be provided by:

(1) pharmacists
(2) pharmacy companies
(3) appliance contractors.

Unless Regulations provide otherwise, arrangements for the dispensing of medicines may only be made with pharmacists or pharmacy companies (section 43). The NHS (Pharmaceutical Services) Regulations 1992 do not provide otherwise.

Supply under Patient Group Protocols is limited to products which already have product licence or marketing authorisation. Dispensing is not defined in the NHS Act. Since supply of medicines under the NHS is allowed by persons who are not pharmacists, it could be argued that the restriction referred to above in section 43b refers only to the making up of medicines. Such an interpretation would however be at odds with the normal use of the term 'dispensing' by the profession.

Unless Regulations provide otherwise, arrangements may not be made with a medical practitioner or dental practitioner under which he agrees to provide or is required to provide pharmaceutical services to any person to whom he is rendering General Medical Services (GMS) or General Dental Services (GDS).

Regulations do provide for General Medical Practitioners (GMPs) to provide pharmaceutical services to:

(1) Patients living in a rural area, more than a mile from a pharmacy,
(2) Patients who have satisfied the HA that they have serious difficulty in obtaining drugs or appliances from a pharmacy because of its distance or the poor communications.

The contract which governs the relationship between the HA and the pharmacy is not contained in any single document, but consists of an amalgam of parts from various documents.

The nature of the arrangements between the HA and those professionals providing the services to patients has been discussed by the courts. In 1968 it was held that the pharmacy had a contract with the Executive Council (a predessessor to the HA) to provide services (*Appleby* v. *Sleep* (1968 2 AER 265)). Other views have since been expressed that there is no contract as such, merely an administrative arrangement set out in Regulations.

Contractors' obligations

Under their contract with an HA pharmacists are obliged to:

(1) Dispense all NHS prescriptions presented to them, within a reasonable time.
(2) Maintain certain minimum hours of opening.
(3) Observe certain other rules.

When a contractor applies to be entered on the list of NHS pharmacies he agrees to the Terms of Service, which are contained in Schedule 2 of the NHS (PS) Regulations 1992.

As a breach of any of these terms may result in a hearing by a discipline committee (see Chapter 8) it is important that they be clearly understood. Each paragraph contains a number of requirements. Failure to comply with any one of them may give rise to a breach.

The requirements of these terms of service are absolute. An error is just as much a breach as is a deliberate fraud. For instance, the supply of the wrong drug, in error, will constitute a breach. However, the terms of service are not all-embracing. For instance, they do not cover errors on dispensing labels, although such an error might give rise to criminal proceedings under the Medicines Act 1968.

Supervision of dispensing

The dispensing of medicines must be by or under the direct supervision of a pharmacist. A company must undertake that all medicines supplied by them under the Act will be dispensed by or under the direct supervision of a pharmacist (section 43 NHS Act 1977).

There are Medicines Act 1968 requirements with respect to supply, but they require only 'supervision'. 'Direct supervision' is probably more onerous than 'supervision'. The courts have discussed this issue in cases brought under the Pharmacy and Poisons Act 1933, and supported the view that there is a distinction. It is difficult to find such a distinction in practice.

The NHS (Pharmaceutical Services) Regulations state in Schedule 2:

'5(1)   Drugs shall be provided by or under the direct supervision of a pharmacist;

Where that pharmacist is an employee, he must not be:

- someone who is held to be unfit to be engaged in the provision of pharmaceutical services, or
- someone who has been suspended by the NHS Tribunal.

Section 46 deals with removal of a pharmacist from a list by the NHS Tribunal.

Fundamental requirements of the terms of service

The fundamental requirement is to supply what is ordered. Schedule 2 of the 1992 Regulations, paragraph 3(1) states:

'Where any person presents on a prescription form:

a) an order for drugs, not being Scheduled drugs, or appliances; or

b) an order for a drug specified in Schedule 11 to the General Medical Services Regulations, signed by and endorsed on its face with the reference 'SLS' by a doctor; or

c) an order for listed drugs and medicines, signed by a dentist or his deputy or assistant; or

d) an order for listed drugs or medicines, or listed appliances, signed by a nurse prescriber;

a chemist shall, with reasonable promptness, provide the drugs or medicines so ordered, and such of the appliances so ordered as he supplies in the normal course of his business.'

There are several requirements here.

Promptness
A pharmacy must supply 'with reasonable promptness'. Discipline Committees have generally taken the view that most medicines should either be supplied from stock in the pharmacy or from the next reasonable wholesaler delivery. They have also taken into account the nature of the condition being treated and the rarity or scarcity of the medicine. The situation which frequently causes problems is where the patient is repeatedly asked to return to the pharmacy to collect an item alleged to be on order but which has not been delivered. This may have resulted from failure to provide an effective system for passing on messages between members of staff, or to 'progress chase' items on order. Breaches

of the requirement to provide promptly have been found where a delay of several days occurred.

Paragraph 3(1A) requires the pharmacy to give, on request, an estimate of the time when the completed prescription will be ready for collection. If the prescription is not ready at that estimated time, a revised estimate must then be given.

Any person

A pharmacy must supply any person who presents a valid form. There is no right to refuse the supply, or to decline to serve the person. Services have to be provided at the premises but it may be possible to exclude a patient from the premises. There may be ethical considerations which require the pharmacist to refuse to dispense a prescription. Such action is not automatically exempt from sanctions under the Terms of Service. The pharmacist has to argue the case.

Such drugs as may be so ordered

A pharmacy must supply any drugs ordered on a prescription form by a doctor except those covered by the Selected List rules. The requirement is to supply the drugs ordered on the form, not any similar drugs. This provision therefore prohibits the supply of generic equivalents. It also prohibits the supply of parallel imports where the name used on the product is different from that on the form. This provision has the somewhat unusual effect of occasionally requiring the pharmacist to supply an import where the doctor's poor spelling has unwittingly produced the foreign name.

Where the wrong drug is supplied in error it will constitute a breach of paragraph 3(1) of Schedule 2 to the NHS (Pharmaceutical Services) Regulations 1992 (the Terms of Service (TOS).

There are additional rules governing the prescribing and supply of Selected List drugs. These are dealt with below under the heading 'Selected List Scheme'.

Dentists may only prescribe from the Secretary of State's list which is in the DT. Although the list is in generic terms, it is accepted that proprietary products fitting those generic descriptions may be ordered and supplied.

Appliances

A pharmacist is only required to supply those appliances which he normally supplies in the course of his business.

Prescription forms

The expression 'prescription form' means a form supplied by the HA or a Trust to enable persons to obtain pharmaceutical services as defined by the NHS Act 1977. All variations are included, e.g. FP10, FP10(HP), FP14.

Signed

Paragraph 3(1) of the 1992 Regulations requires the prescriptions to be signed.

Services may only be provided on receipt of a signed form, except in emergency. Accordingly unless the form is signed no drugs can be supplied. It also follows that an amendment agreed over the telephone with the prescribing doctor does not take effect until either the doctor requests an emergency supply, or he signs the original form again. In some circumstances pharmacists will have to balance the possibility of a service case against the need for the patient to have the medicine.

Forgeries

Paragraph 3(1B) states that a pharmacist may refuse to dispense a form which he believes is stolen or a forgery.

Exemption declaration

Paragraph 3(1C) requires the pharmacist to ask, in most cases, for evidence of entitlement to exemption.

Quality

Paragraph 3(2) of the Terms of Service states that:

'Any drug which is provided as part of pharmaceutical services and included in the DT, British National Formulary (BNF), Dental Practitioners' Formulary (DPF), European Pharmacopoeia, or the British Pharmaceutical Codex (BPC) shall comply with the standard or formula specified therein.'

The Drug Tariff helpfully adds:

'Any drugs which are not included in the DT [or the publications listed in Paragraph 3(2) of the Terms of Service] must be of a grade or quality not lower than that ordinarily used for medical purposes.'

The DT contains a list of galenicals and generic medicines. If he wishes the prescriber can specify a different standard, for example by specifically referring to a foreign pharmacopoeia. Where a prescription calls for a generic drug which is included in a monograph in one of the listed publications the product supplied must comply with the relevant monograph and not just with the generic description.

Quantity

The quantity which is ordered should be supplied, unless the provisions of paragraph 3(3) apply. This sub-paragraph was originally inserted into the Terms of Service (TOS) in 1965 in order to allow for the change-over from the old apothecary system of measures to metric measurements. An agreed system of conversion allowed apothecary measures to be converted into an approximate metric equivalent, e.g. 12 fluid ounces into 300 millilitres.

In practice flexibility is allowed for items which are supplied in special containers to protect the contents, and for creams, etc. supplied in tubes and similar containers.

The DT allows payment to be made on the basis that the total amount has been ordered, but such a supply is strictly outside the requirements of the Medicines Act 1968 (see section on patient packs below).

Missing details on prescription

Paragraphs 3(4) and (5) allow the pharmacist to fill in certain missing details of quantity, strength and dosage.

Where the prescription is for a drug other than a controlled drug (CD), and the quantity, strength or dose is missing, the pharmacist may use his judgment to decide the missing information. He may give up to five days treatment at the appropriate dose. Where the product is a liquid antibiotic, an oral contraceptive or a combination pack he may give the smallest original pack even if that quantity is larger than a five day course.

Paragraph 3(4) states:

'Where an order, not being an order to which the Poisons Rules 1982 or the Misuse of Drugs Regulations 1985 apply, issued by a doctor, a dentist or a nurse prescriber on a prescription form for drugs does not prescribe their quantity, strength or dosage, a chemist may provide the drugs in such strength and dosage as in the exercise of his professional skill, knowledge and care he considers to be appropriate and, subject to the provisions of sub-paragraph (3), in such quantity as he considers to be appropriate for a course of treatment, for the patient to whom the order relates, for a period not exceeding five days.'

Where the strength or dosage are missing the pharmacist has complete free-dom to supply what is appropriate. Note that where the wrong strength is given the pharmacist is not authorised by the Regulations to change it. The PPA interprets the Regulations as requiring the doctor to initial any alteration to the prescription which alters the strength ordered.

Professional practice requires that where an overdose is inadvertently ordered the pharmacist should reduce the dose to a safe one, and discuss his action with the prescriber as soon as possible

Paragraph 3(5) states:

'Where an order to which sub-paragraph (3) applies is for –

  a) an oral contraceptive substance;
  b) a drug which is available for supply as part of pharmaceutical services only together with one or more drugs; or
  c) an antibiotic in a liquid form for oral administration in respect of which pharmaceutical considerations require its provision in an unopened package,

which is not available for supply as part of pharmaceutical services except in such packages that the minimum available package contains a quantity appropriate to a course of treatment for a patient for a period of more than five days, the chemist may provide that minimum available package.'

Patient packs

Although no provision is made for the adoption of patient pack dispensing as a normal procedure, the TOS make special provision for dealing with products which are difficult to dispense from bulk.

Paragraph 3(6) states:

'Where any drug, not being one to which the Misuse of Drugs Regulations 1973 apply, ordered by a doctor, dentist or nurse prescriber on a prescription form, is available for provision by a chemist in a pack in a quantity which is different to the quantity which has been so ordered, and that drug is –

   a) sterile
   b) effervescent or hygroscopic
   c) a liquid preparation for addition to bath water
   d) a coal tar preparation
   e) a viscous preparation; or
   f) packed at the time of its manufacture in a calendar pack or special container,

the chemist shall, subject to sub-paragraph (7) provide the drug in the pack whose quantity is nearest to the quantity which has been so ordered.'

Paragraph 3(7) states:

'A chemist shall not provide, pursuant to sub-paragraph (5), a drug in a calendar pack where, in his opinion, it was the intention of the doctor, dentist or nurse prescriber who ordered the drug that it should be provided only in the exact quantity ordered.'

Paragraph 3(8) provides two definitions as follows:

   'a) 'calendar pack' means a blister or strip pack showing the days of the week or month against each of the several units in the pack
   b) 'special container' means any container with an integral means of application or from which it is not practicable to dispense an exact quantity.'

Emergency NHS supplies

In an emergency a pharmacy may supply a drug if the doctor or nurse prescriber:

(1)   is personally known to the pharmacist
(2)   requests the supply
(3)   undertakes to supply a signed form within 72 hours; *and*
(4)   the drug is not a Scheduled drug
(5)   if a CD the drug is in Schedule 1 to the Misuse of Drugs Regulations.

   The chemist is enabled to supply before the form arrives. He is not obliged to do so. The procedure only applies to a request by a doctor. The procedure does not apply to appliances.
   Paragraph 3(9) states:

'Where in a case of urgency, a doctor or nurse prescriber personally known to a chemist requests him to provide a drug, the chemist may provide that drug before receiving a prescription form, provided that –

   (a) that drug is not a Scheduled drug; and

(b) that drug is not a controlled drug within the meaning of the Misuse of Drugs Act 1971, other than a drug which is for the time being specified in Schedule 4 or 5 to the Misuse of Drugs Regulations 1985; and

(c) the doctor or nurse prescriber undertakes to give the chemist such a prescription form within 72 hours.'

Selected List Scheme (SLS)

In 1985 the government introduced, by means of Regulations, the 'Selected List Scheme' to reduce NHS expenditure by limiting the availability of simple medicines on the NHS. Doctors were prohibited from prescribing, and pharmacists from dispensing a number of medicines in various categories. The categories are:

- indigestion remedies
- laxatives
- analgesics for mild to moderate pain
- bitters and tonics
- vitamins
- benzodiazepine tranquillizers and sedatives.

Most of the medicines in these categories were put on a Schedule to the Regulations. Medicines listed on the Schedule may not be prescribed or dispensed under the NHS. Generic products were unaffected. The current list is in Schedule 10 to the NHS (General Medical Services) Regulations 1992. References in the TOS to 'Scheduled drug' refer to medicines listed on that Schedule.

In December 1992 the DoH announced that the scheme would be extended to an additional 10 categories:

- anti-diarrhoeal drugs
- drugs for allergic disorders
- hypnotics and anxiolytics
- appetite suppressants
- drugs for vaginal and vulval conditions
- contraceptives
- drugs used in anaemia
- topical antirheumatics
- drugs acting on the ear and nose
- drugs acting on the skin.

The list of products is amended from time to time. The latest amendment is in the NHS (GMS) Amendment (No 2) Regulations 2001, SI No. 1178. An up-to-date list is included in the current Drug Tariff.

Schedule 11, referred to in paragraph 3(1) of the TOS contains a list of medicines which can only be prescribed for certain listed conditions, and then only if the prescription form is endorsed *by the doctor* with the initials 'SLS'.

Paragraph 3(10) states:

'Except as provided in sub-paragraph (11), a chemist shall not supply a Scheduled drug, by way of pharmaceutical services or otherwise, in response to an order by name, formula or other description on a prescription form.'

Paragraph 3(11) states:

'Where a drug has an appropriate non-proprietary name (ANPN) and it is ordered on a prescription form either by that name or by its formula, a chemist may supply a drug which has the same specification notwithstanding that it is a Scheduled drug, provided that where a Scheduled drug is a pack which consists of a drug in more than one strength, such provision does not involve the supply of part only of the pack.'

Paragraph 3(11) is intended to restrict the supply of constituent parts of combination packs, which otherwise would not be caught by the rules.

Paragraph 3(12) states:

'Where a drug which is ordered as specified in sub-paragraph (11) combines more than one drug, that paragraph shall apply only if the combination has an appropriate non-proprietary name, whether the individual drugs which it combines do so or not.'

Paragraph 3(12) is similarly intended to catch certain products containing a number of constituent drugs.

Containers

Paragraph 3(13) states:

'A chemist shall provide any drug which he is required to provide under this paragraph in a suitable container.'

The DT expands this requirement as follows:

(1) Capsules, tablets, pills, pulvules, etc. shall be supplied in airtight containers of glass, aluminium or rigid plastics.
(2) Card containers may be used only for foil/strip packed tablets, etc.
(3) Card containers shall not be used for ointments, creams or pastes.
(4) Eye, ear and nasal drops shall be supplied in dropper bottles, or with a separate dropper where appropriate.
(5) When an oral liquid medicine is dispensed, a 5 ml plastics spoon shall be supplied by the pharmacist unless the patient already has a spoon or the manufacturer's pack includes one.

In 1992 the 'dilution convention' agreed between the RPSGB and the British Medical Association (BMA), under which doses of less than 5ml were diluted, was been abandoned. Under the new agreement doses of less than 5 ml are to be measured by the patient using an oral syringe which complies with BS 3221: Part 7: 1986 (or an equivalent European standard). The medicine is to be dispensed undiluted. Patients requiring an oral syringe are to be supplied with one without charge.

Inducements

Paragraph 3(14) states:

> 'A pharmacist shall not give, promise or offer to any person any gift or reward (whether by way of a share of or dividend on the profits of the business or by way of discount or rebate or otherwise) as an inducement to or in consideration of his presenting an order for drugs or appliances on a prescription form.'

This does not prohibit the supply of free controlled dosage systems to users of the pharmacy, nor the availability of collection and delivery systems etc.

Contraceptive services

The supply of contraceptive substances and appliances forms part of the pharmaceutical services to be provided. All contraceptive substances are available, but only those appliances included in the DT. For example, diaphragms are included in the DT, but condoms are not.

Under the provisions of SI 1975 No. 719 a pharmacist could notify the FHSA that he wished to be excluded from the arrangements for the supply of contraceptive substances. It was intended to take account of religious or moral objections to contraception. The provision disappeared from the Regulations in 1987, when an amendment (SI 1987 No. 401) replaced the existing Regulation 26 with a new version which omitted the conscience clause. It is also missing from the 1992 Regulations. When applying for a contract the pharmacist can specify the services he intends to provide. This would seem to be an opportunity to indicate any religious or moral restrictions on the service.

Contractors are only required to supply such appliances as they normally stock, so no problem arises with contraceptive appliances.

Premises and hours

The provisions dealing with hours of service have been extensively altered in the 1992 Regulations in an attempt to introduce flexibility. Those provisions were then amended by SI 1995 No. 644. Paragraphs 4(1) to 4(25) of the main Regulations deal with hours.

Paragraph 4(1) states:

> 'Pharmaceutical services shall be provided at each of the premises from which the chemist has undertaken to provide pharmaceutical services at such times as, following an application in writing by the chemist, shall have been approved in his case by an HA or, on appeal, the Secretary of State, in accordance with the following provisions of this paragraph.'

Paragraph 4(2) states:

'An HA shall not approve any application submitted by a chemist in relation to the times at which he is to provide pharmaceutical services unless it is satisfied that –

a) the times are such that a pharmacist will normally be available –
i) subject to sub-paragraph (3), for no less than 30 hours in any week, and
ii) on 5 days in any such week; and
b) the hours when a pharmacist will normally be available in any week are to be allocated between the days on which he will normally be available in that week in such a manner as is likely to meet the needs of persons in the neighbourhood for pharmaceutical services on working days between the hours of 09.00 and 17.30 (or 13.00 on an early closing day).'

Paragraph 4(3) states:

'In this paragraph "available" means, in relation to a pharmacist, available to provide pharmaceutical services of the kind he has undertaken to provide and "availability" shall be construed accordingly; working day means Monday to Saturday excluding a Good Friday, Christmas Day, 28 December if 26 December is a Saturday, or a bank holiday which falls on any such day; and an early closing day means any working day when most shops in the neighbourhood are habitually closed after the hour of 13.00.'

Paragraph 4(4) states:

'The HA may approve an application to provide pharmaceutical services for less than 30 hours in any week provided that it is satisfied that the provision of pharmaceutical services in the neighbourhood is likely to be adequate to meet the need for such services on working days between the hours of 09.00 and 17.30 (or 13.00 on an early closing day) at times when the pharmacist is not available.'

Paragraphs 4(5) to 4(12) detail the procedure for applying for and appealing against an HA determination on hours.

Notices
Paragraph 4(13) states:

'The premises must display two notices:

a) a notice provided by the Health Authority which shows the opening hours, and
b) when the pharmacy is closed, a notice which indicates the addresses of other pharmacies nearby and their opening hours.'

Illness of pharmacist
Paragraph 4(15) states:

'Where a chemist is prevented by illness or other reasonable cause from complying with his obligations under this paragraph, he shall where practicable, make arrangements with one or more chemists whose premises are situated in the neighbourhood for the provision of pharmaceutical services during that time.'

The obligation to make alternative arrangements is with the affected pharmacy, but only when 'practicable'. The provision applies to illness or 'other reasonable cause'.

Variation of hours
Paragraphs 4(16)–4(17) deal with applications to vary the previous hours.

Changes made by HA
Paragraphs 4(18) to 4(31) deal with review of hours by the HA, in cases where it appears to the HA that the needs of the neighbourhood are not being met. The LPC must be consulted. The changes must be notified to the pharmacy. There is an appeal process.

Supervision

Paragraph 5(1) requires the provision of medicines to be by or under the direct supervision of a pharmacist. This requirement does not apply to the supply of appliances. Some appliances, such as certain medicated dressings, are Prescription Only Medicine (POM). The supply of POM products is subject to the over-riding requirement for supervision in the Medicines Act 1968.

A chemist must make all the necessary arrangements for measuring patients, and for fitting, when the appliance which is ordered requires this.

Particulars of qualified staff

Paragraph 6 states:

'The HA can require the names of any registered pharmacist employed in the provision of drugs.'

Charges

Paragraph 7 deals with the fact that the NHS (Charges for Drugs and Appliances) Regulations 1989, SI 1989 No. 419 are updated each year and contain the charges to be made for the supply of medicines and appliances.

All containers must be provided free to the patient.

Records and inspection

Paragraph 8(1A) allows the HA to inspect the pharmacy to satisfy itself that the 'additional professional services' (practice leaflets, health promotion literature and patient medication records) are being provided.

Remuneration

Paragraph 8(2) requires the HA to pay according to the DT, or the HA determination where appropriate. This facilitates a degree of locally determined remuneration.

Paragraph 8(2A) requires the HA to pay for 'additional professional services'.

Paragraph 8(3) allows the pharmacist to check the way in which his forms have been priced. In practice this service is provided by the PSNC (paragraph 8(4)).

Professional standards

The 1996 Amendments inserted requirements as to professional standards.

Paragraph 8A reads:

'1) A pharmacist whose name is on the pharmaceutical list shall provide pharmaceutical services and exercise any professional judgement in connection with the provision of such services in conformity with the standards generally accepted in the pharmaceutical profession.

2) A chemist who employs a pharmacist in connection with the provision of pharmaceutical services shall secure that the pharmacist complies with the requirements set out in sub-paragraph (1).'

The requirement in sub-paragraph (1) refers to the 'generally accepted standards'. Although it does not specifically refer to the RPSGB Code of Ethics, it is that document which will in most cases set out the generally accepted standards. The second paragraph puts an obligation on an employer to ensure that pharmacist staff comply.

Wages

Paragraph 9, which required the contractor to pay certain minimum rates, was deleted by SI 1995 No. 644.

Withdrawal from the pharmaceutical lists

Paragraph 10 states:

'At any time a pharmacy may give notice to the FHSA requesting removal from the lists. The name must be removed at the expiry of three months from the date of the notice. If the FHSA agrees the removal may be earlier.

The FHSA may make representations to the Tribunal that the continued inclusion of the name of a pharmacy in the lists is prejudicial to the efficiency of the service. Where such a representation has been made the pharmacy cannot avoid the outcome by resigning voluntarily, unless the Secretary of State agrees.'

Complaints procedure

Following the report of a committee chaired by Professor Alan Wilson, the Government introduced changes so that complaints and disciplinary matters are handled by separate procedures.

The aim of the new system is to try and resolve most complaints at pharmacy level.

NHS pharmacies are now required to have in place a system for dealing with 'expressions of dissatisfaction' by users of pharmaceutical services.

Paragraph 10A of the ToS requires the establishment and operation of a 'pharmacy-based' procedure for handling complaints.

Paragraph 10B requires the pharmacy to co-operate with any HA procedure for handling complaints.

See also Chapter 8.

Additional professional services

This term was introduced by the NHS (Pharmaceutical Services) Amendment Regulations 1993, SI 1993 No. 2451. The requirements are now found in Regulation 16A of the 1992 Regulations. Regulation 16A was amended by both the 1995 and 1996 Amendment Regulations. It now reads:

'1) A chemist may, in addition, undertake to provide additional pharmaceutical services.

2) In these Regulations 'additional pharmaceutical services' means:

a) publishing a leaflet ('practice leaflet') which shall include –

i) a list of the pharmaceutical services which the chemist has undertaken to provide and for which his name is included in a pharmaceutical list of the Health Authority,

ii) the name, address and telephone number of the pharmacy from which he provides those services and the hours in each day of the week during which he provides those services from those premises,

iii) the arrangements made by the chemist to provide, or such arrangements as the chemist has made with other chemists to provide, pharmaceutical services to any person who needs those services in an emergency or outside of the normal hours during which the chemist provides pharmaceutical services,

iv) the procedure by which any person may comment upon the provision of pharmaceutical services undertaken by the chemist;

b) displaying such health promotion leaflets as the Health Authority may, in consultation with the Local Pharmaceutical Committee, approve;

c) keeping records in connection with drugs supplied to any person –

i) who claims exemption under regulation 6(1)(c) of the NHS (Charges for Drugs and Appliances) Regulations 1989 [which provides that those aged 60 or over are exempt from prescription charges], or

ii) who, in the opinion of the pharmacist providing the drug, is likely to have difficulty understanding the nature and dosage of the drug provided and the times at which it is to be taken,

in circumstances where the nature of the drug is such that, in the opinion of the pharmacist providing it, the same or a similar drug is likely to be prescribed for that person regularly on future occasions.

3) In paragraph 2(c) above, 'records' includes a record of –

    a) the name and address of the person to whom the drug is supplied

    b) the name, quantity and dosage of the drug supplied

    c) the date on which it is provided.'

The Drug Tariff contains some rules about payment. Payment is only made if a minimum number of records are maintained. There must be records for a minimum of 100 patients. For a pharmacy receiving Essential Small Pharmacy Scheme support the minimum number is 50.

Each record should cover all the drugs supplied to one patient. One or more of the drugs supplied should be long term as described above.

The record system should be suitable for the purpose and provide appropriate levels of security.

Fees are only paid where the pharmacist employed to operate the scheme has a certificate of completion of an approved training course.

Guidance issued by the Department of Health to HAs asks them to monitor the provision of additional professional services by pharmacists. In order to do this officers of the HA need access to the records. They are required to check that the pharmacy is keeping the requisite number of records for payment. They are also to check that the records contain the required information.

Paragraph 8(1A) of the TOS states that pharmacists will be required to make all records kept as additional professional services available to the HA for inspection on request.

Incorporation of other provisions

The following are incorporated in the Terms of Service:

(a)   The Regulations

(b)   The Drug Tariff, so far as it lists drugs and appliances for the purposes of section 41 of the NHS Act 1977

(c)   The discipline committee procedure

(d)   The tribunal procedure

(e)   Any appeals procedure.

Chapter 6

The Drug Tariff

Form and content of the Drug Tariff

Every month the Secretary of State approves and the PPA publishes the Drug Tariff (DT). It contains a list of drug prices, detailed information on appliances, sets the standards of and payments for drugs and appliances, and details what can and cannot be prescribed on NHS prescriptions and by which class of practitioner (that is doctor, dentist, or nurse). Separate Drug Tariffs are produced for England and Wales, Scotland, and Northern Ireland.

Regulation 18(1) of the NHS (Pharmaceutical Services) Regulations 1992 states:

'For the purpose of enabling arrangements to be made for the provision of pharmaceutical services, the Secretary of State shall compile and publish a statement (in these regulations referred to as "the Drug Tariff") which he may amend from time to time and which shall include ...

a) the list of appliances for the time being approved by the Secretary of State for the purposes of section 41 of the Act

b) the list of chemical reagents for the time being approved by the Secretary of State for the purposes of section 41 of the Act

c) the list of drugs for the time being approved by the Secretary of State for the purposes of section 41 of the Act

d) the prices on the basis of which the payment for drugs and appliances ordinarily supplied is to be calculated

e) the method of calculating the payment for drugs not mentioned in the Drug Tariff

f) the method of calculating the payment for containers and medicine measures

g) the dispensing or other fees payable in respect of the supply of drugs and appliances and of supplemental services

h) arrangements for claiming fees, allowances and other remuneration for the provision of pharmaeutical services

i) the method by which a claim may be made for compensation for financial loss in respect of oxygen equipment.'

Regulation 18(1A) The Drug Tariff may state in respect of any specified fee falling within paragraph (1)(g), or any other specified fee, allowance or other remuneration in respect of the provision of pharmaceutical services by chemists included in the pharmaceutical list of an FHSA, that the determining authority for that fee, allowance or other remuneration for those chemists is the HA, and in such a case paragraphs (4) and (5) shall apply.

Regulation 18(2) states:

'The prices referred to in paragraph (1)(d) may be fixed prices or may be subject to monthly or other periodic variations to be determined by reference to fluctuations in the cost of drugs and appliances.'

Besides the list included in the Regulations the DT also contains many other items of information useful to pharmacists and prescribers.

By virtue of paragraph 2 of Schedule 2 of the NHS (PS) Regulations 1992 the DT lists of drugs and appliances are incorporated into the TOS. In other words whatever is in the DT about prices to be paid for drugs and appliances is considered to be something which is agreed to by the pharmacist on taking up the contract.

The DT is produced on a monthly basis and the amendments for the month are listed in the preface. The preface bears the words 'Pursuant to Regulation 18(1) of the NHS (PS) Regulations 1992 the Secretary of State for Health as respects England and the National Assembly for Wales as respects Wales has amended the Drug Tariff with effect from [date]'. Amendments, including prices, come into effect on the date specified, regardless of whether the DT has been received by the pharmacist and regardless of whether the particular amendment has actually been printed in the DT.

Part I – Requirements for the supply of drugs, appliances and chemical reagents

The Drug Tariff sets out much of the arrangement for prescribing and dispensing for NHS patients. The basic principles of prescribing under the NHS are that:

(1) Doctors may prescribe any medicine, unless its use at NHS expense is specifically prohibited by the Secretary of State, or its use is restricted to specified circumstances.
(2) Doctors may prescribe an appliance or chemical reagent, only if its use at NHS expense is approved by the Secretary of State, and only in the circumstances specified.
(3) Doctors may prescribe a 'borderline substance' only if its use at NHS expense is approved by the Secretary of State, and only in the circumstances specified.

Clause 1 requires that any drugs supplied must comply with the standard specified in the DT (if any such standard is included). Otherwise the drug must comply with the relevant standard in the BNF, DPF, EP, the British Pharmacopoeia (BP) or BPC. The prescriber may indicate that he requires some other standard. If the prescriber has not indicated the standard, and the drug does not appear in one of the relevant publications, then the grade or quality must be no lower than that ordinarily used for medicinal purposes.

Clause 2 states that only the appliances listed in the DT may be supplied, and that they must comply with the specifications listed in the DT.

In practice the Technical Specifications of the DT were last issued as a separate document in 1981, although they are available on request from the Department of Health. However, many of the individual entries contain details which in effect are specifications, e.g. the size of a bandage. Dressings are included in the category 'appliances'. Neither the NHS Act 1977 nor the 1992 Regulations refer to dressings as such except to define them as appliances.

Since June 1998, 'medical devices' (as defined in the Medical Devices Regulation 1994) which are supplied on prescription have to bear a CE mark.

Clause 3 states that only the chemical reagents listed may be supplied.

Pharmacists are not required to ascertain the purpose for which prescribed items are to be used. All drugs may be supplied except those on Schedule 10. Pure chemical compounds, organic or inorganic, may be supplied as drugs. Chemical reagents other than those listed could therefore be supplied, and the pharmacist would be paid for their supply. If they were prescribed as reagents the doctor would be liable to pay the cost if action were brought under Regulation 36 of the NHS (General Medical Services) Regulations 1992, SI 1992 No. 635 (determination of whether a substance is a drug).

Clause 4 states that the requirements for the Domiciliary Oxygen Therapy service are in Part X of the DT.

Part II – Requirements enabling payments to be made

The DT contains a number of rules about how prescription forms are to be handled in order for the correct payments to be made.

Sorting and despatch of forms

At the end of each month the forms have to be sorted as instructed by the HA, and despatched, together with the claim forms, by the fifth day of the following month.

Where contractors have failed to despatch the forms on time, HAs have held this to be a breach of the TOS. Occasional lateness is not considered to be a problem, but persistent and serious lateness is. The late submission of forms to the PPA causes extra costs and disrupts the PPA system. HAs take these factors into account when considering the penalty.

Zero Discount List

Clause 6 contains a brief description of the payment system and a reference to the 'zero discount' lists. See later in this chapter.

Calculating payments

Clause 7 contains a more detailed description of the way payments are calculated for drugs. There is also a statement that if, after being requested to endorse a form properly the contractor fails to do so, then the Secretary of State may decide the price.

Clause 7D is unusual in nature. It is a deeming provision. If the contractor's overall use of a particular product would seem to justify the use of a larger pack size than that endorsed, then the endorsement will be ignored and the price paid will be based on the appropriate larger size. The actual words refer to 'that normally required pursuant to orders on prescription forms' which is a remarkably unclear phrase. Further there is no indication of the criteria for determining that a larger size ought to have been used.

Clause 8

The basic price for drugs, appliances and chemical reagents listed in Parts VIII and IX of the DT is the price in the DT. For other generic and branded drugs it is the manufacturer's list price.

The PPA may, under specified circumstances, accept an endorsement that a price higher than the 'statutory maximum price' has been paid.

Endorsement

The forms must be endorsed as required. The intention of endorsement is to ensure that the PPA has sufficient information to price accurately. The principle is that as far as possible the actual price paid by the pharmacist is paid by the NHS. Account is taken of the discounts obtained on purchases by averaging them and deducting an average discount from the totals of list prices.

Additional rules for endorsement are found in Clauses 9–13, the remainder of Part II, in Part III, and in Part III and in the Notes to Part VIII.

Clause 9 contains the main endorsement requirements. For generic drugs listed in Part VIII; for appliances listed in Part IX; for chemical reagents listed in Part IX, no endorsement is needed except for 'broken bulk' or where the quantity supplied differs from the order. The pack size and name of the maker or wholesaler is needed for orders for generic drugs not in the DT.

Where no product is available to contractors at the Part VIII price, the prescription may be specially endorsed. This concession is only allowed when the Secretary of State has agreed that the product is not available. The contractor must have made all reasonable efforts to obtain the product at the DT price. The endorsement must include the brand name or manufacturer or wholesaler of the product, the pack size, the phrase 'no cheaper stock obtainable' or 'NCSO') and be signed and dated on behalf of the contractor.

The PPA may request additional information in order to price the prescription.

Clause 10 allows what is supplied to deviate from the exact quantity ordered only in specified circumstances. These are where it is particularly difficult to open the container and dispense a part of its contents. (See also Chapter 5, Terms of Service.)

'Broken bulk'

Clause 11 sets out the rules whereby a contractor may be paid for the whole amount of a drug when less has been supplied. The rules appear to set out an objective test, *viz.* that the remainder cannot readily be disposed of, whereas in practice a subjective test is used. The contractor may claim if he believes he will not readily dispose of the remainder. Subsequent supplies are deemed to have been made from the remainder for the next six months, or until the remainder would in any event have been used up.

The Prescription Pricing Authority interpret the 'broken bulk' facility by using a 'two-thirds' rule. If a contractor receives two or more prescriptions in the same calendar month, totalling more than two-thirds of a pack, the PPA assume that this establishes usage and so consider the broken bulk claims as invalid.

In a service case where a contractor made a large number of broken bulk claims which were unjustified, the FHSA decided that that constituted a breach of the TOS and recommended a very large withholding. The conduct was also regarded as fraud by the Crown Court, resulting in a heavy fine.

Miscellaneous matters

Clause 12 provides that out of pocket expenses over 10 pence may be claimed in certain circumstances.

Clause 13 extends the broken bulk rules in Clause 11 to allow for payment of the full cost of using reconstituted products with a short life.

Urgent prescriptions

Extra fees are payable when a prescription is dispensed:

- when the pharmacy is not open for dispensing
- the prescription is dispensed on the day it was written or on the following day (if dispensed after midnight)
- the prescriber marked the form 'urgent' and it was dispensed between closing time and opening time

or

- when the pharmacy is not open for dispensing
- the prescription is dispensed on the day it was written or on the following day (if dispensed after midnight)
- the contractor marked the form 'dispensed urgently'
- the patient or the patient's representative signed the form
- it was dispensed between 11 pm and opening time, or on Sundays or on public holidays.

Two different rates of fees are payable, depending on whether or not the contractor is resident 'on his business premises'. To qualify for the non-resident rate, the contractor must:

- normally live elsewhere
- have left the business premises; and
- have returned to open them to dispense an urgent prescription.

This formulation of the rules is not very clear. First, very few contractors actually live on the business premises. Many live *above* the business premises, with a separate entrance. It is not clear if the presence of common access is a necessary requirement.

Secondly, it is the residence of the contractor which is referred to, not that of the pharmacist who dispenses the prescription.

Thirdly, the non-resident must 'normally' live elsewhere. What constitutes 'normally'? If a non-resident contractor is snowbound but is able to leave the business premises to go next door, on his return to dispense an urgent prescription is he entitled to the higher fee?

Fourthly, returning to make an urgent sale of medicine and then dispensing an urgent prescription brought in by another customer attracts a resident fee, since the return was not for the purpose of dispensing the urgent prescription but for the sale. Moreover if the first transaction was not a sale but the dispensing of a non-urgent prescription, no urgent fee at all is payable, since the premises were open for dispensing when the 'urgent' prescription was brought in.

What may be supplied?

Pharmacists will be paid for any medicines (including over-the-counter medicines, homoeopathic preparations and herbal products) provided the item does not appear in Schedule 10 of the NHS (GMS) Regulations, which is reproduced in the DT as Part XVIIIA.

Quantity
Clause 10 allows what is supplied to deviate from the exact quantity ordered only in specified circumstances. These are where it is particularly difficult to open the container and dispense a part of its contents.

Quality
Drugs and medicines supplied must comply with the standards in the appropriate book, the BNF, DPF, EP, BP, BPC or the DT itself. Where a drug or medicine does not appear in one of those then the grade or quality supplied should be the ordinary medicinal grade. For appliances, the quality will be determined either by an official standard referred to in the name, e.g. absorbent lint BPC, or by a specification in the DT itself. The specification section of the DT is obtainable as a separate volume.

Type
Any drug or medicine which is ordered may be supplied provided it is not included in Schedule 10 (printed as Part XVIIIA of the DT). Drugs or medicines included in Schedule 11 may only be supplied when the prescription bears the endorsement 'SLS' inserted by the prescriber. Additionally the conditions referred to in the Schedule must be complied with, although the pharmacist is under no obligation to verify these.

There is no requirement that the drugs or medicines supplied are to be licensed medicinal products (i.e. licensed under the Medicines Act 1968).

Only the appliances listed in Part IXA, B, and C may be supplied. The only chemical reagents which may be supplied are those listed in Part IXR.

Diagnostic reagents

Some diagnostic reagents are regarded as drugs. Neither the NHS Act 1977 nor the NHS (PS) Regulations refer specifically to diagnostic reagents. The effect of sections 41 and 128 of the Act together with Regulation 18 is that the DT can make provision for diagnostic reagents only if they are drugs, chemical reagents, medicines or appliances. Since it is difficult to regard something used for determining whether an illness exists to be the means of treating that illness, diagnostic reagents might not be regarded as medicines. The definition of a medicinal product in the Medicines Act 1968 specifically includes a substance used in 'diagnosing disease or ascertaining the existence, degree or extent of a physiological condition'. For NHS purposes, however, the matter is clarified by a notice, ECL 80/1953 (ECN 132), which states that the Minister is prepared to regard certain diagnostic reagents as drugs for the purposes of the NHS Regulations. The list comprises:

- Dick Test
- Protein Sensitisation Test Solution
- Schick Test; and
- certain Tuberculin Tests (Koch Test, Mantoux Test, Patch Test, Diagnostic Jelly).

How are payments made?

The DT lays down the basic rules which will be followed by the PPA when calculating the payments to be made in respect of the drugs, etc. supplied on Forms FP10 and variants.

Basically payment is made for the quantity supplied on the prescription. The price paid is calculated from the normal wholesale price of the product for supply to community pharmacists. This price is normally set out by the manufacturer in price lists.

A discount is deducted from the total due to each contractor for each month's dispensing. The discount is calculated according to the total amount due, on a sliding scale constructed to reflect the discounts generally achieved by contractors in their purchasing.

How must the forms be endorsed?

Rules for endorsing the forms are found in Clauses 9, 10 and 11, Part III and the Notes to Part VIII.

At the end of each calendar month the contractor must sort the prescription forms in a manner directed by the HA. They must then be despatched, together with the appropriate claim form, not later than the fifth day of the next month. The claim form is standard, and also contains the instructions for sorting.

Containers

Part IV specifies that card containers may only be used to dispense foil or strip packed tablets, capsules etc. All other medicines, including creams and ointments must be supplied in airtight containers of glass, aluminium or rigid plastic. Where appropriate, a dropper bottle or separate dropper is to be used.

Appliances and dressings

Part IX of the DT lists the appliances and dressings which may be supplied. The list is very specific and in some instances only certain sizes may be supplied although others are made; for example, only 10 cm Non-Sterile Gauze Swabs, packed in 100s, may be supplied.

In some entries, where a general specification is given, any make which meets the specification may be supplied, e.g. crêpe bandage BP. In others only the specified makes may be supplied. This is particularly noticeable where items for incontinence are concerned, where the detail extends to the model number.

Borderline substances

Under the NHS a general medical practitioner may prescribe (and the NHS may pay for) only drugs, medicines and certain appliances. Drugs and medicines are not clearly defined, but the category does not include food or cosmetics. Hospitals are not restricted in the same way and are able to provide anything needed for the care of the patient.

Note that the NHS Acts use the terms 'drugs' and 'medicines' whereas the Medicines Act 1968 uses the term 'medicinal product'. The two terms 'medicine' and 'medicinal product' are not synonymous. 'Medicinal product' is defined in the Medicines Act as a substance which is made or sold for use in treating, diagnosing or preventing disease or otherwise altering the normal physiological state. 'Drug' is a wider term which includes pure chemicals which are not produced for any particular purpose, e.g., glucose, but which are used in therapeutics. 'Medicines' refers to the product ready for administration, e.g., tablets.

There are circumstances where a patient will benefit from the prescribing of food or cosmetics. Certain metabolic disorders are best treated by the supply of special foods which do not contain a particular amino acid. Photosensitivity reactions caused by drugs can be minimised by the use of sunscreens.

Prescribers are requested to endorse prescriptions for borderline substances, which are written in accordance with the advice of the ACBS, with the letters 'ACBS'.

Prescriptions are monitored by the PPA, which may refer them to HAs. Where a HA receives a prescription for a product which it does not believe is a drug, it may refer the matter to a Local Medical Committee (LMC) under procedures provided by Regulation 36 of the NHS (General Medical Services) Regulations 1992. If the LMC agrees that in the circumstances the product was not a drug, the cost may be recovered by the HA from the doctor's remuneration. There is provision for an appeal.

The Advisory Committee on Borderline Substances (ACBS)

The ACBS exists to provide the S of S with expert independent medical advice on those substances which, although not drugs or medicines, are used in a similar manner. The Committee advises on classification and on whether or not they should be prescribed by GPs at NHS expense or prescribed only for patients with specified medical conditions.

Terms of reference and membership

The terms of reference which were announced in December 1992 are:

'To advise UK Health Ministers as to whether particular substances, preparations or items should not be treated as drugs for the purpose of the GMS Regulations; and to advise on appropriate amendments to Schedules 10 and 11 to the NHS (GMS) Regulations 1992 and the corresponding schedules in the regulations in Scotland and Northern Ireland accordingly.

In considering whether a particular substance, preparation or item should be included in such schedules, the Committee will have regard to the need to ensure that substances etc. which have therapeutic use in the treatment of disease in the community can be provided as economically as possible under the NHS.'

The Committee itself contains experts from many disciplines and is advised by medical and pharmaceutical assessors within the Department of Health. The members are appointed by the Secretary of State for Health in England, and the Secretaries of State for Scotland and Wales, after consultation with professional bodies. Members are appointed for a period of three years.

The Committee is a non-statutory body. Its existence has no basis in law and depends only upon the need for advice from an authoritative independent body.

Requests for consideration

It is open to doctors, manufacturers or the Health Departments to request the Committee to consider any substance or product of a borderline nature. The manufacturers are asked to provide the following information about the product:

(1) the indications for use
(2) details of formulation
(3) relevant clinical trials
(4) promotional policy
(5) confirmation that the product will be available for dispensing by community pharmacies
(6) applicability of the Medicines Act (e.g. exemption under the Food and Cosmetics Order)
(7) descriptive literature, samples, packaging.

ACBS advises manufacturers in writing of proposed unfavourable recommendations, giving them at least 30 days in which to make representations. An oral hearing may be granted if the case is complex. The manufacturer may be represented at the oral hearing, either legally or by other experts.

The Committee considers all relevant information provided by the manufacturer of the substance concerned.

If the Secretary of State accepts the decision of the Committee that a product should not be regarded as a drug, he may place the product on Schedule 10 to the NHS (GMS) Regulations. This is the list of products which may not be prescribed by GPs.

Medical Foods Regulations

The Medical Foods Regulations (England) 2000 SI No. 845 implement European Commission Directive 99/21/EC, which was developed to meet the Commission's requirement under framework Directive 89/398/EC to introduce specific rules for dietary foods for special medical purposes.

Corresponding regulations have been introduced in Wales, Northern Ireland and Scotland.

Medical foods are a unique group of foods used in the dietary management of specific diseases or medical conditions. The government considered that the population group for whom these products are intended is particularly vulnerable, and therefore specific controls, in addition to the general provisions of the Food Safety Act, are appropriate.

The Regulations define foodstuffs which may be sold as 'Food(s) for Special Medical Purposes' (FSMPs); lay down specific compositional and labelling requirements for them; and introduce a notification system to facilitate efficient monitoring of new products.

Maximum and minimum vitamin, mineral and trace element levels for specific categories of FSMPs are set by the Regulations.

The labelling requirements supplement those required by the Food Labelling Regulations 1996 (as amended) and are intended to provide sufficient nutritional and other information to health professionals and consumers to ensure the appropriate and effective use of these products under medical supervision.

The Regulations introduce a formal obligation to notify new products when first placed on the market.

Statutory procedure for classifying borderline substances for licensing

The Medicines for Human Use (Marketing Authorisations, Etc.) Amendment Regulations, SI 2000/No. 292 amend the 1994 Marketing Authorisations Regulations to give power to stop a company selling a product, which the licensing authority believes is a medicine, without a marketing authority. The licensing authority must explain why they consider the product to be a medicine. There is an appeal to a review panel.

Maximum price legislation

The basic price for a generic medicine listed in parts VIII and IX of the DT is the price stated in the DT.

However, maximum prices are set by the Department of Health. The list is available on their website www.doh.gov.uk/generic.

An exemption allows contractors to claim a higher price in certain circumstances as set out in Clause 8.

The prices of medicines supplied for NHS use are controlled in a number of ways.

Pharmaceutical Price Regulation Scheme

The majority of branded medicine manufacturers belong to a voluntary price regulation scheme. The current scheme, called the Pharmaceutical Price Regulation Scheme (PPRS) was agreed between the Department of Health and the Association of the British Pharmaceutical Industry (the trade organization for the pharmaceutical industry). It came into effect on 1 October 1999 and is scheduled to run for five years. It covers those medicines which are manufactured by scheme members and which:

(a)   have EC or UK marketing authorizations and
(b)   are sold as branded products and
(c)   are supplied to the NHS.

The scheme includes branded medicines regardless of whether patent protection is in force, and medicines supplied on tender or on contract. Over-the-counter (OTC) medicines dispensed against an NHS prescription are included. Generic medicines and OTC medicines sold directly to the public are not included.

Under this scheme prices are controlled indirectly. The control is exerted by limiting the profits made by manufacturers. Target profits are set as a percentage of capital invested. If the figure is exceeded the company is required to reduce its prices or to make a repayment to the DoH. However, prices may only be raised with the approval of DoH. A company has freedom to set the price for new products within the constraint of the profit target.

Statutory control of prices

Membership of the PPRS is voluntary. The Health Act 1999 gives powers to impose statutory price and profit controls on companies which are not scheme members.

Control of branded medicine prices

The Health Service Medicines (Control of Prices of Branded Medicines) Regulations 2000, SI No 123, came into force on 14 February 2000.

The Regulations, which apply to the UK, control the price of branded medicines sold for national health service purposes. They apply only to medicines which:

(a)   have EC or UK marketing authorizations and
(b)   are sold as branded products and
(c)   are supplied to the NHS and
(d)   are supplied by companies which are not scheme members within the meaning of Section (33(4) of the Health Act 1999.

Under the Regulations, the maximum price which may be charged for the supply for health service purposes of a branded health service medicine of a particular presentation shall not exceed '(a) 95.5 per cent of the 1999 price and for newer products the initial price'. Financial information must be provided to the DoH. There are penalties for failing to supply information, and for supplying above the specified price.

Control of generic medicine prices

The Health Service Medicines (Control of Prices of Specified Generic Medicines) Regulations 2000 SI No. 1763 came into effect on 3 August 2000.

These Regulations allow the Department of Health to control the prices of generic medicines which are sold 'for the purposes of the national health services in England and Wales, Scotland and Northern Ireland'.

Under the Regulations, the maximum price which is charged by a manufacturer or supplier for the supply of a specified generic medicine for health service use shall not exceed the 'specified price'.

'Supply' means supply by way of sale to a person lawfully conducting a retail pharmacy business or to a registered medical practitioner, in order to enable that person or practitioner (as the case may be) to provide pharmaceutical services within the meaning of:

(a)   section 41 of the National Health Service Act 1977[6] in England or Wales
(b)   section 27 of the National Health Service (Scotland) Act 1978[7] in Scotland;

and

(c)   article 63 of the Health and Personal Social Services (Northern Ireland) Order 1972[8] in Northern Ireland.

The 'specified price' is the price specified in the list. Provision is made for the maximum price to be increased.

The Regulations apply only to the medicines specified in the list of controlled prices, which is published on the World Wide Web at http://www.doh.gov.uk/generics. Printed copies of the list are available from the DoH. They apply only to medicines that have marketing authorizations.

The manufacturers and wholesalers must provide sales information to the Secretary of State. There are penalties for failing to supply information, and for supplying above the specified price.

Appeals
A manufacturer or supplier affected by price controls made under the statutory provisions has a right of appeal in accordance with The Health Service Medicines (Price Control Appeals) Regulations 2000 SI No. 124.

OTC prices
Following a decision of the Restrictive Practices Court on 15 May 2001, there are no longer any controls on the prices of OTC medicines sold to the public.

Chapter 7

Prescription Charges

The basic principle expressed in the National Health Service Act 1977 is that services are to be free unless there is some statement to the contrary. Section 1(2) states:

'The services so provided shall be free of charge except in so far as the making and recovery of charges is expressly provided for by or under any enactment, whenever passed.'

Section 77 provides the power for making charges for pharmaceutical services:

'Regulations may provide for the making and recovery in such manner as may be prescribed of such charges as may be prescribed in respect of —

a) the supply under this Act (otherwise than under Part II) of drugs, medicines or appliances (including the replacement and repair of those appliances)

b) such of the pharmaceutical services referred to in Part II as may be prescribed.'

The effect of section 77 is that charges may be made for the supply both in hospital and in the community, of medicines and appliances. Section 77 also gives Ministers power to charge for the supply of contraceptive substances and appliances, although the Regulations themselves specifically exclude contraceptive substances and appliances from charges.

The Regulations

The current Regulations are the NHS (Charges for Drugs and Appliances) Regulations 1989, SI 1989 No. 419. These substantive Regulations are amended each year as new charges are announced.

Charges for drugs

The Regulations require that, subject to the exemptions, a pharmacist must make and recover from a patient the specified charge in respect of the supply of 'each quantity of a drug'. The term 'drug' includes 'medicine'. The interpretations given in the DT are that, e.g.:

(1) The supply of water for injection with an antibiotic, or in accordance with the BNF, is not charged.
(2) The supply of different strengths of the same tablet results in only one charge.
(3) The supply of both tablets and capsules of the same strength of the same drug would be two charges.

Definitions

The 1989 Regulations include a number of definitions which are specific to the Charges Regulations and important to their meaning. In the 1989 regulations:

(1) Appliance means a 'listed appliance', but excludes contraceptive appliances.
(2) Chemist means any person who provides pharmaceutical services (other than a doctor).
(3) Drugs include medicines, but do not include contraceptive substances.
(4) Elastic hosiery means anklet, legging, knee-cap, above-knee, below-knee or thigh stocking.

What is a patient?

Patient means:

- any person for whose treatment a doctor is responsible under his terms of service; *or*
- any person who applies to a chemist for the provision of pharmaceutical services including a person who applies on behalf of another person; *or*
- a person who pays or undertakes to pay on behalf of another person a charge for which these Regulations provide, *or*
- any person who seeks information or treatment from a walk-in centre, i.e. a centre at which information and treatment for minor conditions is provided to the public under arrangements made by or on behalf of the Secretary of State.

This last definition is added by The National Health Service (Charges for Drugs and Appliances) Amendment Regulations 2000, SI No. 122, which has the effect of making prescription charges applicable to supplies of drugs and appliances made from walk-in centres.

When the Regulations refer to a 'patient' the word also includes someone acting on behalf of the patient, such as a parent and also, say, someone collecting the prescription for a neighbour. That parent or neighbour must pay the charge on demand. Pharmacists are under no obligation to dispense a prescription until after the appropriate charges have been paid. They are entitled to collect the charge when the prescription is handed over for dispensing.

How many charges?

Provided the order is on one form, the supply of the same medicine in more than one container (whether ordered by the prescriber in that way or not) is treated as the supply of one quantity. Detailed guidance on what constitutes 'each quantity of a drug' is found in the DT.

Appliances

There is only one charge payable for the supply of two or more appliances of the same type (excluding elastic hosiery). The supply of two or more component parts of the same appliance also attracts only one charge.

Elastic hosiery and tights
Each piece of hosiery, e.g. a stocking, is treated as one appliance and attracts a separate charge.

Prescription form

Prescription form means a form provided by a HA, a Health Board constituted under section 2 of the National Health Service (Scotland) Act 1978[4], a Health and Social Services Board constituted under the Health and Personal Social Services (Northern Ireland) Order 1972[5], or an NHS Trust and issued by a doctor, dentist or nurse prescriber to enable a person to obtain pharmaceutical services.

Hospital patients

The general rule is that treatment in hospital is free. Hospitals can only charge for medicines which are provided to a patient for administration outside the hospital. That means that medicines for the following are free:

- inpatients
- day patients whose medicines are administered to them whilst they are in the hospital; and
- patients attending accident and emergency departments whose medicines are administered while they are in the hospital.

Charges for medicines and appliances are the same as in community pharmacies, except for certain appliances which are only supplied under the NHS by hospitals. These appliances are surgical brassières, abdominal or spinal supports, and wigs.

Instalment prescribing

Where a medicine is ordered on a single prescription form, and it is supplied in instalments, the standard charge is payable when the first instalment is supplied. Only one charge is made, regardless of the number of instalments.

Receipts

Patients are entitled to a receipt if they ask for one. This must be on the form provided by the HA.

Exemptions

The following persons are exempt from charges:

(1)   persons under 16 years
(2)   persons under 18 years in fulltime education
(3)   a person aged 60 years or over
(4)   a woman holding a maternity exemption certificate (expectant women and those who have given birth within the last 12 months)
(5)   a person holding a medical exemption certificate
(6)   a person holding a prescription prepayment certificate
(7)   a person holding a War Pension exemption certificate (exemption only for prescriptions to treat their accepted disabilities)
(8)   a person named on a current HC2 charges certificate (low income)
(9)   a person receiving free-of-charge contraceptives
(10) a person who is themselves or whose partner is receiving various Social Security and similar allowances and payments. These are: income support, income-based jobseekers allowance, disability working allowance, full working families tax credit or credit reduced by £70 or less and full disabled persons tax credit or credit reduced by £70 or less.

Different categories apply in Wales.

Exemption certificates
Exemption certificates are supplied to the patient by HAs. They are valid for five years. An application form must be completed by the patient and sent to the HA (or the Department of Social Security in the case of (10) above).
  The following medical conditions entitle the person to exemption:

● a permanent fistula requiring continuous dressing or an appliance. Fistula includes caecostomy, colostomy, laryngostomy and ileostoma
● with epilepsy requiring continuous anti-convulsive therapy
● diabetes mellitus except where treatment is by diet alone
● myxodema or other conditions which require supplemental thyroid hormone
● hypoparathyroidism
● diabetes insipidus and other forms of hypopituitarism
● forms of hypoadrenalism (including Addison's disease) for which specific substitution therapy is essential
● myasthenia gravis
● a continuing physical disability which prevents the patient leaving his residence without the help of another person.

Pre-payment certificates

Pre-payment certificates are supplied by the HA. The regulations state the amount to be paid for the four month and the 12 month certificate.

All exemptions, and the pre-payment certificate, apply to all drugs and appliances provided to that patient. The exemption is not limited to treatment specifically for the condition for which exemption was granted.

Accuracy of exemption statement

Paragraph 3(1C) of the Terms of Service requires the pharmacist to ask any person who fills in the exemption section on the back of the prescription form for evidence of entitlement to exemption. The question need not be asked if the exemption is claimed by virtue of sub-paragraphs d, e, f of reg. 6(1) of the Charges Regulations and at the time the pharmacist had such evidence available to him.

If no satisfactory evidence is produced the pharmacist must endorse the form to that effect.

Declaration on prescription form

The declaration of entitlement to exemption or remission which appears on the prescription form must be duly completed, by or on behalf of the patient, in order for the exemption to be valid.

The amended Regulations require that where a person pays a prescription charge he shall sign the declaration on the prescription form that the relevant charge has been paid.

Penalty charges

The National Health Service (Penalty Charge) Regulations 1999 came into force on 1 November 1999. They provide that a penalty notice may be served on any person who fails to pay a required prescription charge (or a charge for dental treatment and appliances, optical services, or any other appliances).

A penalty notice requires payment of the amount that the person has failed to pay plus an additional penalty charge calculated according to the Regulations.

Where the amount required to be paid under the penalty notice is not paid within 28 days, a further sum by way of penalty ('a surcharge' equal to 50% of the penalty charge) must be paid.

A person is not liable to a penalty charge, or a surcharge, if he shows that he did not act wrongfully, or with any lack of care, in respect of the original charge.

These Regulations are administered by a section of the PPA.

Additionally a person who fails to pay a charge when not exempt *may* be prosecuted for the new criminal offence of evading a prescription charge. (Guidance issued by the DoH restricts this to repeat offenders. The Guidance also indicates that either a penalty charge or a prosecution may be appropriate but not both.)

A patient's representative is jointly and severally liable with the patient for unpaid charges in a manner specific to this Act and *may* be issued with a penalty charge notice. The Guidance states that where a representative has signed the declaration of exemption, they are to be the initial recipient of any penalty notice and debt recovery action with the patient only being joined in that action if the representative enters a defence or otherwise fails to pay.

County Court judges should be asked to apportion liability between patients and representatives. (There is some debate as to how likely it is that a judge will be prepared to do this.)

Bulk prescribing is only allowed on NHS forms FP10NC and FP10C.

Bulk prescriptions

No charges are payable for bulk prescriptions. A bulk prescription is: an order for two or more patients bearing the name of a school or institution in which at least 20 persons normally reside, and where a particular doctor is responsible for the treatment of at least 10 of those persons. The order must be for non-POM medicines or for prescribable dressings which do not contain POM products. Bulk prescribing is only allowed on NHS forms FP10NC and FP10C.

Contraceptives

There are no charges for contraceptive substances, or for those contraceptive appliances which are listed in the DT. Section 77 gives Ministers power to charge for the supply of contraceptive substances and appliances, although the Regulations themselves specifically exclude contraceptive substances and appliances from charges.

Dispensing doctors

Dispensing doctors must charge patients for medicines and appliances in exactly the same way as pharmacists. There are similar obligations in respect of the evidence of exemption.

Emergency supplies made by the doctor

No charges are payable where the medicine or appliance is supplied by the doctor (e.g. after normal hours) for immediate treatment, and no order is written on a prescription form.

'Personally administered' medicines or appliances

Similarly no charge is payable for items administered or applied to the patient by the doctor personally. Although the Regulations state 'personally', this also applies when a nurse acts on behalf of the doctor.

Reward scheme

There are two types of reward made available under the Pharmacy Reward Scheme, set up under Regulation 18B of the NHS (PS) Regulations 1992. The scheme allows pharmacists to claim a financial reward when they have identified fraudulent prescription forms and thereby prevented fraud. Participation is voluntary. It is not a requirement of the Terms of Service.

The Basic Reward, payable when a fraudulent prescription form is identified and the items have not been dispensed, is 10% of the price of the items on the form, or £10, whichever is the greater.

The Bonus Reward is payable when the identification of a fraudulent form contributes to the detection and prevention of a fraud, or the recovery for the NHS of sums lost through fraud, regardless of whether items have been dispensed. It is 5% of the total savings resulting from the information provided, up to a maximum of £10,000.

Chapter 8

Complaints and Discipline in the NHS

The report of a review committee, chaired by Professor Alan Wilson, on NHS complaints procedures was published in 1994. Most of its recommendations, in particular the separation of the complaints and discipline procedures, were accepted by the Department of Health.

The changes are intended to make the systems more accessible, speedier and fairer to everyone. The same systems for handling complaints will be in place across the whole of the NHS.

The aim of the changes to the complaints procedures is to try and resolve most complaints at pharmacy level. NHS pharmacies are required to have in place a system for dealing with 'expressions of dissatisfaction' by users of pharmaceutical services.

Pharmacy-based complaints procedure

The 1996 Amendment Regulations inserted new paragraphs 10A and 10B into the Terms of Service.

Paragraph 10A requires the establishment and operation of a 'pharmacy-based' procedure for handling complaints.

Paragraph 10B requires the pharmacy to co-operate with any HA procedure for handling complaints.

The complaint may relate to:

'Any matter reasonably connected with the chemist's provision of pharmaceutical services and within the responsibility or control of:

    (a) the chemist
    (b) any directors or former directors of a body corporate
    (c) a former partner of the chemist
    (d) any pharmacist employed by the chemist
    (e) any other employee of the chemist.'

Complaints may be made by the person affected, or by someone acting on their behalf.

The complaints procedure established by the pharmacy must comply with the following requirements:

(1)   The pharmacy must specify a person who is responsible for receiving and investigating complaints. The person need not be connected with the

pharmacy. The person can be specified by a job title, e.g. Director of Complaints Procedures.

(2) All complaints must be recorded in writing.

(3) All complaints must be acknowledged within three working days, or as soon as is reasonably practicable.

(4) All complaints must be properly investigated.

(5) The complainant must be given a written summary of the investigation and its conclusions within 10 days, or as soon as is reasonably practicable.

(6) The complainant must be informed if the investigation will disclose information contained in records to a person other than the pharmacist, directors or staff of the pharmacy.

(7) The pharmacy must keep a record of complaints, and copies of all correspondence relating to complaints. These records are to be kept separate from any records relating to the complainant.

Information about the complaints procedure must be provided at all the pharmacy premises. The information must also be provided to any person in charge of a home which is receiving supplemental services.

No time limits are set within which a complaint must be made to a pharmacy.

Complaint handling in Health Authorities

The HA can still be asked by the complainant to investigate a complaint. Time limits are set for complaints made directly to HAs – the complaint must be made within six months of the incident, or within six months of discovering the problem (provided that is within 12 months of the incident).

HAs have set up internal procedures to handle complaints, in accordance with Directions from the NHS Executive. These Directions were issued under powers given by section 17 of the NHS Act 1977, and are dated 28 March 1996.

A copy of the arrangements made by the HA for dealing with complaints must be given to anyone who requests it.

Two levels of complaint handling are created in HAs – 'Conciliation' and 'Independent Review'.

Every HA is required to appoint a Complaints Manager to handle the complaints procedure.

Within the HA, one of the non-executive directors will be designated as 'Convenor', and will be responsible for looking at complaints and deciding whether to agree to an Independent Review.

Options available to the Convenor include:

(a) No further action

(b) Referral back to the pharmacy for further action

(c) Conciliation

(d) Independent review

(e) Advising the complainant of the right to approach the NHS Ombudsman.

Advice is available to the Convenor from independent practitioners nominated by LPCs and based outside the HA area, and from an independent lay chairperson nominated by the Secretary of State from a list held by the NHS Executive Regional Office.

Conciliation

After consulting with the LPC, the HA is required to appoint one or more conciliators, for a period of not more than a year at a time. The conciliator must not be or have been a doctor, dentist, optician, pharmacist or registered nurse.

After consulting with the LPC, the HA is required to set up a list of pharmacists to assist the conciliator.

Conciliation must be provided by the HA:

where the complainant and the person subject to the complaint both agree to conciliation
and

(a) A person wishes to complain under a practice based procedure, but the HA believe it would be unreasonable for the complaint to be made direct to the pharmacist *or*

(b) A complaint is being investigated under the pharmacist's in-house scheme *or*

(c) The complainant is dissatisfied with the results of the in-house investigation *or*

(d) The convenor has decided conciliation is the appropriate course of action for dealing with a complaint which requests an independent review.

Independent Review

The Independent Review Panel is composed of:

(a) The Convenor
(b) An independent lay chairperson
(c) An independent lay member.

If the complaint is a clinical one, then two independent clinical assessors nominated by the LPC will be appointed also.

The Panel must conduct its proceedings in private. The procedure is not specified in detail in the Regulations, allowing for considerable flexibility. Anyone interviewed by the Panel may be accompanied by a person of their choosing, who may speak to the Panel if the Chair permits. However, where the accompanying person is legally qualified he may not act as an advocate.

The Panel will report to:

(a) The complainant
(b) The pharmacy
(c) The HA.

It may comment about possible service improvements.

Where a complaint indicates a possible need for disciplinary investigation it is for the HA to decide whether any further action is appropriate. The Panel will make no recommendations about disciplinary procedures.

Disciplinary procedures

The investigation by HAs of allegations that family practitioners have breached their terms of service is now governed by the NHS (Service Committees and Tribunals) Regulations 1992, SI 1992 No. 664, which were substantially amended by the NHS (Service Committees and Tribunals) Amendment Regulations 1996. These amended regulations came into force on 1 April 1996.

Discipline Committees

The NHS (SC & T) Regulations require a HA to establish a 'Discipline Committee' for each of the services – dental, medical, optical and pharmaceutical (Reg. 3).

Three or more HAs may appoint discipline committees jointly.

Schedule 2 deals with the constitution of the discipline committee.

The pharmaceutical discipline committee consists of:

- a legally qualified chairman
- up to three lay members appointed by the HA, and
- up to three members who are pharmacists appointed by the HA from a list of nominees provided by the LPC.

Deputies
At least three lay persons, and at least three pharmacists have to be appointed to act as deputies. They can act in place of a member of the same category who is absent.

Chairman
The chairman is appointed by the HA, but subject to the approval of the Discipline Committee. If a majority of either the lay or professional members object in writing within 14 days of the appointment, then the matter must be referred to the Secretary of State. The S of S may alter or confirm the appointment.

What is a 'lay member'?
Lay member means someone who is not, and never has been:

- a doctor, a dentist, an ophthalmic medical practitioner or a chemist
- a registered dispensing optician within the meaning of the Opticians Act 1989
- a registered nurse, a registered midwife or a registered health visitor
- an officer of, or otherwise an employee of any HA or a Community Health Council (CHC).

'Chemist' here means a person who is in the pharmaceutical list and is:

- a registered pharmacist
- a person lawfully conducting a retail pharmacy business
- a supplier of appliances.

Quorum

The quorum is five: the chairman, two lay members and two professional members. A quorum must be maintained for the whole hearing (Schedule 4). In addition there must be a balance between lay and professional members: either two of each or three of each.

Function

The main function of the Pharmaceutical Disciplinary Committee (PDC) is to investigate allegations that pharmacists have failed to comply with the terms of service.

The PDC also investigates allegations made against appliance contractors. These regulations refer to both pharmacy contractors and appliance contractors as 'chemists'.

The PDC shall investigate any matter referred to it.

Where a HA receives information which it considers could amount to an allegation that a pharmacist has failed to comply with his terms of service, that HA may decide either to take no action, or to take one or both of the following actions:

(1) Refer the matter to another HA for investigation by that HA's Disciplinary Committee.
(2) Refer the information, as appropriate to:

- The Family Health Services Appeal Authority
- the RPSGB
- the local police authority.

Procedure

Schedule 4 sets out the procedure for investigations. Time limits for exchange of statements, notifications, etc. are given.

Where the detail is not laid down in the regulations the PDC may set out its own procedure. The DoH guidance document contains a model procedure.

HA's statement of case

Where a disciplinary matter is referred to a discipline committee the appropriate HA must send:

(1) Notice of the referral to the pharmacist within two working days of the referral.
(2) A statement of case to the pharmacist within 28 days.
(3) A statement of case to the discipline committee within 28 days.
(4) Any necessary notice to an employee within two working days.

The statement of case must include:

(1) Details of each provision of the terms of service which are alleged to have been broken.
(2) The details of each alleged breach.
(3) Copies of all relevant documentary evidence.
(4) Names and addresses of any witnesses to be called by the HA.
(5) Copies of any statements made by the witnesses.

Extension of time limits
The 28 day time limit may be extended by the Chair of the disciplinary committee for another 28 days.

Employee pharmacists
The disciplinary procedure bites on the contractor. Where complaints are made about an employee pharmacist, the HA must send that employee pharmacist a notice asking if he wishes to be a party to the investigation.

The employee pharmacist may send his written comments on the matter, even if he does not wish to be a party at the investigation.

Who may be present at a hearing
The proceedings are private. The only persons allowed to be present are:

(a) The pharmacist against whom the allegation is made.
(b) If appropriate, an employee pharmacist.
(c) A duly authorized officer or member of the LPC.
(d) Witnesses.
(e) One member of the HA making the allegation.

In addition the pharmacist may be assisted in the presentation of the case by one other person. If that person is a barrister or solicitor then he may not address the committee or put questions to witnesses. If either the complainant or the pharmacist is also qualified as a barrister or solicitor, he may still conduct his own case.

Members of the Council on Tribunals are entitled to be present at any service case (although their presence is very occasional) (Reg. 33).

Procedure at the hearing
Both sides are heard, starting with the HA making the allegation. The member or officer of the HA making the allegation, the pharmacist, and anyone assisting him who is not a barrister or solicitor can address the committee, and can question witnesses.

The standard of proof required is not specified, but appears to be a 'civil' standard, i.e. the matter is decided on the balance of probabilities.

Decision
The job of the PDC is to investigate the complaint and report to the HA which made the allegation.

The HA has to accept the findings of fact and the inferences from those facts made by the PDC in its report.

The HA must then determine what action, if any, it will take. It must have regard to the recommendations of the PDC. If the HA does not follow those recommendations then it must record in writing the reasons for that decision.

Options when a breach has been found
When a breach has been found by the HA it may then take the following action:

(1) Determine that an amount shall be recovered from the contractor, either by deduction from remuneration or otherwise.
(2) Give a warning to the contractor that in future he comply more closely with his terms of service.

Account may be taken of previous breaches by the same contractor at the same premises, provided these are no more than six years old.

After a decision has been made the HA must then, and as soon as may be practicable, send a copy of the PDC report and of the HA decision, to:

(1) The pharmacy contractor.
(2) The Secretary of State.
(3) If appropriate, an employee pharmacist.

The parties must be informed of their right of appeal to the FHS Appeal Authority.

Appeals

A contractor may appeal to the FHS Appeal Authority against:

(1) A finding of fact or an inference which is adverse to him.
(2) A determination by a HA to take action against him.
(3) A determination that he repay money overpaid to him by the HA.

Time limits on appeals
Notification of appeals must be made within one month, and the notice must contain a concise statement of the grounds of appeal.

Nature of the appeal
The FHS Appeal Authority may dismiss appeals which it considers as vexatious, frivolous, or which disclose no reasonable grounds. An oral hearing must be held, unless a practitioner appealing the determination but not the facts has stated in writing that he does not want an oral hearing.

Who must be notified
The FHS Appeal Authority must send a copy of the notice of appeal and any further particulars given by the appellant to the HA.

The HA has 28 days to respond. Any response must be copied to the practitioner, who then has 21 days to comment.

Withdrawal of appeals

An appeal may be withdrawn at any time before it is determined, with the consent of the FHS Appeal Authority. Written notice of intent to withdraw must be given.

Oral hearings

The FHS Appeal Authority appoints three people to hold an oral hearing on its behalf. The Chairman must be a barrister or solicitor. Where the appeal concerns a pharmacy contractor, then the two other persons appointed to hear the appeal are to be pharmacists.

Who may take part in the appeal

Oral hearings are held in private. The practitioner, a HA representative, and witnesses are the only persons allowed into the hearing.

The parties may be represented by a barrister, solicitor or any other person. This is in contrast to the rules at a PDC hearing.

Procedure

The persons holding an inquiry report their findings and recommendations to the FHS Appeal Authority.

They may make such findings of fact as they see fit, draw such inferences as they see fit, and determine action to be taken.

If the appeal was only against the determination, and the facts were not contested then the inquiry must accept the facts and inferences as found by the PDC.

The FHS Appeal Authority considers the report and determines the appeal. It must notify the parties of its decision, and the reason for it. Its decision is final and conclusive.

What may the FHS Appeal Authority do on appeal?

If the FHS Appeal Authority finds that, after considering the report, the contractor was in breach, it may direct the HA to make a withholding. This may be done by deduction from the pharmacist's remuneration. If the money is not recovered in this way, the amount becomes a debt due to the HA, which may be recovered in the courts.

New arrangements for dealing with serious allegations

HA lists of practitioners

The Health and Social Care Act 2001 introduced new arrangements covering the regulation of family health service practitioners. The details will be set out in Regulations.

HAs are required to maintain lists of all practitioners who undertake to provide services in their area. This list system was extended by the HSC Act 2001 to cover those who assist in the provision of primary care services (e.g. deputies or locums) as well as those practitioners performing personal pharmaceutical services.

Declaration of convictions
The intention is that persons will have to declare any criminal convictions, bindings-over following a criminal conviction and cautions in order to be admitted to a list or remain on it. HAs will verify the information that they are given, using the Criminal Records Bureau.

Grounds for refusal to admit to list
HAs may refuse a practitioner admission to the appropriate list on the grounds of unsuitability, prejudice to efficiency or because of previous fraudulent behaviour. Regulations may be made allowing the HA to set conditions for inclusion in a list.

Under the new system:

- Only practitioners, including deputies and locums, who are included in lists maintained by HAs will be able to deliver family health services.
- Criteria to be admitted to (and to remain on) a list include probity and positive evidence of good professional behaviour and practice. This will involve a system of declarations, annual appraisal and participation in clinical audit.
- HAs may refuse to include a practitioner on the relevant medical, dental, ophthalmic or pharmaceutical list on the grounds of unsuitability, prejudice to efficiency or because of previous fraudulent behaviour.

Removal or suspension of practitioners
Under the new arrangements HAs may suspend and remove practitioners from the relevant lists on the grounds of inefficiency, fraud or unsuitability.

Hearings
The regulations will include provision for a practitioner to be given notice of any allegations against him; for him to put his case at a hearing before a HA makes a decision; and for him to be informed of a HA's decision, the reasons for it and his right of appeal.

Appeals
The Act sets up a right of appeal to the FHSAA against a HA's decision to impose conditions, to vary a condition, to vary terms of service or to remove a person from a list for a breach of condition. The regulations may provide for a HA decision not to have effect until the FHSAA has determined the appeal (and must do so in relation to a decision to remove the person from a list).

If a HA suspends a practitioner, it must specify the period of suspension unless the Regulations provide otherwise.

National disqualification
A HA may apply to the FHSAA for the national disqualification of a practitioner that it has removed from one of its lists.

Referral to the Royal Pharmaceutical Society

The Regulations allow an HA or the S of S to bring a matter to the attention of the

RPSGB. Any relevant documents may be passed to the RPSGB. Since discipline committee hearings are in private this is often the only way for the RPSGB to obtain details of matters of professional misconduct.

A HA may refer a matter to the RPSGB instead of a referral to a disciplinary committee, or as well.

The Secretary of State may also refer a matter to the RPSGB when he receives a decision of the Tribunal.

The FHS Appeal Authority

Certain functions of the S of S have been devolved to the FHS Appeal Authority. The functions are to provide an appeal mechanism from decisions of HAs in relation to discipline committee hearings, pharmacy contract applications and rural dispensing matters.

Family Health Services Appeals Authority

The Family Health Services Appeals Authority was reconstituted by the HSC Act 2001 as an independent body under the Lord Chancellor's Department, whose functions will include dealing with appeals by these practitioners against HA decisions. Consequently the NHS Tribunal, which previously carried out these functions, has been abolished.

The FHSSA will consist of a President, one or more Deputy Presidents, and a number of other members, all to be appointed by the Lord Chancellor on terms to be determined by him. The membership must include people with a lay background as well as those with relevant professional expertise.

Pharmacy appeals dealt with by the FHS Appeal Authority
(1) Inclusion in list.
(2) Refusal to allow amended application.
(3) Refusal to extend time limits for opening.
(4) Rurality.
(5) Applications to dispense in controlled localities.
(6) Removal of name from list.
(7) HA decision to require GP to dispense.
(8) Hours of service.
(9) Discipline committee decisions.

Chapter 9

Retail Pharmacy

The operation of a pharmacy is subject to a number of laws, which deal with ownership and with the activities carried on in the premises. There are more than 200 different pieces of relevant legislation but this chapter deals only with those directly relevant to the establishment of the professional practice.

History

The Pharmacy Act 1852 established a system of control over the practice of pharmacy by requiring registration as a 'chemist and druggist' or a 'pharmaceutical chemist'. Passing an exam entitled the person to registration and to the right to sell poisons.

The Pharmacy and Poisons Act 1933 compelled all pharmacists to become members of the then PSGB. (It acquired 'Royal' in its title in 1988.) The statutory committee system was established to disqualify persons from membership and hence from being an 'authorised seller of poisons'.

The Pharmacy Act 1954 removed the connection between poisons and pharmacy (which had been present since the Arsenic Act 1851) and dealt only with the profession of pharmacy. The 1954 Act is still extant, covering the registration process applicable to individual pharmacists.

The current legislation dealing with premises is the Medicines Act (MA) 1968. Subject to certain exceptions, the MA 1968 requires that the sale of medicinal products to the public takes place in registered premises and that the sale is by or under the supervision of a pharmacist. The MA 1968 lists the persons who can operate a pharmacy.

Who may own a pharmacy?

A retail pharmacy business may be lawfully carried on by:

- a pharmacist
- a partnership of pharmacists
- a 'body corporate'
- a 'representative' of a pharmacist.

There are a number of additional conditions for each circumstance outlined above.

Pharmacist

The part of the retail pharmacy business (RPB) which concerns the retail sale of medicines (whether or not they are General Sale List (GSL)) must be under the personal control of the pharmacist owner or of another pharmacist. The meaning of 'personal control' is dealt with in Chapter 17.

Partnerships

In England, Wales and Northern Ireland partnerships can only carry on a pharmacy if all the partners are registered pharmacists. In Scotland the partnership running the pharmacy must have one partner who is a pharmacist, but the rest need not be qualified as pharmacists.

The part of the business concerned with the sale or supply of Pharmacy Only Medicine (P) and Prescription Only Medicine (POM), and the dispensing of medicines must be under the personal control of one of the partners who is a pharmacist, or under the personal control of another pharmacist.

The general law relating to partnerships is discussed in Chapter 33.

The Limited Liability Partnership Act 2000 came into force on 6 April 2001. The limited liability partnership is a hybrid of partnerships and companies. Limited liability partnerships are treated by the Medicines Act (MA) as companies rather than partnerships and therefore they may include non-pharmacist members. They will need to appoint a superintendent pharmacist.

Body corporate

This is a term applied to any association of individuals which is so constituted as to acquire a collective legal personality. The law recognises that some groups of people ought to be treated as a single individual, which is a separate legal entity from those who make up the group.

There are two types of body corporate. First, there is a corporation sole. The Crown, Ministers and an Archbishop are examples. The idea of a body corporate enables the post to be sued instead of the person who holds the post for the time being. Secondly, there is a corporation aggregate. There are various types including public corporations, cooperative societies, mutual building societies, and private and public limited companies.

The most important and numerous are private limited companies. Generally speaking, where the term 'body corporate' is used, the term 'company' can replace it.

The business of keeping, preparing and dispensing P and POM in a company must be under the management of a superintendent pharmacist.

The sale or supply of P and POM by retail or as dispensed medicines must be:

- under the personal control of the superintendent, *or*
- under the personal control of another pharmacist who is subject to direction by the superintendent.

Superintendent

The superintendent must be a pharmacist. He must not act in a similar capacity for any other body corporate. He must send a statement to the registrar of the RPSGB stating whether or not he is a member of the board of the body corporate. The statement must be in writing, signed by him and signed on behalf of the body corporate.

Representative

A representative of a pharmacist may carry on the pharmacy in certain circumstances (section 72). These are:

(1) Where the pharmacist has died.
(2) Where he has become bankrupt.
(3) Where he has become mentally unfit and a receiver has been appointed under the Mental Health Act 1983.

The representative is:

(1) The executor or administrator of a deceased pharmacist. For the first three months after the death any person beneficially interested in the estate may carry on the business.
(2) The trustee in bankruptcy (or similar).
(3) The receiver (or similar) of a mentally unfit pharmacist.

The representative may carry on business for a period of five years after the death of a pharmacist, or for three years in any other case.

The name and address must be notified to the registrar of the RPSGB. At all premises where the retail sale or supply of P and POM occurs, the sale of all medicines must be under the personal control of a pharmacist.

Retail pharmacy business

The MA 1968 does not use the term 'pharmacy' but 'retail pharmacy business'. This is defined as:

'a business (not being a professional practice carried on by a practitioner) which consists of or includes the retail sale of medicinal products other than medicinal products on a general sale list (whether medicinal products on such a list are sold in the course of that business or not).'

In other words, a business is an RPB if it is:

- a business which consists of the retail sale of POM or P, or
- a business which includes the retail sale of POM or P, and
- it is not part of the professional practice of a practitioner, which in this instance means a doctor, dentist or vet.

The words in brackets at the end of the definition do not appear to add anything at all to the meaning.

Registered pharmacy

Section 74(1) defines a registered pharmacy as the premises where a person is lawfully conducting an RPB. The Registrar of the RPSGB is required to keep a register of premises where a person is lawfully conducting a retail pharmacy business (section 75).

Applications to enter premises in the register of premises are made in writing to the Registrar. The RPSGB provides a printed form for convenience, but its use is not mandatory provided the specified details are given. According to SI 1973, No. 1822, all applications must be accompanied by a plan of the premises.

The phrase 'registered pharmacy' refers to the premises, and the phrase 'RPB' refers to the professional practice of a pharmacist or body corporate selling medicines and dispensing prescriptions.

Transactions covered

Wholesale dealing – This is a sale to a person who buys the substance in order to sell it, supply it, administer it or cause it to be administered in the course of business.

Retail sale – Section 131 of the MA 1968 defines 'retail sale' as the sale of a substance or article to a person who buys it other than to sell it, supply it, administer it or cause it to be administered in the course of business.

Supply in circumstances corresponding to retail sale – Section 131 defines this as a supply *otherwise than a sale* of a substance or article to a person who buys it other than to sell it, supply it, administer it or cause it to be administered in the course of business.

Between them these definitions cover almost all possible kinds of transactions. One kind remains, i.e. a supply, without being a sale, which is for the same purpose as a wholesale transaction. Such a supply does not seem to have been envisaged by the Act and no provisions are made to control the transaction.

Supply of NHS medicines

Legally, the supply of medicines on an NHS prescription is not a sale. This has been considered by the courts on two occasions. In 1965, the House of Lords considered whether the Minister of Health could import medicines for which the Pfizer Corporation held patents in this country. In dealing with this, they decided that there was no sale of medicines by a hospital to a patient (*Pfizer Corporation* v. *Minister of Health* (1965)).

In 1968 a court had to deal with contaminated medicine supplied to a patient. The case was brought under the Food and Drugs Act 1955, which required that the medicine had been *sold* to the complainant. The court decided that the pharmacy had a contract with the then Executive Council for the supply of services. The pharmacy was paid remuneration for the services, and there was not a *sale* of medicine to the Executive Council (*Appleby* v. *Sleep* (1968)).

Dispensing-only pharmacies

The definition of a retail pharmacy business, taken from section 132 of the MA 1968 suggests that a business where no retail sales took place (that is which only dispensed NHS prescriptions) would not be a RPB. But section 52 also restricts supply in 'circumstances corresponding to retail sale' to a retail pharmacy business in a registered pharmacy. This clumsy phrase 'supply in circumstances corresponding to retail sale' covers the supply of dispensed medicines in the NHS. Therefore even dispensing-only pharmacies have to be registered, because the operation of such pharmacies can only be as part of an RPB. The Act does not envisage a pharmacy where no retail sales occur.

Register of Pharmaceutical Chemists

A pharmacist is a person whose name is entered in the Register of Pharmaceutical Chemists. This was established originally by the Pharmacy Act 1852, but now exists, in England, Wales and Scotland, as a result of section 2(1) of the Pharmacy Act 1954. For Northern Ireland the Register is maintained under a requirement in section 9 of the Pharmacy and Poisons Act (Northern Ireland) 1925. The register is computer-based and is kept by the Registrar of the RPSGB (and the Registrar of the Pharmaceutical Society of Northern Ireland (PSNI)). A printed version is produced every year for reference, but the definitive version is the up-dated computerized list.

Restricted titles

The use of some professional titles is restricted to a pharmacist. Only pharmacists may 'take or use' any of the following titles:

- pharmacist
- pharmaceutical chemist
- pharmaceutist
- member of the Royal Pharmaceutical Society
- fellow of the Royal Pharmaceutical Society.

Unqualified persons may not use the above titles. The abbreviations MRPharmS and FRPharmS are the approved abbreviations indicating membership and fellowship of the Society. The older forms MPS and FPS are still used occasionally.

Additionally, the MA 1968 specifies that no one may use any of those titles in connection with a retail business (or a business which consists of or includes a supply in circumstances corresponding to retail sale) unless the premises are a registered pharmacy or a hospital.

Pharmacy

The use of the term 'pharmacy' is restricted to a registered pharmacy or the pharmacy department of a hospital.

Its use in circumstances which cannot be confused with the operation of a pharmacy, for instance a restaurant is still unclear. In 1998, the Society considered whether or not to instigate proceedings against a restaurant called 'Pharmacy', but it did not take any action in court, and at the date of writing the restaurant is still open.

Companies

Companies operating an RPB may use the title 'pharmacy' in connection with the premises. Companies may also use the following titles, as may pharmacists:

- chemist and druggist
- druggist
- dispensing chemist
- dispensing druggist.

A body corporate may only use the title 'chemist' if the superintendent is a member of the board. It may use 'pharmacy' even though the superintendent is not on the board.

Representatives may use any title which the pharmacist was entitled to use.

European Union nationals

Article 7 of EC Directive 85/433 (which deals with the mutual recognition of the qualifications of European Community (EC) (now European Union) pharmacists) allows nationals of member states of the European Union (EU) to use the lawful academic titles of their home state. They may do this if they are registered with the RPSGB.

Display of certificate of registration

The certificate of registration of the pharmacist in personal control at each premises must be conspicuously exhibited (sections 70 and 71 of the MA 1968).

Chapter 10

Manufacture and Licensing of Medicinal Products

The Medicines Act 1968 and other controls

In this chapter we deal with the licensing of the product, and of its manufacturer.

The Medicines Act 1968, together with the Medicines for Human Use (Marketing Authorisations, etc.) Regulations 1994, lays down a general framework for controlling dealings in medicinal products by way of a licensing system. This requires persons responsible for the composition of a product to hold a licence. Licences are also required by wholesale dealers and by manufacturers. It is unlawful for the products concerned to be manufactured, sold or supplied in, or imported into, the UK (and certain biological products may not be exported) except with the appropriate licences, certificates or exemptions.

The legislative basis for the controls on the manufacture and supply of medicines is the Medicines Act 1968 (MA 1968).

A number of general remarks about the Medicines Act 1968 (MA 1968) are appropriate at this point.

The Act was produced in response to two main factors: the Thalidomide tragedy in the early 1960s and the Directives issued by the European Economic Community (as it was then called). Although the UK had not yet joined, the intention to do so was well known. In many ways the MA 1968 was a consumer safety Act, concerned with protecting the public from faulty products by introducing a licensing system.

The opportunity was taken to include controls on the operation of pharmacies.

The Act was written against a background of Crown exemption, i.e. the doctrine that institutions of the Crown, meaning in effect institutions of the government, were not bound by the laws that affected the rest of us. Unless a law contained a specific provision that the Crown was bound, then that law did not apply to government institutions. The NHS hospitals were such institutions until their immunity was removed in 1990.

The MA 1968 is written in a difficult style. It starts off by prohibiting almost all dealings with medicines, referred to as 'medicinal products'. It continues by setting out a number of exemptions to the general rules, thereby allowing, for instance, the sale and manufacture of medicines. The first set of exemptions relates to licences. The second set refers to various activities done by professionals, i.e. practitioners. The third set removes some types of products from some controls, e.g. the General Sale List (GSL).

In order to discover the rules governing an activity it is usually necessary to read a number of inter-related sections of the Act. For example, section 8 prohibits the manufacture of any medicinal product except in accordance with a licence. Section 10 exempts pharmacists from the provisions of section 8, but only for certain activities done in certain places in certain ways.

The Act allows for secondary legislation (Orders or Regulations) to modify the provisions of the Act itself very considerably.

Since 1968 the EU has issued several Directives which establish a community-wide system of control on medicines.

The EU also set up a centralized procedure for licensing high-technology products.

Medicines for Human use (Marketing Authorisations, etc.) Regulations 1994

The Medicines for Human Use (Marketing Authorisations, etc.) Regulations 1994, SI 1994 No. 3144 (MAR 1994) Regulations) replace the provisions of the Medicines Act 1968 which deal with the licensing, labelling and supply of leaflets with products. These Regulations also replace a mass of subordinate legislation which previously covered the same areas. They follow the same style as the main Act, but refer to 'relevant Community provisions'.

They apply to all medicinal products to which Chapters II to V of Directive 65/65/EEC apply, which are described in the Regulations as 'relevant medicinal products'.

Medicinal products

A medicinal product is defined by Directive 65/65/EEC as:

(1)   any substance or combination of substances presented for treating or preventing disease in human beings or animals
(2)   any substance or combination of substances which may be administered to human beings or animals with a view to making a medical diagnosis or to restoring, correcting or modifying physiological functions in human beings or animals is likewise considered a medicinal product.

Certain products used outside the human body, such as preservation agents for transplant organs are also included.

Relevant medicinal products

The MAR 1994 Regulations apply to all medicinal products to which Chapters II–V of Directive 65/65/EEC apply, which are described in the Regulations as relevant medicinal products.

'Relevant medicinal products' are all medicinal products for human use, except

(a)   those prepared on the basis of a magistral or official formula
(b)   medicinal products intended for research
(c)   intermediate products intended for further processing by an authorised manufacturer.

Magistral refers to a medicine made in a pharmacy in accordance with a prescription for an individual patient.

Official formula refers to a medicine made in a pharmacy to a pharmacopoeial formula for direct supply to patients.

In practice most medicines which are sold or supplied in the UK are covered by the EEC Directive definition.

Medicines Act definition

Section 130 of the MA 1968 defines a 'medicinal product' as any substance or article which is manufactured, sold, supplied, imported or exported for use wholly or mainly as something which is administered, or is an ingredient of something which is administered, for a medicinal purpose.

Medicinal purpose

A 'medicinal purpose' is:

- treating disease
- preventing disease
- diagnosing disease
- ascertaining the existence, degree or extent of a physiological condition
- contraception
- anesthesia
- preventing or interfering with the normal operation of a physiological function in any other way.

Administration

Administer means to give to someone as a medicine. This may be: orally, by injection, by introduction into the body in any other way, by external application. There may be direct contact with the body, e.g. a cream, or indirect, e.g. inhalation.

European Directives

A number of Directives cover the licensing of medicines. The most important is Directive 65/65 which lays down the basic requirements for the licensing system to be operated in each member state. Several later directives have extended the scope of this directive, in particular Directive 93/39 EEC.

The Licensing Authority

Legally speaking, licences are issued by the 'Licensing Authority' which for human medicines consists of the Health Ministers of the UK. In practice, the licensing of human medicines is handled by the Medicines Control Agency of the DoH. The licensing of veterinary products is generally dealt with by the Ministry of Agriculture, Fisheries and Food (MAFF).

The European Medicines Evaluation Agency

The European Medicines Evaluation Agency is a part of the European Commission (EC) bureaucracy. Its function is to handle the EC centralized procedure, which is used for new active substances and certain high-technology and biotechnology products. The EMEA is advised by the Committee for Proprietary Medicinal Products (CPMP) whose members are drawn from the EU's Member States.

The advisory machinery

A number of committees of experts were set up under the Act, to advise Ministers about the matters dealt with by the MA 1968.

The Medicines Commission

Section 2 of the Act established the Medicines Commission to give advice on general matters of policy relating to medicines control. In certain circumstances it also considers applications for licences. It reports to the licensing authority which must take account of its report in determining an application.

The specific duties of the Medicines Commission are set out in the Act:

(1)   It must make recommendations as to the constitution and functions of the other committees to be set up under the Act.
(2)   It must recommend people to serve on those committees.
(3)   It must review the functions of the committees.
(4)   It must receive representations, in certain cases, from applicants for licences or certificates.
(5)   It must act as an advisory committee if no other committee is set up specifically to deal with the problem.
(6)   It must direct the preparation of publications such as the BP.

Composition
The Medicines Commission is a body corporate, whose members generally hold office for four years. They must include:

● a doctor
● a vet
● a pharmacist
● a chemist and
● a member with experience in the pharmaceutical industry.

Their experience in their field must be 'wide and recent' and they must have shown 'capacity' in that activity.

Committee on Safety of Medicines
This committee advises on the safety, quality and efficacy of new medicines for humans. It is also responsible for collecting and investigating reports of adverse reactions to medicines.

Veterinary Products Committee
The VPC advises MAFF on veterinary products.

British Pharmacopoeia Commission
The BP Commission is responsible for preparing the BP, which contains standards for human medicines. It is also responsible for selecting non-proprietary names for medicinal substances.

The Advisory Board on the Registration of Homoeopathic Products
The Advisory Board on the Registration of Homoeopathic Products (ABRHP) was established in 1994 to give advice on the safety and quality of homoeopathic medicinal product for human and veterinary use, for which a certificate of registration could be granted.

Medicinal claims
The MCA will generally regard a product as a 'medicinal product' if medicinal claims are made for it.

Marketing Authorization

The MAR 1994 Regulations prohibit the placing on the market of most medical products, unless they have an EC or UK marketing authorization.

Regulation 3(1) states:

> 'except in accordance with any exception or exemption set out in the relevant Community provisions and subject to paragraphs 1 and 3 of Schedule 1 —
>
> a) no relevant medicinal product shall be placed on the market; and
> b) no such product shall be distributed by way of wholesale dealing,
>
> unless a marketing authorization in respect of that product has been granted ... and is in force ...'

In effect a marketing authorization is required by the person responsible for the composition of the product, i.e. either the manufacturer or the person to whose order the product is manufactured.

Prior to 1994 the marketing authorization was termed a 'product licence'. These were designated on the product label with the initials PL and a number. This 'PL' designation is still used for marketing authorizations.

Placed on the market

A product is 'placed on the market' when it is first made available in return for payment or free of charge with a view to distribution, use or both on the Community market.

The term 'made available' means the transfer of the ownership of the product, or the passing of the product to the final consumer or user in a commercial transaction. It may be for payment or free of charge. The legal instrument by which the transfer is achieved, e.g. sale, loan, lease, gift, etc. is irrelevant.

A product is not 'placed on the market' if it is made in a hospital pharmacy and then used elsewhere in the same hospital to treat patients.

Exemption in section 7 of MA 1968

Section 7 of the MA 1968 only applies to products which are not covered by the MAR 1994 Regulations.

Section 7 of the Act states that, except where exempted by provisions in the Act or in Regulations, a marketing authorization is required by any person who in the course of his business sells, supplies, exports, imports, or procures the sale, supply, export, manufacture or assembly of a medicinal product.

Conditions for granting a 'marketing authorization'

Applications must be in writing, comply with relevant E provisions and be accompanied by the correct fee. Details of the necessary accompanying material are set out in a series of EC Directives, mainly in 65/65/EEC, 75/319/EEC and 75/318/EEC.

There must be a Summary of Product Characteristics (SPC) which contains certain required information about the therapeutic indications, contra-indications and side-effects of the product. Other information includes dosage, method and route of administration, shelf life, storage precautions and the results of clinical trials and tests.

Twenty-six copies of the application and accompanying material are required for a new application.

The application must be accompanied by a statement indicating whether the product should be a POM, P or GSL medicine.

The licensing authority has to be satisfied as to the safety, quality and efficacy of a product before it may grant a marketing authorization. The appropriate committee (CSM, VPC or ACRHP) must be consulted where the authority intends to refuse a licence.

Safety includes consideration of the extent to which the product:

(a) if used without proper safeguards, is capable of causing danger to the health of the community; or
(b) may interfere with the treatment, prevention or diagnosis of disease; or
(c) may be harmful to the person administering it (section 132 MA 1968).

Section 28 states the grounds for suspending, revoking or varying a licence. The most important is the availability of new factual information relevant to the licence. Other reasons include failure to keep to conditions in the licence, e.g. standards of quality.

Manufacturers' Licence

Section 8 of the MA 1968 provides that subject to exceptions, every person who makes or packs a medicinal product in the course of business must have a manufacturers' licence (ML).

Specials licence

A pharmacist or a doctor may ask a pharmaceutical manufacturer to prepare a medicinal product for him. No product licence is necessary provided the manufacturer holds an ML specifically authorizing him to produce 'specials'. The manufacturer is prohibited from advertising the products or from soliciting the orders (SI 1994 No. 3144).

Assembly

This term is used to include various packaging activities, e.g. enclosing the product in a container which is then labelled before sale or supply, labelling the container of medicine. A container is the box, bottle or carton, etc. in which the product is contained. It does not mean the capsule, etc. in which the product is to be administered.

The assembly of a medicine is an activity which requires a manufacturers' licence, or an exemption.

Wholesaling

Section 8 also requires that everyone who wholesales, or offers for sale by wholesale, a medicinal product must hold a 'wholesale dealers' licence'. Persons holding a manufacturers' licence do not need a separate licence for the wholesale supply of the products they manufacture. Pharmacies are also exempt provided the volume of wholesaling is insignificant (less than 5% of turnover is used by the Medicines Control Agency (MCA)).

Appeal process

An aggrieved applicant for a licence may first take his case to the CSM, VPC or ARCHP. He may then appeal to the Medicines Commission (MC). The final appeal is to an independent person appointed by the licensing authority.

Medicinal claims

The MCA will generally regard a product as a medicinal product if medicinal claims are made for it. Medicinal claims are claims to treat or prevent disease, or to interfere with normal operation of a physiological function of the human body.

Statutory procedure for classifying borderline substances

The Medicines for Human Use (Marketing Authorisations, etc.) Amendment Regulations, SI No. 2000/292 amend the MAR 1994 Regs to give power to stop a company selling a product, which the licensing authority believes is a medicine, without a marketing authority. The licensing authority must explain why they consider the product to be a medicine. There is an appeal to a review panel.

Medical Foods Regulations

The Medical Food Regulations 2000 SI No. 845 implement Directive 99/21/EC which introduces specific rules for foods used for the dietary management of specific diseases or medical conditions. Maximum and minimum vitamin, mineral and trace element levels for specific categories of FSMPs are set by the Regulations. There is an obligation to notify new products when first placed on the market.

Medical devices

Prior to 1994 many medical devices were controlled under the MA 1968. They are now controlled under consumer safety legislation, specifically The Medical Devices Regulations 1994 SI No. 3017.

A medical device is

'an instrument, apparatus, appliance, material or other article, whether used alone or in combination, together with any software necessary for its proper application which:

1) is intended by the manufacturer to be used for human beings for the purpose of
   a) diagnosis, prevention, monitoring, treatment or alleviation of disease
   b) diagnosis, prevention, monitoring, treatment or alleviation of or compensation for an injury or handicap
   c) investigation, replacement or modification of the anatomy or of any physiological process *or*
   d) control of contraception; *and*
2) does not achieve its principal intended action in or on the human body by pharmacological, immunological or metabolic means, even if it is assisted in its function by such means.'

The definition includes devices which are intended to administer a medicinal product or which incorporate a substance which would be a medicinal product if used on its own.

Such devices include intra-uterine devices, diaphragms, dental fillings, contact lens care products, non-medicated dressings, sutures and ligatures.

Medical devices must comply with the regulations and with the 'essential requirements' set out in Directive 93/42/EEC. There are specific labelling requirements. The Medical Devices Agency (MDA) administers the legislation.

Exemptions from the need to hold licences

Pharmacists

Section 10 provides that no licence is required for the normal activities of a pharmacist.

Some activities are covered simply because they are done by a pharmacist, whereas others are covered only if the activities take place in a registered pharmacy.

Doctors, dentists, vets

Section 9 exempts doctors, dentists and vets from the need to have MLs and marketing authorisations. They may prepare, import, order the preparation or importation, manufacture, assemble, sell, supply or procure the manufacture, sale or supply of a medicinal product for administration to a patient.

What can a pharmacist do?

The Act allows certain activities to be done by pharmacists which would otherwise require the holding of a licence.

(1) All pharmacists are allowed to procure the assembly of a medicinal product. The activity may also be done under the supervision of a pharmacist (section 10).
(2) Where the activity takes place in a registered pharmacy, a hospital or a health centre a pharmacist may assemble a medicinal product (section 10).
(3) Where the activity takes place in a registered pharmacy, a hospital or a health centre, *and* it is done in accordance with a prescription given by a practitioner, a pharmacist may prepare or dispense a medicinal product (section 10).

The terms 'prepare' and 'dispense' are not defined in the Act, and therefore take their normal meaning. However, section 10 provides exemptions from sections 7 and 8, which although they do not refer to preparation or dispensing, do refer to manufacturing. Section 10 does not use 'manufacturing', leading to the conclusion that preparation and dispensing are activities which are similar to but less than manufacture. In 2000 the MCA issued Guidance Note No. 14 'The Supply of unlicensed relevant medicinal products for individual patients', which indicates how in practice the MCA will determine whether an activity is 'preparation' or 'manufacture'. Criteria include the location of the process, the nature of the activity and the scale of the activity.

(4) Where all the following conditions apply, a pharmacist may prepare or dispense a medicinal product. It must be done:
    - in a registered pharmacy
    - by or under the supervision of a pharmacist
    - in accordance with a specification furnished by the person to whom the product is or is to be sold or supplied
    - the person is going to administer the product to himself or to someone under his care (section 10).
(5) A pharmacist may prepare a stock of medicinal products in a hospital or health centre ready for dispensing them in accordance with a prescription given by a practitioner (section 10).
(6) A pharmacist may prepare or dispense a medicinal product in a registered pharmacy, if the following conditions are satisfied:

- the product is for administration to a person
- the pharmacist was requested by or on behalf of that person to exercise his judgment as to the treatment required
- the person was present in the pharmacy at the time of the request (section 10).

(7) A pharmacist can prepare a stock of medicinal products in a registered pharmacy:

- with a view to dispensing them in accordance with a prescription given by a practitioner, *or*
- with a view to dispensing them in accordance with a specification from a person who is going to administer them to himself or to someone under his care.

Chapter 11

Control of Sales of Medicines

Various sections of the MA 1968 place restrictions on the supply of medicines by restricting who may sell medicines and where they may be sold.

Control of retail sales

The underlying principle of MA control on the retail sales of medicines is that they should normally be supplied through pharmacies. There are three main exceptions to that. First, certain medicines are designated by statutory instruments as ones which may be sold to the public by an ordinary shop. Secondly, medicines may be sold by a hospital or health centre even where there is no pharmacy if the products are sold or supplied in the course of the business of the hospital or health centre, *and* they are for the purpose of being administered in accordance with the directions of a doctor or dentist. The 'directions of a doctor' need not comply with the requirements for a prescription set out in the POM order.

It does not matter whether they are to be administered in the hospital or health centre or elsewhere. The doctor or dentist is not required to be an employee of the hospital, or to be associated with it in any way.

Thirdly, Patient Group Directions may empower certain health professionals to supply medicines to the public in accordance with protocols. This supply may take place anywhere.

Legal categories of medicines

The EC Directive on Legal Classification (92/26/EC) came into effect on 1 January 1993. This Directive required Member States to classify medicines into those which may only be sold or supplied on prescription, and those which may be obtained without a prescription.

The Directive lays down the criteria which must be used to determine whether a product should be subject to prescription control. These criteria have been incorporated into the Medicines Act by The Medicines Act 1968 (Amendment) (No. 2) Regulations 1992, SI 1992 No. 3271. This introduced a new section 58A into the Act.

Marketing authorization

Regulation 4 of the MAR 1994 Regs requires each application for the grant of an MA to indicate whether the product is one that should be available:

(a) only on prescription
(b) only from a pharmacy
(c) on general sale.

The application must also indicate whether the authorization should include any other restrictions on the sale or supply of the product, for example a restriction on promotion.

Where the community marketing authorization contains such restrictions, Ministers are required to include the product in the POM Order.

General Sale List

This is a list of medicines which can be sold, with reasonable safety, without the supervision of a pharmacist. The sales have to take place from proper shops, i.e. ones which can be closed so as to exclude the public. This prohibits sales being made from vans or other vehicles, or from open market stalls.

There is a separate list of products which may be sold from automatic vending machines.

To sum up GSL medicines may be sold:

- without the supervision of a pharmacist
- from any ordinary shop (not a pharmacy)
- from a shop which must be capable of being closed up
- *not* from a vehicle or market stall.

Pharmacy medicines

Pharmacy medicines (P) may be sold only in a registered pharmacy by or under the supervision of a pharmacist. This is the default category into which all medicines fall, unless placed by legislation into either of the other two categories.

Pharmacy medicines may only be sold:

- in a registered pharmacy
- by or under the supervision of a pharmacist.

Prescription Only medicines

POM may only be sold or supplied in a registered pharmacy, by or under the supervision of a pharmacist, in accordance with the prescription of a doctor, dentist or veterinary practitioner. A nurse prescriber can write prescriptions for the POM medicines listed in the Nurse Prescribers' Formulary.

Section 58A requires that a product is to be designated as a POM medicine if

(a) it needs medical supervision in use to prevent a direct or indirect danger to human health *or*
(b) it is widely and frequently misused, and so presents a danger to health *or*
(c) it is a new active substance *or*
(d) it is for parenteral administration.

The POM Order

The list of POM medicines for human use is contained in the POM Order, properly called the Prescription Only Medicines (Human Use) Order 1997, SI No. 1830.

This Order has been amended a number of times, by Prescription Only Medicines (Human Use) Amendment Orders in the following years:

- 1997, SI No. 2044
- 1998, SI No. 108
- 1998, SI No. 1178
- 1998, SI No. 2081
- 1999, SI No. 3463
- 2000, SI No. 1917
- 2000, SI No. 2899.

Medicinal products on prescription only

Generally the following medicinal products are POM:

(a) medicinal products consisting of or containing a substance listed in column 1 or Schedule 1
(b) controlled drugs
(c) medicinal products that are for parenteral administration
(d) cyanogenetic substances, other than preparations for external use
(e) radiopharmaceuticals and generators
(f) medicinal products for human use which are licensed by the EU and classed as prescription only.

There are a number of exceptions.

Schedule 1 sets out a list of medicines together with the conditions which make a product exempt from POM.

Four categories of exemptions are set out in Schedule 1. They are based on:

(a) maximum strength
(b) route of administration, use of pharmaceutical form
(c) treatment limitations
(d) maximum quantity.

Schedule 2 excludes some controlled drugs from POM when the preparation complies with the conditions.

Schedule 3 sets out the POM medicines which may be prescribed by nurses.

Schedule 4 lists a number of substances which may not be contained in a POM sold or supplied by a pharmacist under the emergency supply provisions.

Schedule 5 sets out exemptions for certain persons from the POM provisions on sale, supply or administration.

Injections

All parenteral products are POM.

Water for injection
Sterile water for injection is POM.

Administration of POMs
Section 58(2)(b) of the Act states that no one can administer a POM, except to himself, unless he is either a practitioner, or (Article 9) a person acting in accordance with the directions of a practitioner.

The POM Order makes three exceptions to this blanket prohibition. The first one exempts all medicines which are not for parenteral administration. Thus, effectively, anyone can administer to anyone else any medicines which are not injections.

Secondly, some injections are specifically exempted from the blanket prohibition (Article 7). They are ones which might be needed in an emergency:

Adrenaline injection	Hydrocortisone injection
Atropine sulphate injection	Mepyramine injection
Chlorpheniramine injection	Promethazine hydrochloride
Cobalt edetate injection	Sodium nitrite injection
Dextrose injection strong BPC	Snake venom antiserum
Diphenhydramine injection	Sodium thiosulphate injection
Glucagon injection	Sterile pralidoxime.

Thirdly, ambulance paramedics may administer a range of injections (Article II and Schedule 5 Pt.III). See Chapter 21.

A number of exceptions are made to allow the supply and use of POMs for research, business and in various unusual circumstances.

Prescription requirements
POM may only be supplied on prescription. The conditions which a prescription for POM must meet are laid out in the POM Order (Article 15).

(1)   All prescriptions must be signed in ink, with his own name, by the practitioner.
(2)   Private prescriptions must be written in ink, or otherwise be indelible.
(3)   NHS prescriptions, other than for Schedule 1, 2 or 3 of the Misuse of Drugs Act (MDA) Regulations, may be written by means of carbon paper or similar material.
(4)   No prescription may be dispensed more than six months after the date on which it was signed, except:

    (a)   NHS prescriptions may bear a date before which they may not be dispensed. The six months runs from that date if it is later than the date of signing.

    (b)   Where a prescription contains a direction that it may be dispensed more than once, then the first dispensing must be within the six month period.

(5)   Where a prescription contains directions that it may be dispensed more than once, those directions must be followed. If the number of repeats is not

specified, only one repeat is allowed, except oral contraceptives may be dispensed six times in total before the end of the six month period.

(6) All prescriptions shall contain the following particulars:

    (a) Address of the practitioner giving it.

    (b) The date of signing (or start date).

    (c) An indication of whether the prescriber is a doctor, dentist, veterinary surgeon, veterinary practitioner or nurse practitioner.

    (d) For prescriptions from doctors, dentists or nurse practitioners: name of patient, address of patient, age of patient (if under 12 years).

    (e) For vet prescriptions: name and address of person in charge of the animal, declaration by vet that the medicine is for an animal or herd under his care.

Due diligence clause

The Order states that if the person making the sale or supply has exercised due diligence and accordingly believes on reasonable grounds that the conditions are fulfilled, he will not commit an offence if it turns out that the practitioner did not in fact fulfil the conditions (Article 14).

Records of transactions

Records must be kept of the retail sale or supply of POM. Entries must be made in a register kept for that purpose. The entry must be made on the day of the transaction, or on the next day.

Records are not required for:

(1) The sale or supply on a NHS prescription.

(2) The sale or supply of oral contraceptives.

(3) Where records are made in the CD register.

(4) Sale or supply to persons in respect of a drug testing scheme.

(5) Sale or supply in Scotland, to a doctor under the Stock Order scheme.

(6) Sale or supply in Northern Ireland to a doctor for NHS use by way of immediate administration.

What details of prescriptions must be recorded?

For sale or supply of POM on a prescription, the following details are required:

(1) Date of transaction.

(2) Name and quantity of medicine.

(3) Form and strength of medicine (unless obvious).

(4) Date of script.

(5) Name and address of prescriber.

(6) Name and address of patient (or of owner of animal).

Repeat prescriptions

When second or third, etc. supplies are made on repeat prescriptions, a shortened record may be made. The date of supply must be recorded together with a reference to the original entry.

How long must the records be kept?

The POM register must be kept for two years from the date of the last entry. Prescriptions must be retained for two years from the date of last dispensing. The owner of the RPB is responsible for preserving the records.

Facsimile transmission of prescriptions

The requirements for a valid prescription are set out above. A fax does not comply because it is not itself 'signed' by the practitioner. The RPSGB view at the time of writing is that a fax can confirm the existence of a valid prescription. The POM order does not require that the prescription itself be in the possession of the pharmacist at the time of dispensing the medicine. The Misuse of Drugs Regulations 1985 contain more stringent requirements for prescriptions for Schedule 2 and 3 medicines, in particular that the prescription must be in the handwriting of the prescriber. Accordingly the RPSGB advise that such medicines cannot be dispensed against a fax.

Retail sales staff

The terms 'supervision', 'direct supervision', and 'personal control' are used in the legislation. They have similar, but not identical meanings.

Supervision

This term is used in the MA 1968. The sale or supply of P and POM medicines must take place by or under the supervision of a pharmacist (section 52).

The case of *Roberts* v. *Littlewoods Mail Order Stores Ltd* (1943) is usually quoted as the source of the meaning attributed to this term. The case concerned the sale of a Part 1 poison, under the provisions of the Pharmacy and Poisons Act 1933. Section 18(1) stated:

> '... it shall not be lawful for a person to sell any poison in Part 1 of the Poisons List unless ... the sale is effected by, or under the supervision of, a registered pharmacist.'

The sale of the poison occurred while the pharmacist was upstairs and unaware that the sale was taking place.

The court held that the statute required that the qualified person must be aware of each individual sale. The court rejected the contention that the words were sufficiently complied with by having a pharmacist in general control of the department.

In the judgment Lord Caldecote said:

> '... the man who was upstairs might have been a person who was exercising personal control of a business, but I do not think that, while he was upstairs and therefore absent, he could be a person who was supervising a particular sale. It has been suggested that a man can supervise a sale without being bodily present. I do not accept that contention ... each individual sale must be, not necessarily effected by the qualified person, but something which is shown

by the evidence to be under his supervision in the sense that he must be aware of what is going on at the counter, and in a position to supervise or superintend the activities of the young woman by whom each individual sale is effected.'

The judge also quoted from an earlier case, *Pharmaceutical Society* v. *Wheeldon* (1890), which concerned the Pharmacy Act 1868:

'nothing to our understanding can be clearer than that the object of the Act was beyond all other considerations to provide for the safety of the public, and to guard, as far as possible, all members of the community from the disastrous consequences, so frequent in occurrence, arising from the sale of poisons by persons inadequately acquainted with their baneful properties.'

Although the words of the MA are slightly different, and the legislation is concerned with medicinal products rather than poisons, the meaning given above is accepted today as the law.

Direct supervision

The NHS (PS) Regulations 1992 also use the term 'direct supervision'. The Regulations state: 'Drugs shall be provided by or under the direct supervision of a pharmacist...'. Given the meaning of 'supervision' as outlined above, it is difficult to see how the word 'direct' adds anything to the meaning.

Personal control

The meaning attributed to this phrase is usually based upon the judgment in the case of *Hygenic Stores Ltd* v. *Coombs* (1937). In this case the company sold drugs at 13 of its 16 shops, although there were no pharmacists employed at these shops. The company did employ three pharmacists, who worked long hours at the other three shops. The court found that there were no pharmacists in personal control at the 13 shops, and consequently the conditions for sale of drugs were not met. The Pharmacy and Poisons Act 1933 required that:

'... in each set of premises the business must, so far as concerns the retail sale of drugs, if not under the personal control of the superintendent, be carried on subject to the direction of the superintendent, under the personal control of a manager or assistant who is a registered pharmacist'.

The court did not define what constitutes personal control. It only decided that the circumstances outlined above did not constitute personal control.

The Statutory Committee has considered the question on a number of occasions, and its views are summarized in the following sentences. It is a matter of degree. A pharmacist does not cease to be in personal control because he leaves the pharmacy for a few minutes. At the other end of the scale, a pharmacist is not in personal control if he puts in only an occasional appearance. A pharmacist was held not to be in personal control when he was absent for one and a half hours a day on weekdays, and six hours at the weekend.

The most recent interpretation can be found in the *Pharmaceutical Journal* of 3 September 1994.

Protocols and medicines counter assistants

From 1 January 1995 it has been a requirement of the RPSGB that all pharmacies have a written protocol which specifies the procedure to be followed when a medicine is supplied, and when advice on treatment is requested.

From 1 January 1996, the RPSGB has required that all staff whose work regularly involves the sale of medicines must have either completed, or be undertaking, an approved course of training. A number of such courses have been approved covering the knowledge syllabus of the National Vocational Qualification Level 2 in retail training.

Wholesaling of medicines

A Wholesale Dealers Licence (WDL) is required by any person who distributes a medicinal product by way of wholesale dealing. The person may be a real person, a body of persons or a limited company. There are certain exceptions.

What is wholesaling?

The Medicines Act 1968 Amendment Regulations 1993, SI No. 834 altered section 8 (7) of the MA to define 'distribution by way of wholesale dealing' as meaning: selling or supplying it *or* procuring, holding or exporting it for the purposes of sale or supply to a person who receives it for the purposes of selling or supplying it, or administering it, or causing it to be administered to one or more human beings in the course of business.

The term 'business' includes a professional practice, such as that of a medical practitioner. Thus sales to a medical or dental practitioner 'for use in his practice' will be wholesale sales. Moreover, the provision of services under the National Health Service is considered to be the carrying on of a business by the appropriate Minister (section 131 Medicines Act 1968).

Certain medicinal products are outside the definition of 'relevant medicinal product'. Distribution of these products, for example, exempt herbal remedies, certain homoeopathic medicines, investigational medicinal products and unlicensed medicinal products for export to third countries, remains subject to the wholesale dealing controls of the Medicines Act.

Veterinary medicinal products are subject to specific legislation.

The legislation

Wholesale dealing is controlled by a combination of the MA 1968, sections 8, 9, 10 and 61, (which allows for Regulations to be made limiting the persons to whom products may be sold by wholesale) and Regulations, mainly SI 1980 No. 1923. SI

1971 No. 1445 amended section 10 of the MA 1968 by adding a number of sub-sections.

The result of the interplay of this legislation is as follows.

Who may wholesale medicinal products?

Wholesaling of medicinal products may be carried out by:

(1) the holder of a WDL, *or*
(2) the holder of a Product Licence (PL), *or*
(3) an RPB or hospital pharmacy, provided the wholesale sales constitute 'no more than an inconsiderable part' of the business (section 10(7), MA 1968). (This last phrase has been interpreted by MCA as meaning the sales by wholesale of no more than 5% of the purchases of medicinal products.)
(4) a wholesale dealer handling only GSL medicated confectionery.

No licence is required where a person merely acts as a carrier. No licence is required where an import agent imports a product to the order of another person who intends to distribute it. No licence is required for export from the UK direct to companies outside the EU.

Who may buy?

Pharmacy only medicines

P medicines may be sold by way of wholesale dealing to:

(1) Doctors, dentists, vets.
(2) Any person conducting an RPB.
(3) Persons carrying on the business of a hospital or health centre.
(4) Licensed wholesale dealers.
(5) Persons who are exempt from holding a WDL.
(6) Ministers of the Crown, government departments and their officers.
(7) NHS Trusts.
(8) Any person who requires P to administer them to human beings in the course of a business where the medicines are for the purpose of being so administered.
(9) Any person who may sell or supply in circumstances corresponding to retail sale:

   - P as specified in SI 1980 No. 1924
   - certain herbal remedies
   - veterinary drugs.

(10) Persons supplying under a Patient Group Direction (PGD).

Category (7) was added by the Medicines (Sale or Supply) (Miscellaneous Provisions) Amendment Regulations 1992, SI No. 2938 to enable P and POM to be sold to ambulance trusts for use by the paramedic staff.

Prescription only medicines

POM may be sold by way of wholesale dealing to:

(1)   Categories (1) to (6) in respect of P above.
(2)   For the specified products, persons exempted by Schedule 5 of The POM Order.
(3)   Registered ophthalmic opticians, for certain POM.
(4)   Suppliers of homoeopathic preparations.
(5)   Those practising homoeopathy.
(6)   Persons supplying under a PGD.

Licence types

(a)   Manufacture and assembly. Allows the holder to manufacture and assemble (package) medicinal products.
(b)   Assembly only. Allows the holder to assemble (package) medicinal products.
(c)   Manufacturer 'specials' (MS). Allows the holder to manufacture unlicensed medicinal products (commonly referred to as 'specials').
(d)   Full wholesale dealer. Allows the holder to wholesale deal pharmacy (P), prescription only (POM) and General Sale List (GSL) medicines.
(e)   Wholesale dealer (GSL). Allows the holder to wholesale deal General Sale List (GSL) medicines only.
(f)   Wholesale dealer's import. Allows the holder to wholesale deal medicines imported from countries outside the EEA.

Requirements for wholesalers

The Medicines (Applications for Manufacturers and Wholesale Dealers Licences) Regulations 1971, SI No. 974 set out the information to be given on the applications for a licence.

Applicants must specify the classes of products; give the address of each site of business; a description of the facilities available; details of record keeping; details of plans for recalling defective products; and the name of a 'Responsible Person'.

Schedule 3 of the Medicines (Standard Provisions for Licences and Certificates) Regulations 1971, SI No. 972 (as amended) sets out the Standard Provisions for wholesalers.

The wholesaler must maintain suitable staff, premises and facilities; provide information as required; record transactions; have an emergency recall plan; only buy from licensed manufacturers and wholesalers or exempt persons and only sell to those who may lawfully handle the products.

When supplied for retail sale or supply the wholesaler must provide an invoice detailing the date of transaction, the name and pharmaceutical form of the product, the quantity supplied and the name and address of the supplier.

The Responsible Person

The RP is responsible for ensuring good distribution practice. The RP must ensure that the licence conditions the Guidelines on Good Distribution Practice are complied with.

The RP does not have to be an employee of the wholesaler, and need not be a pharmacist. If not a pharmacist then he must have relevant knowledge and experience.

Records

WDL and PL holders must keep sufficient records to enable the recall of defective medicines. Pharmacies which wholesale POM must retain for two years the order or invoice relating to the transaction.

'Pseudo'-wholesale transactions

Some transactions appear on the surface to be wholesale, but on closer examination are seen not to be.

The supply of vaccines by HAs to GPs

HAs may make various vaccines available to general medical practitioners in their area. Where no charge is made by the HA to the GP for these supplies the transaction is not a wholesale transaction. There is no charge and hence no sale, an essential element in the definition of 'wholesale'. Equally the transaction is not a retail sale, because it is not a sale. Neither is it a supply 'in circumstances corresponding to retail sale', since section 132 requires that such a supply be made to persons who 'receive the product for purposes other than that of administering it or causing it to be administered...'.

Such a transaction may fall within the ambit of section 55, which exempts from certain controls '... supply ... in the course of the business of a hospital or health centre, where the product is ... supplied for the purpose of being administered (whether in the hospital or health centre or elsewhere) in accordance with the directions of a doctor or dentist'.

For section 55 to apply the actual supply must be made by a hospital, not just by the HA itself.

The supply by one hospital to another hospital unit owned by the same authority or trust

Again there is no sale, because although a nominal book charge may be made for accounting purposes, the units belong to the same body. One cannot sell to oneself.

Supply by a hospital pharmacy to wards, for administration to patients in that ward by nursing staff or doctor

There is no sale, even though the condition of supply for the purpose of administration is fulfilled.

Co-operatives

Sometimes groups of pharmacists are formed for the purpose of buying goods for subsequent retail sale by the individual members. Where the orders are simply bulked together the group will not normally require a WDL. However, if the group has a separate legal identity, e.g. as a limited company, then a licence may be required. If the group sells its purchases to persons who buy in order to sell on (whether those persons are members of the group or not), then a licence will be required.

Importers

A person who distributes, other than by way of sale, a proprietary medicinal product for human use which is imported from a non-EU source, must be the holder of a WDL (SI 1977 No. 1050). There is no need for a WDL where the only activity in relation to the product is:

(1) The provision of transport facilities.
(2) The business of an import agent who imports for another person who intends to deal with it by wholesale or otherwise to distribute it.

Parallel imports

Parallel imports are medicines imported from another member state of the European Union. They may have been manufactured in this country, or elsewhere. They are sold in parallel to the brands marketed in this country by the manufacturers. The parallel imports may bear the same English brand name, a foreign language version or a completely different name.

Market prices for pharmaceuticals differ considerably between the countries in the EU. The price differences are due mainly to the following factors:

- The degree of price control exerted in some form by the government.
- The pricing policies adopted by manufacturers to meet the competition from similar products.
- Different margins at wholesale and retail level.

Legal basis for the trade

The Treaty of Rome promotes free trade between EU countries. Articles 30–34 generally prohibit restrictions on imports. The Treaty does not allow either direct restrictions such as a complete ban, or indirect restrictions such as laws which favour the sale of home produced products rather than imported ones.

Article 36 allows import restrictions if they are justified on grounds of protection of health and life of humans, animals and plants.

In 1976 the European Court of Justice (ECJ) ruled that 'national restrictions on parallel imports within the Community would be against Community rules on freedom of trade' (case 104/75: *Re De Peijper*).

The ECJ has considered parallel imports on a number of occasions since then. Parallel imports must be allowed if:

(1) The imported product is therapeutically equivalent to the domestic product.
(2) It is manufactured in accordance with correct quality control standards.
(3) It is manufactured within the same company or group of companies, *or*

(4) Subject to some conditions, it is manufactured under licence from the original manufacturer.

The medicines regulatory agency in the importing country is responsible for verifying that the imports satisfy the criteria. This is done in the UK by the Medicines Control Agency (MCA).

Product licence (parallel import) (PL(PI))

As only products for which a PL has been issued may be marketed in the UK, the MCA issues a version for parallel imports known as the Product Licence (parallel import) or PL(PI). This is issued subject to the following conditions:

(1) The product must be imported from an EU member state.
(2) It must be a product which is already the subject of a standard marketing authorization issued by an EU Member State.
(3) The imported product must be a 'proprietary medicinal product' which is not a vaccine, toxin, serum, human blood product, radio-active isotope or homoeopathic product.
(4) It must have the same therapeutic effect as the UK product.
(5) It must be made by, or under licence from, the manufacturer of the UK product.
(6) The importer must prove that the import conforms with the specifications for the product.

Other requirements for the importer
- If the product is repacked the importer will need a ML for assembly.
- A WDL is required to distribute the product.
- Sufficient records to enable batch recalls must be kept.

Labelling

The Labelling Regulations require all medicinal products to be labelled in English. Labels in other languages may be present as well, provided the required information is in English.

Products with different name

In 1986 both the DoH and the RPSGB stated that pharmacists must not dispense a parallel import bearing a different brand name from that which the doctor had prescribed. The rule was challenged and the ECJ decided in 1989 that the rule was justified on public health grounds (cases 266 and 267/87: *R* v. *Royal Pharmaceutical Society of Great Britain*).

The rule applies even where the difference in name is small and due to language problems. The rule applies to the written names. Names which are spelt differently but which sound the same are treated as different names. It makes no difference that the therapeutic effect and quality of the products are identical.

Advertising and sales promotion

The advertising of medicines is controlled by the MA 1968, and by Regulations made under the Act. There are specific prohibitions on the advertising of treatments for various diseases. The Code of Ethics of the RPSGB deals with advertising by pharmacists. The use of certain titles, e.g. 'pharmacist', is also restricted by law. Some consumer law carries restrictions which are applicable to pharmacy.

The main Regulations dealing with the advertising of medicines are the Medicines (Advertising) Regulations 1994, SI No. 1932 – referred to as the Advertising Regulations, and the Medicines (Monitoring of Advertising) Regulations 1994, SI No. 1933 – referred to as the Monitoring Regulations. The Regulations implement the European Community Directive 92/28/EC, which concerned the advertising of medicinal products.

Both the above Regulations have been amended, mainly by The Medicines (Advertising and Monitoring of Advertising) Regulations 1999, SI No. 267.

The Regulations apply to 'relevant medicinal products', i.e. those to which Chapters II to V of the 1965 Directive 65/65/EC apply, which will be products with a 'marketing authorization'. The previous regulations on advertising, the Medicines (Labelling and Advertising to the Public) Regulations 1978, SI 1978 No. 41 remain in force for those products which fall outside the 65/65/EC definition:

- Products authorized for clinical trials;
- Products controlled by section 104 or section 105 orders;
- Products prepared in a pharmacy in accordance with a pharmacopoeia for direct supply to patients, or products made up in accordance with a prescription for an individual patient.

Medicines (Advertising) Regulations 1994

The Advertising Regulations are wide-ranging:

(1) It is an offence to advertise a medicinal product for which there is no marketing authorization.
(2) Holders of marketing authorizations have certain duties:

- to monitor information received about their product
- to provide information about adverts to regulatory authorities on request
- to comply with directions given by regulatory authorities about advertisements
- to provide adequate training for sales representatives.

(3) The Regulations make it an offence to offer or receive an inducement to prescribe or supply particular medicinal products.

What is an 'advertisement'?

For the purposes of the MA, an advertisement includes every form of advertising:

- in a publication
- by display of a notice
- by means of a catalogue or price list
- circular letters
- letters addressed to particular people
- in any other document
- words inscribed on an article
- photographs
- cinema film
- sound recording
- radio and television
- or in any other way.

It does not include spoken words which are not part of a recording or broadcast on radio or television, or the supply of a medicine in a labelled container.

Under the Regulations, price lists, trade catalogues, reference materials and factual informative statements or announcements are not advertisements unless they make a product claim.

Consent of marketing authorization holder

Advertisements may only be issued by product licence holders, or with their consent.

Advertisements to the public

The Regulations differentiate between advertising directed to the public and advertising aimed at health professionals.

POM medicines may not be advertised directly to the public. Where the retail sale of products has been restricted by a 'safety order' under section 62, then those products may not be advertised either.

Products subject to the Narcotic Drugs Convention cannot be advertised.

All advertisements must clearly be such, and the product must clearly be identified as a medicine. The advertisement must include:

- the name of the product
- the common name of the ingredient of a single active ingredient product
- how to use it
- an invitation to read the instructions.

Prohibitions

Some claims for licensed medicinal products are prohibited in adverts:

(1) Claims which give an impression that a medical consultation or a surgical operation might be unnecessary.

(2) Unsubstantiated claims of superiority, both made directly and through the use of literature, quotations and references.
(3) Suggestions that health might be affected by taking or by not taking the product.
(4) Advertisements aimed at children.
(5) The use of celebrity endorsement.
(6) Suggestions that safety or efficacy are due to the product being 'natural'.
(7) Case histories leading to false self-diagnosis.
(8) Misleading claims of recovery.
(9) Misleading or alarming illustrations of changes in the human body as a consequence of disease or the action of a product.

The advertisement must not mention that the product has been granted a product licence.

The advertisement must not suggest that a medicinal product is a foodstuff, cosmetic or other consumer product.

Schedule 1 of the 1994 Regulations prohibits advertisement to the public in respect of the following diseases:

- bone diseases
- cardiovascular diseases
- chronic insomnia
- diabetes and other metabolic diseases
- diseases of the liver, biliary system and pancreas
- endocrine diseases
- genetic disorders
- malignant diseases
- psychiatric diseases
- serious disorders of the eye and ear
- serious gastro-intestinal diseases
- serious infectious diseases including HIV related diseases and TB
- serious neurological and muscular diseases
- serious renal disease
- serious respiratory diseases
- serious skin disorders
- sexually transmitted diseases.

Specific exemptions are made for medicinal products for the treatment of the symptoms of sprains or strains; the relief of pain or stiffness of rheumatic or non-serious arthritic conditions or for the prevention of neural tube defects.

The advertising to the public of medicines containing psychotropic or narcotic substances controlled under the Narcotics Drugs Convention 1961 or the Psychotropic Substances Convention 1971 is prohibited (except for those products containing very small amounts) (Reg. 8).

Contraceptive products
Oral contraceptive products are POM and hence cannot be advertised to the public (Reg. 7).

Abortion

Products for abortion cannot be advertised to the public (Reg. 6).

Promotional sales to the public

Manufacturers, wholesalers and marketing authorisation holders are prohibited from selling or supplying medicinal products for promotional purposes to the public (Reg. 12). Small-sized packs may be sold on normal business terms through normal trade outlets.

Registered homoeopathic medicinal products

These are products marketed in the UK in accordance with the procedure in the Medicines (Homoeopathic Medicinal Products for Human Use) Regulations 1994, SI 1994 No. 105.

Advertisements for these products must contain only the following details:

- name of the stock and the dilution
- name and address of the certificate holder/manufacturer
- certificate number
- administration details
- form, expiry date and storage details
- warnings
- batch number
- content of the sales presentation
- the words 'homoeopathic medicinal product without approved therapeutic indications'
- warning to user to consult a doctor if symptoms persist.

Advertisements to health professionals

The Regulations lay down certain specified particulars to be included in advertisements which are wholly or mainly directed at health professionals who prescribe or supply the products.

The advertisements must include for instance the licence number and details of the marketing authorization holder, lists of active ingredients, one or more of the licensed indications for use, the side-effects, cautions and contra-indications from the summary of product characteristics (SPC), warnings and cost.

Small, abbreviated advertisements in professional publications are allowed which need only contain name of product, legal classification, name of marketing authorization holder, ingredients and an indication of where further information may be found.

Medical sales representatives must on each visit give a copy of the SPC for the product they are promoting.

Free samples

Free samples may only be supplied to people qualified to prescribe. There are a number of conditions laid down. Failure to comply may be punished by a fine.

- Samples may only be supplied in limited numbers;
- There must be a signed dated written request;
- There must be a system of control and accountability;
- Only small size packs are allowed;
- Each pack must be marked 'free medical sample – not for resale';
- Each sample must be accompanied by a copy of the SPC.

Samples of medicines containing psychotropic or narcotic substances controlled under the Narcotics Drugs Convention 1961 or the Psychotropic Substances Convention 1971 are prohibited (except for those products containing very small amounts).

Promotional aids

The Regulations allow for 'promotional aids' such as pens and mugs to carry the name of the product and the company without any other information. 'Promotional aid' means a non-monetary gift made for a promotional purpose by a commercially interested party. It should be relevant to the practice of medicine or pharmacy. The value should be less than £5.

Inducements

Generally it is an offence to promote a medicinal product by supplying, offering or promising any 'gift, pecuniary advantage or benefit in kind' to persons qualified to prescribe or supply medicines. The offences are serious, carrying the possibility of a two year prison term. 'Persons qualified to prescribe or supply' includes doctors, dentists, pharmacists and nurses.

There are a number of exceptions:

- Inexpensive gifts or benefits which are relevant to the practice of medicine or pharmacy are allowed.
- Reasonable hospitality at scientific or professional meetings is allowed.
- Any 'trade practices' relating to prices, margins or discounts which were in existence on 1 January 1993 are allowed to continue.

It is also an offence for any person qualified to prescribe or supply relevant medicinal products to 'solicit or accept any gift, pecuniary advantage, benefit in kind, hospitality or sponsorship prohibited by these Regulations', for which the penalty is a fine.

Medical representatives

Medical representatives must receive adequate training. They must provide information which is as precise and complete as possible about the products. On each visit, medical representatives must give a copy of the Summary of Product Characteristics (SPC) for the product they are promoting.

Summary of Product Characteristics

The SPC is a document prepared by the holder of the marketing authorization. It must contain the information laid down in regulations (MAR Regs 1994 as amended). Details of typesize and layout are also specified.

The SPC may be distributed in the form of a compendium. The Association of the British Pharmaceutical Industry (ABPI) produces an annual compendium of Summary of Product Characteristics for products on the UK market.

Monitoring

The Medicines (Monitoring of Advertising) Regulations 1994 give powers to monitor the form and content of advertisements, and deal with the handling of complaints. Control is based on a system of self-regulation.

Complaints about the content of advertisements may be referred by the Medicines Control Agency to a suitable self-regulatory body for investigation and action. The three most important self-regulatory bodies are the Advertising Standards Authority, the Prescription Medicines Code of Practice Authority and the Proprietary Association of Great Britain. The Monitoring Regulations also set out formal procedures which allow the MCA to take enforcement action in both civil and criminal courts.

Ministers are able to seek court injunctions prohibiting advertisements which do not comply. Those responsible for the advertising can be compelled to issue correction statements.

Advertising of NHS pharmaceutical services

Prior to 1992 the TOS prohibited the advertising of NHS services. Any advertising which is done is subject to the RPSGB Code of Ethics.

RPSGB Code of Ethics
The 2001 Code states:

'Publicity for professional services is permitted provided that such publicity does not create an invidious distinction between pharmacists or pharmacies, is dignified and does not bring the profession into disrepute.'

- Any information or publicity material regarding pharmacy services must be accurate and honest.
- All information and publicity for goods and services must be legal, decent and truthful; be presented and distributed in a manner so as not to bring the profession into disrepute; and not abuse the trust or lack of knowledge of the public.
- Pharmacists should not make any unsolicited approach for promotional purposes directly to the public.
- Promotions for medicines aimed at the public must emphasize the special nature of medicines; must not promote inappropriate use, must not make any medicinal claim which cannot be substantiated; be consistent with the SPC; not promote a product by way of a pharmacist endorsement; and must not offer an inducement by way of free samples, price reductions, etc.

Chapter 12

Special Circumstances

Supply of medicines in an emergency

In an emergency a pharmacist can lawfully sell or supply most POMs, provided certain conditions are satisfied.

Section 58(2)(a) of the Medicines Act 1968 generally requires a prescription for the sale or supply of POMs. Paragraph 8 of the POM Order 1997 allows exemptions from this requirement in certain circumstances. The supply must be made by a person lawfully conducting a retail pharmacy business.

Two situations are envisaged:

- a request made by a doctor
- a request made by a patient.

Supply made at the request of a doctor

The conditions that apply are:

(a)   that pharmacist must be satisfied that the sale or supply has been requested by a doctor who by reason of an emergency is unable to furnish a prescription immediately
(b)   the doctor has undertaken to furnish the pharmacy with a prescription within 72 hours
(c)   the POM is sold or supplied in accordance with the directions of the doctor requesting it
(d)   the POM is not a Controlled Drug in Schedule 1, 2 or 3 of the Misuse of Drugs Regulations 1985
(e)   an entry must be made in the Prescription Book or on the computerised record stating:

    (i)   name and address of the patient
    (ii)   date on the prescription
    (iii)   the date on which the prescription is received.

Controlled Drugs

In an emergency a practitioner can personally obtain a Schedule 2 or 3 drug if he cannot immediately supply a signed requisition. This does not authorize supply direct to the patient. The practitioner must undertake to deliver a signed requisition within 24 hours of receiving the drug.

Supply made at the request of the patient

The conditions that apply are:

(a) The sale or supply must be made by or under the supervision of a pharmacist.
(b) That pharmacist must have interviewed the patient and satisfied himself:

  (i) that there is an immediate need for the POM, and that it is impracticable in the circumstances to obtain a prescription without undue delay
  (ii) that treatment with the POM requested has been previously prescribed by a doctor for the patient
  (iii) that the dose is appropriate.

(c) Up to 5 days treatment may be sold or supplied except:

  (i) the smallest pack that the pharmacist has available may be supplied where the medicine is an original pack of an ointment or cream, an asthma aerosol, or an insulin preparation
  (ii) a full cycle of an oral contraceptive may be supplied
  (iii) the smallest quantity which provides a full course of treatment may be supplied of a liquid oral antibiotic.

(d) The pharmacist makes an entry in the Prescription Book stating:

  (i) the date of the transaction
  (ii) the name, quantity, pharmaceutical form and strength of the medicine supplied
  (iii) the name and address of the patient
  (iv) the nature of the emergency.

(e) The container or package must be labelled to show:

  (i) the date of supply
  (ii) the name, quantity, form and strength of the medicine
  (iii) the name of the patient
  (iv) the words 'Emergency Supply'.

(f) Schedule 4 to the POM Order 1997 contains a list of drugs which may not be supplied at the request of a patient.

Despite inclusion in Schedule 3 of the Misuse of Drugs Regulations 1985, and in the above Schedule, a supply of Phenobarbitone or Phenobarbitone sodium may be made where it is supplied for the treatment of epilepsy. (Para 8 (5) of the POM Order 1997.)

RPSGB has issued Guidelines, which are more stringent than the law requires:

(1) the pharmacist should consider the medical consequences, if any, of not supplying
(2) the pharmacist should identify the patient through means of documentary evidence and/or personal knowledge

(3) the doctor who prescribed on a previous occasion should preferably be identified and contacted, if possible
(4) the question should be asked of the patient as to whether the doctor has stopped the treatment
(5) enquiries should be made as to whether any other medicine is being taken at the same time to check any drug reactions
(6) an emergency supply should not be made if the item requested was prescribed previously more than six months prior to the request. Variations may be made in the case of those illnesses which occur infrequently, for example, hay fever, asthma attack or migraine
(7) consideration should be given to providing less than five days quantity if this is justified in the circumstances
(8) labelling should be clear and legible and there should be some suitable identification of emergency supply entries in the prescription book.

Supplies under the NHS

The NHS (Pharmaceutical Service) Regulations 1992 allow a doctor may request a supply to be made to a patient in an emergency. The doctor must be known to the pharmacist. He must promise to give a prescription in 72 hours. The request must not be for a CD, except one in Schedules 4 or 5 (see Chapter 18). There is no procedure for a patient to request an emergency NHS supply.

Collection and delivery schemes

Certain types of collection and delivery schemes are given special exemption from the general Medicines Act requirement that the supply of medicines must be from a pharmacy.

The Medicines (Collection and Delivery Arrangements – Exemption) Order 1978, SI No. 1421 states that the restrictions of sections 52 and 53 of the Medicines Act 1968 do not apply where the medicine:

- is for human use
- is supplied in accordance with a prescription from a doctor or dentist
- and where the supply is as part of a collection and delivery arrangement used by a pharmacy.

Section 52 restricts supply of POM and P medicines to pharmacy premises. Section 53 restricts the supply of GSL medicines to premises which can 'be closed so as to exclude the public'.

A 'collection and delivery arrangement' means any arrangement whereby a person takes or sends a prescription to premises other than a pharmacy, and later collects the dispensed medicine from those premises. A common example is where a grocery shop in an isolated village acts as a collecting point for scripts written by visiting GPs. After dispensing they are held in the shop until the patient collects them.

The script must have been dispensed at a registered pharmacy, by or under the supervision of a pharmacist. The premises used must be capable of being closed so as to exclude the public.

The arrangements are not limited to the NHS. There are no other formal legal requirements.

Delivery direct from the pharmacy

Many pharmacists have a service where they collect prescriptions from a doctor, dispense them and deliver the medicines to the patient's home. These arrangements are not covered by the restrictions outlined above. They are subject to normal legal requirements in that the dispensing must be under the supervision of a pharmacist, etc. In addition the RPSGB Code of Ethics makes specific mention of such schemes.

Prescription collection
- Prescriptions must be collected by individuals acting on the instructions of the pharmacist.
- Pharmacists must ensure confidentiality and security.
- The request for the service must come from the patient or carer.
- The initial request should be recorded.
- Requests to the doctor for repeat prescriptions should be made by the patient or carer unless the pharmacy offers a repeat medication scheme complying with Service Specification 6.
- Wrongly directed prescriptions should be returned to the surgery or authorized pharmacy.

Delivery services
- On each occasion the pharmacist must use his professional judgement to decide whether a direct face-to-face consultation is appropriate.
- Pharmacists must ensure safe delivery of medicine.
- Pharmacists must ensure appropriate storage conditions.
- There must be a verifiable audit trail identifying the initial request for the service, and each delivery or attempted delivery.

Named-patient supplies

The Medicines Act requires that marketing authorizations be held in respect of substances which are marketed as medicines. Some substances, e.g. raw chemicals may on occasions be prescribed as medicines, although they are not marketed as such. This prescribing is perfectly legal – the Medicines Act does not prohibit it.

Unlicensed medicines may be obtained in three ways:

(1) prepared extemporaneously in the pharmacy
(2) obtained from a Specials manufacturer
(3) imported from another country via a wholesaler.

Exemptions for unlicensed medicines

Section 10 of the MA 1968 contains exemptions from licensing which allow the normal activities of a pharmacist.

Section 9 of the Medicines Act 1968 states that the restrictions imposed by Sections 7 and 8 of the Act (which generally require licences) do not apply to anything which is done by a doctor or dentist which: 'relates to a medicinal product specially prepared or specially imported by him, or to his order for administration to a particular patient of his'. This allows a doctor to order an unlicensed product.

Section 7 does not apply to 'relevant medicinal products' by virtue of Regulation 9 of the MAR 1994 Regulations. 'Relevant medicinal products' are subject to the MAR 1994 Regulations.

Regulation 3 of the MAR 1994 Regulations prohibits the placing on the market or the wholesale distribution of a relevant medicinal product unless it has a marketing authorization. Products specially made for a particular patient will not have a marketing authorization.

Schedule 1, paragraph 3 allows a pharmacist to prepare or obtain a stock of an unlicensed product so that it may be supplied on prescription. The product must be prepared under the supervision of a pharmacist, and in a pharmacy, hospital or a health centre.

Extemporaneous preparation in the pharmacy

Pharmacists may carry out the preparation of an unlicensed medicine to a formula specified in a prescription in the pharmacy. Following a case where a mixture was wrongly dispensed, resulting in the death of a child, the pharmacist and postgraduate trainee involved were both found guilty of a breach of Section 64 of the MA 1968. The RPSGB issued guidance. Pharmacists are advised to check carefully all calculations, paying particular attention to the decimal points, and to either carry out the preparation themselves or to delegate to suitably trained staff. In all cases the pharmacist should verify the formula used, the weightings or other measurements, and the calculations. Where possible an independent check is advisable. The pharmacist should always undertake a final review before the product is supplied to the patient.

Specials

The term 'named-patient medicine' is usually used to refer to an unlicensed medicine specially ordered from a manufacturer. It is usually a medicine available ready-made from the manufacturer, not made up to a recipe supplied by the pharmacy or the doctor.

According to the MAR Regulations, medicinal products which have no marketing authorization may be 'placed on the market' in the following circumstances:

- the company must hold a special manufacturer's licence
- orders must be unsolicited
- the manufacture must be properly supervised
- records must be kept
- the product must be formulated in accordance with the specification of a doctor or dentist
- the product is supplied for use by a doctor or dentist, by his individual patients, on his direct responsibility

- the supply must be to a doctor or dentist, or for use under the supervision of a pharmacist in a pharmacy, hospital or health centre
- the product must be distributed by a licensed wholesaler.

Record keeping

The 'Specials' manufacturer, the pharmacist and any practitioner who sells or supplies a 'special' must keep records for at least five years, which show:

(a) the source of the product
(b) the name of the person who obtained the product
(c) the date of the transaction
(d) the quantity of each sale or supply
(e) the batch number
(f) details of any adverse reaction to the product which he knows about.

He must notify the licensing authority of any serious adverse reactions (Schedule 1, para 6, MAR Regs 1994).

Imports

A further exemption allows importation of unlicensed products. The Medicines (Standard Provisions for Licences and Certificates) Regulations 1971, SI No. 972 was amended by the Medicines (Standard Provisions for Licences and Certificates) Amendment Regulations 1999 SI No. 4 to allow a licensed wholesaler to import an unlicensed product:

- in response to a *bona fide* unsolicited order to fulfil special needs
- formulated in accordance with the specification of a doctor or dentist and
- for use by his individual patients under his direct personal responsibility.

There are conditions laid down in the Regulations:

(1) the importer must give notice in writing to the MCA of intention to import, with details
(2) written undertaking that:
    (a) the quantity imported will not exceed 25 single doses or 25 therapeutic courses (each not to exceed 3 months)
    (b) the MCA will be told of new safety concerns
    (c) the product will not be promoted
    (d) records will be kept for five years
(3) MCA must not have objected. They have 28 days to do so
(4) no equivalent product with a UK Product Licence is available on the UK market.

Counter-prescribing and customers own formula

The exemptions allow a pharmacist to:

- prepare or dispense a product against a prescription
- prepare a stock in anticipation of dispensing
- prepare or dispense a medicinal product against a specification given by the intended purchaser, where the product is to be administered to that purchaser or to someone under his care
- prepare a product for counter prescribing.

Conditions for counter-prescribing
The pharmacist is requested by or on behalf of the patient to use his own judgement as to the treatment required and the patient is present in the pharmacy at the time of the request.

Chemist's Nostrums
The pharmacist may prepare a medicinal product (or a stock of such products) with a view to retail sale rather than to supply against an order. The sale must be from the registered pharmacy where the product was prepared. The product may not be advertised (Advertising Regulations 1994). The label must contain the standard labelling particulars.

Packing from bulk
The requirements of the Leaflet Regulations prevent a pharmacist packing small sizes of product from bulk containers.

Doctors' or dentists' personal exemption certificate

The Medicines (Exemptions from Licences) (Special Cases and Miscellaneous Provisions) Order 1972, SI No.1200 provides a procedure for a doctor or dentist to order medicine for use by them in their practice. A form is sent to the MCA, which has 21 days to object to the import. The procedure is detailed in MAL 31.

Chapter 13

Hospitals and the Medicines Act

Crown immunity

Under the doctrine of Crown immunity (also called Crown exemption) the Crown and its servants or agents are not bound by any Act of Parliament unless that Act specifically states that it applies to the Crown. The idea developed from the view that all laws are made in the name of the Crown.

The MA 1968 was drafted at a time when all NHS hospitals were considered to be Crown property and the Act was not intended to apply to them. In practice the NHS generally agreed to behave in accordance with the Act.

In 1990 Crown Immunity for NHS hospitals was abolished by section 60 of the NHS and Community Care Act 1990. As a consequence the MA 1968 now applies to NHS hospitals in exactly the same way as it does to private hospitals.

Exemptions in the Medicines Act for hospitals

The MA 1968 specifies that certain activities are lawful when they are done by or in a hospital. The Act contains no clear definition of a 'hospital', although section 132 helpfully states 'hospital includes a clinic, nursing home or similar institution'.

The following activities may be done by or under the supervision of a pharmacist in hospital:

(1) Preparing a medicine in accordance with a prescription given by a practitioner.
(2) Dispensing a medicine in accordance with a prescription given by a practitioner.
(3) Assembling a medicine.
(4) Preparing a stock of medicines with a view to dispensing them in accordance with a prescription given by a practitioner.

Where there is a registered pharmacy in the hospital, the person lawfully conducting the retail pharmacy business may:

- sell by retail, *or*
- offer or expose for sale by retail, *or*
- supply in circumstances corresponding to retail sale,

any POM, P or GSL medicine, provided the transaction is made:

- on registered pharmacy premises, *and*
- by or under the supervision of a pharmacist.

In the course of business of a hospital

Section 55 of the MA 1968 provides an exception to the previous paragraph. Thus certain transactions are lawful if they take place 'in the course of the business of a hospital'. The presence or supervision of a pharmacist is not required.

A hospital may sell by retail, *or* offer for sale, *or* supply in circumstances corresponding to retail sale, any POM, P or GSL medicine provided the transaction is made in the course of the business of the hospital, *and* for the purpose of the product being administered (whether in the hospital or elsewhere) in accordance with the directions of a doctor or dentist.

This provision allows, for example, the sale of oral contraceptives in a family planning clinic, by a nurse or a member of the administrative staff. Most situations which would have been dealt with in this way will now be covered by PGDs.

Movement of medicinal products within a hospital

The movement of medicines within a hospital, e.g. supply from the pharmacy to wards, is not regarded by the MCA as requiring a licence. Similarly, prescribing by hospital doctors for inpatients is regarded as instructions to nurses to administer the medicine.

A corporate body, e.g. an NHS Trust, may have more than one hospital on different sites. Movement within the corporate body, even between sites, is not regarded as licensable.

Wholesaling

In the hospital situation, an activity will be a wholesale transaction if:

(1)   there is a sale, *and*
(2)   the transaction is between two separate legal persons *and*
(3)   the medicinal product is bought:

>   (a)   for the purpose of administering it in the course of business, *or*
>   (b)   for the purpose of causing it to be administered in the course of business, *or*
>   (c)   for selling or supplying it to another in the course of business.

Section 10 of the MA 1968 allows wholesale transactions to take place without a WDL if:

(1)   The sale is by a pharmacist or under his supervision.
(2)   The activity takes place in a hospital or health centre.
(3)   It is in accordance with a prescription or order of a doctor or dentist (or vet).
(4)   The medicine is supplied to a person who is authorized to administer the medicine or cause it to be administered.

This exemption allows hospitals to supply one another, and to supply hospices, clinics, etc.

Procurement

Section 7 restricts certain activities to PL holders. These activities include: procuring the sale, supply or exportation of any medicinal product, and procuring the manufacture or assembly of any medicinal product for sale, supply or exportation.

Section 10 exempts a pharmacist from certain of the restrictions in sections 7 and 8. A pharmacist or someone acting under his supervision may: procure the preparation of a medicinal product, *or* procure the dispensing of a medicinal product, *or* procure the assembly of a medicinal product. The procurement of preparation or dispensing must be in accordance with a prescription given by a practitioner.

Clinical trials

Section 31 MA 1968 defines a clinical trial as an investigation or series of investigations consisting of the administration of one or more medicinal products, by or under the direction of one or more doctors or dentists, to one or more of their patients, where there is evidence that:

(a)   medicinal products of that type have effects which may be beneficial to the patient or patients in question; and
(b)   the administration of the product is for the purpose of ascertaining whether, or to what extent, the products have beneficial or harmful effects.

Hospitals may conduct clinical trials. Certain activities in relation to clinic trials do not require a PL or a clinical trial certificate if done:

- by or under the supervision of a pharmacist, *and*
- in a hospital, *and*
- in accordance with a prescription given by a doctor or dentist.

The activities are selling, supplying or procuring the sale or supply of a medicine, and procuring the manufacture or assembly of a medicine.

Further details are available in *Guidance to the NHS on the Licensing Requirements of the MA 1968*, issued by the MCA in September 1992.

Chapter 14

Traditional and Alternative Medicines

The MA makes special provision for two difficult areas: homoeopathy and herbal medicines. Both present problems for the licensing system. Both represent traditional forms of treatment which have numbers of practitioners who are unable to use the exemptions from control provided for doctors and pharmacists.

The arrangements enable specified groups of medicines to be sold or supplied only by practitioners who do so after using their own judgment as to the treatment required for persons who are physically present in the premises where the supply takes place.

Additionally certain groups of medicines may be sold in non-pharmacy outlets. Herbal products which make no medicinal claims (even if they may have a medicinal use) can be sold as foods, e.g. parsley, or as food supplements. Where an ingredient has no use other than a medicinal use the product will fall within the medicines controls.

Herbal remedies

A herbal remedy is a medicinal product consisting of:

- a substance produced by subjecting a plant or plants to drying, crushing or any other process, *or*
- a mixture whose sole ingredients are two or more substances so produced, *or*
- a mixture of one or more such substances and water or some other inert substance.

Special arrangements were made to enable herbal practitioners to continue to practise and to enable the sale of simple herbs to continue. It would be impracticable to list all herbs.

Herbal practitioners
The MA 1968 generally requires the manufacture of, and dealing in medicinal products to be licensed. Section 12 of the Act exempts herbal remedies from some of these requirements. The restrictions do not apply to the sale, supply, manufacture or assembly of any herbal remedy:

- in the course of business of a herbal practitioner *and*
- where the remedy is manufactured or assembled on premises of which the

person carrying on the business is the occupier *and* which are able to be closed to the public.

The herbal practitioner (the person carrying on the business) may only sell or supply the herbal remedy in this way for administration to a particular person and after being requested by that person to use his own judgment as to the treatment required. The person being treated must be present on the premises, but another person may make the request on his behalf.

Remedies sold under section 12 exemption

The licensing restrictions also do not apply where the herbal remedy is sold or supplied in a simple way without any written recommendation as to use. In this case only the processes of drying, crushing or comminuting the plant or plants may be used to produce the herbal remedy.

Remedies sold under this section:

- must not contain non-herbal ingredients, other than inert substances such as water
- must not be accompanied by any written recommendations in the absence of a personal consultation
- must not be given names other than designations specifying the plants used and the processes they have undergone.

Section 52 restricts the sale of non-GSL products to pharmacies. Section 53 lists the general conditions for the sale of GSL medicines. Section 56 lists the situations when the restrictions in sections 52 and 53 do not apply to herbal remedies. Section 53(3) allows Ministers to make an Order which narrows the effect of the exemptions in section 56. The relevant order is the Medicines (Retail Sale or Supply of Herbal Remedies) Order 1977, SI 1977 No. 2130. The Order contains a three-part schedule of substances.

The effect of this interplay of the MA 1968 and the Order is:

(1) Those herbal remedies which contain any of the substances listed in Parts I and II of the Schedule are restricted to pharmacies.
(2) Herbal practitioners may sell remedies containing the substances in Part III of the Schedule.
(3) Herbal practitioners may also sell GSL herbal remedies.
(4) Any shopkeeper can sell dried, crushed or comminuted herbs which are not in the Schedule, provided:

    (a) he has a manufacturing licence, *or*
    (b) he has notified the RPSGB.

(5) Herbs may be sold as in (4) even if they have been tabletted, compressed, diluted with water, or made into pills.
(6) Any shopkeeper may sell GSL herbal remedies.
(7) Any shopkeeper may sell dried, crushed or comminuted herbs without a written recommendation provided the herbs are not listed in the Schedule

Certain potent plants, e.g. Digitalis are restricted to use by medical practitioners and are classified as POM.

Nature and quality
Section 64 of the MA 1968 provides that no person shall, to the prejudice of the purchaser, sell any medicinal product which is not of the nature or quality demanded by the purchaser. Thus although there are often no applicable official standards for herbal medicines, poor quality or unsafe medicines are illegal.

Marketing Authorisations Regulations
Regulation 1(3) of the Medicines for Human Use (Marketing Authorisations, etc.) Regulations 1994, SI No. 3144 excludes herbal remedies which are manufactured or sold or supplied in accordance with Section 12 from the definition of 'relevant medicinal product'. Hence the 1994 Regulations do not apply.

Homoeopathic medicines

Homoeopathy is a system of treatment elaborated by Samuel Hahnemann (1755–1843), a German physician. Its basis is treatment with minute quantities of the drugs capable of producing the symptoms of the disease treated. Conventional medicine is referred to as allopathy.

Homoeopathic medicines are the preparations used in homoeopathy. The high dilutions are prepared from 'unit preparations' which are defined as:

'a preparation, including a mother tincture, prepared by a process of solution, extraction or trituration with a view to being further diluted tenfold, or serially in multiple powers of ten, in an inert diluent, and then used either in this diluted form or where applicable, by impregnating tablets, granules, powders, or other inert substances for the purpose of being administered to human beings'

Homoeopathic medicines are generally included in the GSL, although parenteral homoeopathic medicines and certain strengths of some substances are restricted to POM.

Licensing

When the Medicines Act came into force, existing homoeopathic products were issued with 'product licences of right'. These were given without any evidence of quality, safety or efficacy. Products licensed under this system continue to be covered by licences of right and remain available.

A new scheme was set up when Directive 92/73/EEC ('the Homoeopathic Directive') was implemented. Under this scheme a homoeopathic product may be given a 'certificate of registration' if it meets quality and safety standards. It is not necessary to show efficacy. Because there are no demonstrations of efficacy, medical claims may not be made for the products. Certificates of registration last for five years.

The Medicines (Advisory Board on the Registration of Homoeopathic

Products) Order 1995, SI No. 309 established the Advisory Board in 1
function of the Advisory Board is to give advice to the Licensing Auth
the safety and quality of homoeopathic medicinal products.

The Medicines (Homoeopathic Medicinal Products for Human Use) Regulations 1994, SI No. 105 sets out the law governing certain over the counter (OTC)
homoeopathic products. The safety criteria were classified in SI 1994 No. 899.

It applies to all homoeopathic products except those which are made to a
'magistral or officinal' formula as defined in the 65/65/EEC.

Products which fall into this system are:

- for oral or external use
- contain not more than 1 part in 10,000 of the mother tincture *or*
- if the active principle is a POM, contain not more than 1 part in 100 of the
  smallest allopathic dose
- are prepared in accordance with a homoeopathic manufacturing procedure
  described in the European Pharmacopoeia or an official pharmacopoeia of a
  Member State.

Products may not use a brand name or be labelled with a specific therapeutic
indication.

The Medicines Act 1968 (Amendment) (No. 2) Regulations 1994, SI No. 276
contain a definition of a homoeopathic medicinal product:

'any medicinal product (which may contain a number of principles) prepared
from products, substances or compositions called homoeopathic stocks in
accordance with a homoeopathic manufacturing procedure described by the
European Pharmacopoeia or, in the absence thereof, by any pharmacopoeia used
officially in a member state.'

These regulations mainly amend sections 7 and 8 of the MA 1968, so that the
Medicines (HMPHU) Regulations 1994 apply to products with a certificate of
registration, and the existing MA 1968 provisions apply to any other homoeopathic product.

Sale, supply or administration of homoeopathic medicines

Many of the drugs used in homoeopathy are restricted to POM when used at
conventional strengths. Sale and supply is controlled by the inclusion of such
drugs in the POM Order, with exceptions for diluted products.

Section 58(2)a of the MA 1968 generally restricts the sale, supply or administration of medicines containing substances specified in the POM Order (Parts I
and II) to prescription.

The POM Order makes specific exemption for medicine which contains, or
consists of one or more unit preparations of highly diluted substances on the
lists.

Conditions for sale (1)
Each unit preparation has been diluted to at least one part in one million (6x).

The person who sells, supplies or administers the product was requested to do so. The person who requested the product was present when the seller, etc. made a judgment to supply, etc.

Conditions for sale (2)
Each unit preparation has been diluted to at least one part in one million million (6c).

It should be remembered that although homoeopathic practitioners claim that the more highly diluted products have greater potency, these are subject to restrictions based on conventional thinking, i.e. the lower restriction applies to the more dilute.

Standard labelling requirements for containers and packages of homoeopathic products marketed under a certificate of registration

(1) The scientific name of the stock or stocks followed by the degree of dilution, making use of the symbols of the pharmacopoeia used in relation to the homoeopathic manufacturing procedure described therein for that stock or stocks.
(2) The name and address of the holder of the certificate of registration and, where different, the name and address of the manufacturer.
(3) The method of administration and, if necessary, route.
(4) The expiry date of the product in clear terms, stating the month and year.
(5) The pharmaceutical form.
(6) The contents of the sales presentation.
(7) Any special storage precautions.
(8) Any special warning necessary for the product concerned.
(9) The manufacturer's batch number.
(10) The registration number allocated by the licensing authority preceded by the letters 'HR' in capital letters.
(11) The words 'homoeopathic medicinal product without approved therapeutic indications'.
(12) A warning advising the user to consult a doctor if the symptoms persist during the use of the product.

Leaflets for homoeopathic products

The Medicines (Labelling and Leaflets) Amendment Regulations 1994, SI No. 104 also set out the requirements for Patient Information Leaflets to be supplied with homoeopathic medicines. These apply to any product placed on the market with a certificate of registration. A new Regulation 3B is inserted into the Leaflet Regulations.

Standard requirements relating to leaflets for homoeopathic products

Subject to the following provisions of these regulations, any leaflet which is enclosed in or supplied with the packaging of a proprietary medicinal product which is a homoeopathic product to which Council Directive 92/73/EEC applies and which is placed on the market in the UK in accordance with a certificate of registration, shall, in addition to clear mention of the words 'homoeopathic medicinal product', contain the particulars set out in Schedule 3 to these regulations and no other particulars.

The detailed requirements are set out in Schedule 3.

Restrictions on sale for safety reasons

The MA provides various mechanisms for restricting the sale of substances considered to be harmful. The more important products, and the relevant legislation are listed below.

Substances

Laetrile

A substance known variously as laetrile, amygdalin or Vitamin B17 has been used as a possible treatment for cancer. It is claimed to work by releasing cyanide in the tissues. Laetrile is a naturally occurring substance found especially in the kernels of apricots, peaches, plums and almonds. After several deaths were attributed to use of the compound it was decided that it should no longer be available freely over the counter.

The prohibition was achieved by the Medicines (Cyanogenetic Substances) Order 1984, SI 1984 No. 187 which was made pursuant to section 104 of the MA 1968. This section allows Ministers to extend the provisions of the Act to substances which do not ordinarily fit the definition of medicinal product. In the case of laetrile products the parts of the Act which are applied by the Order are mainly concerned with sale, supply, importing and promotion. In conjunction with the POM Order the effect is to restrict the sale to prescription.

The POM Order 1997:

(1) defines 'cyanogenetic substances' as preparations which:

   (a) are presented for sale or supply under the name of amygdalin, laetrile or vitamin B_{17}
   (b) are presented for sale or supply as containing amygdalin, laetrile or vitamin B_{17}
   (c) contain more than 0.1% by weight of any substance having the formula either: alpha-cyanobenzyl-6-ortho-beta-D-glucopyranosyl-beta-D-glucopyranoside *or* alpha-cyanobenzyl-beta-D-glucopyranosiduronic acid

(2) includes 'cyanogenetic substances' in the categories of products which are on prescription.

The 0.1% figure corresponds with the maximum level of cyanide regarded by the DoH as acceptable in food, such as marzipan.

The title of the Order refers to 'cyanogenetic' substances. This is an interesting example of the wrong word used in legislation. 'Cyanogenetic' means 'from cyanide' and not 'cyanide-creating' (cyanogenic) as was presumably intended.

Chloroform

The Medicines (Chloroform Prohibition) Order 1979, SI 1979 No. 382 generally prohibits the sale or supply of medicinal products for human use which contain chloroform. There are a number of exemptions:

(1) Sales and supplies by doctors, dentists, pharmacies and hospitals. The sale or supply must be to a patient. The product must have been made by a doctor or dentist *or* to his prescription.
(2) Sale or supply as an anaesthetic. The supply must be to a doctor, dentist or hospital, *or* to a wholesaler for supply as above.
(3) Sale for use solely in dental surgery.
(4) Where the medicinal product contains not more than 0.5%.
(5) Where the product is for external use, but not for use on mucous membranes, the mouth or teeth.
(6) Where the product is to be used as an ingredient in the preparation of a substance in a pharmacy or hospital, or by a doctor or dentist.
(7) For export.

This Order interacts with the POM and GSL Orders so that only items in categories (4) and (5) may be sold by retail to the public.

Bal Jivan Chamcho

Bal Jivan Chamcho is an Asian baby tonic containing high levels of lead. The product has been banned from sale, supply or importation by the Medicines (Bal Jivan Chamcho Prohibition) (No. 2) Order 1977, SI 1977 No. 670.

Aristolochia

Following concerns about the quality of various herbal products sold as aristolochia, a series of temporary orders severely restricted its sale and supply.

Following a consultation exercise the ban is to be made permanent with effect from 1 July 2001, by The Medicines (Aristolochia and Mu Tong, etc.) (Prohibition) Order 2001.

This Order prohibits the sale, supply, and importation, of any medicinal product for human use which

(a) consists of or contains a plant belonging to a species of the genus Aristolochia or belonging to any of the species: *Akebia quinata, Akebia trifoliata, Clematis armandii, Clematis montana, Cocculus laurifolius, Cocculus orbiculatus, Cocculus trilobus, Stephania tetrandra,* or an extract from such a plant; or
(b) is presented as consisting of or containing Mu Tong or Fangji, a plant belonging to any of the species *Akebia quinata, Akebia trifoliata, Clematis armandii, Clematis montana, Cocculus laurifolius, Cocculus orbiculatus, Cocculus trilobus, Stephania tetrandra,* or an extract from such a plant.

These prohibitions are subject to the following exceptions:

(i) where the sale or supply is to, or the importation is made by or on behalf of, a person exercising functions in relation to the enforcement of food or medicines legislation

(ii)   in the case of the prohibitions on importation, where the product is imported from a Member State of the EU, or, where the product originates in the European Economic Area, from a State Party to the European Economic Area Agreement which is not also a Member State;

(iii) where the product is the subject of a marketing authorization or homoeopathic certificate of registration.

Alkyl nitrites or 'poppers'

Alkyl nitrites such as butyl nitrite and amyl nitrite have long been used as recreational drugs, collectively known as 'poppers'. The RPSGB won a test case in 1996, which established that their retail sale was illegal. The court took the view that the products were medicines and hence they could not be sold without being licensed, and could not be sold from ordinary retail outlets.

On 13 January 1997 amyl nitrite was made a POM, by being included in the Medicines (Products Other than Veterinary drugs) (Prescription Only) Amendment No. 2 Order 1996. A pharmacist may still sell amyl nitrite to a person to whom cyanide salts may legally be sold, if the sale is to provide an antidote to cyanide poisoning.

Other products

Some other groups of products fall within the MA 1968 by regulations made under Section 104.

The Medicines (Specified Articles and Substances) Order 1976, SI No. 968, as amended by SI 1994 No. 3119 brings under control contact lenses, contact lens fluids and similar products, and intra-uterine contraceptive devices.

The Medicines (Radioactive Substances) Order 1978 SI No. 1004, together with the Medicines Act 1968 (Application to Radiopharmaceutical-associated Products) Regulations 1992, SI No. 605 applies to radiopharmaceuticals.

HIV testing kits

Section 23 of the Health and Medicines Act 1988 gave the Secretary of State power to make Regulations controlling the sale or supply of HIV testing kits and the provision of HIV testing services.

HIV means Human Immunodeficiency Virus of any type.

An 'HIV test kit' is any diagnostic kit which is for detecting the presence of HIV or HIV antibodies.

'HIV testing services' means diagnostic services which are for the purpose of detecting the presence of HIV or HIV antibodies in identifiable individuals.

Contravention of the Regulations makes a person liable on conviction to a fine and imprisonment for two years.

The HIV Testing Kits and Services Regulations 1992 SI 1992 No. 460

The Regulations are intended to prevent 'do-it-yourself' testing for HIV or antibodies. The Regulations prohibit the sale or supply of HIV testing kits to members of the public. They allow people to buy or receive kits for use in the course of business. Exporters are allowed to supply kits for use abroad. An exception is made to allow charities to receive or supply kits.

Pharmacies may receive kits, as may doctors. Pharmacies may sell kits either by wholesale, or to other professionals.

The Regulations place restrictions on the use of kits. Any service provided must be provided either by a doctor, or at the request of a doctor.

There are controls on the advertising of kits and services, and on the labelling on kits.

Paragraph 2 of the Regulations makes it an offence to sell or supply a kit, or a component part of a kit, to the public. A member of the public is any person who buys or receives a kit other than in the course of his business.

Paragraph 3 requires certain warnings with the kits. There must be statements that the kits are not to be supplied to the public, and warnings that the test results should be confirmed by at least one other test. There is also a warning against 'false negatives' (where antibodies to the infection have not yet developed).

Paragraph 4 limits the provision of testing services to doctors, and to persons providing the test on a doctor's request or for ensuring the quality of blood transfusions or other blood products.

Paragraph 5 prohibits the advertising of the sale of kits to the public. It also requires advertisements for the availability of testing services to state that the service may only be provided on the request of a doctor.

Chapter 15

Labelling and Containers

Various Regulations and Orders have been issued under the MA 1968 to deal with the labelling of medicinal products.

Section 85 enables Ministers to regulate labelling in order to ensure descriptions are correct, to ensure that suitable instructions are given, and to promote safety. The section provides that it is an offence not to comply. Section 86 deals with leaflets relating to medicinal products.

The main Regulations

The main Regulations are the Medicines (Labelling) Regulations 1976, SI No. 1726, which have been amended a number of times, and which were substantially altered by:

(a) Medicines (Labelling) Amendment Regulations 1992, SI No. 3273.
(b) Medicines (Leaflets) Amendment Regulations 1992, SI No. 3274, and
(c) Medicines for Human Use (Marketing Authorisations, etc.) Regulations 1994, SI No. 3144 [the MAR Regs].

These 1992 Amendment Regulations implemented Directive 92/27/EC, which set out the EC requirements for labels and leaflets as part of the move to a single market.

They apply to 'relevant medicinal products' which constitute the vast majority of products. Relevant medicinal products are those to which Chapters II–V of Directive 65/65/EEC apply, and constitute all products for human use except those prepared on the basis of a magistral or official formula, products intended for research or development trials, and intermediate products intended for further processing.

General provisions for labelling

(1) All labelling of containers and packages of relevant medicinal products shall be:

(a) legible and indelible
(b) comprehensible; and
(c) either in the English language only or in English and in one or more other languages provided that the same particulars appear in all the languages used.

Symbols or pictograms may be used to clarify the standard labelling requirements.

Strength of product

In any case where there is more than one pharmaceutical form or more than one strength of a product, a statement of the pharmaceutical form or strength of that product must appear on the label. This can be as part of the name of that product, but otherwise must be added immediately after the name, in the same style and size of letters as the name. 'Strength' means the suitability of the product for a baby, child or adult.

The requirement for a container or package of a relevant medicinal product to be labelled to show its name is not met by the container or package being labelled to show an invented name which is liable to be confused with the common name.

Additional information useful for health education may appear on the label so long as it is not of a promotional nature.

Labelling details must be approved by the licensing authority, and any changes notified to them. The licensing authority has a 90 day period during which it may object to any changes.

The standard labelling requirements for medicinal products for human use

(1) The name of the product followed, where the product contains one active ingredient and its name is an invented name, by the common name.

(2) A statement of the active ingredients of the product expressed qualitatively and quantitatively per dosage unit or according to the form of administration for a given volume or weight, using the common names of the ingredients.

(3) The pharmaceutical form of the product.

(4) The contents of the product by weight, by volume or by number of doses of the product.

(5) A list of excipients known to have a recognised action or effect. In relation to products which are injectable or are topical or eye preparations, all excipients.

(6) The method, and if necessary, the route of administration of the product.

(7) A special warning that the product must be stored out of reach of children.

(8) Any special warning required by the marketing authorization for the product concerned.

(9) The expiry date of the product (stating the month and year) in clear terms.

(10) Any special storage precautions for the product.

(11) Any special precautions for the disposal of any unused products or waste materials derived from such products.

(12) The name of the holder of the marketing authorization of the product.

(13) The address of the holder of the marketing authorization.

(14) Any licence number as allocated by the licensing authority which relates to

the product, preceded by the letters 'PL' in capital letters or other abbreviation of the expression 'marketing authorization'.

(15) The manufacturer's batch reference.

(16) Where a product is intended for self-medication, any instruction on the use of the product.

Appropriate non-proprietary name

Appropriate non-proprietary name means:

(1) Any name, or abbreviation of such a name, at the head of a monograph in one of the publications listed in section 103 of the MA 1968. The publications listed there are:

    (a) The European Pharmacopoeia (EP).
    (b) The British Pharmacopoeia (BP).
    (c) The British Pharmaceutical Codex (BPC).
    (d) The British Veterinary Codex.
    (e) The British National Formulary (BNF).
    (f) The Dental Practitioners' Formulary.
    (g) Any other compendium published under the MA 1968.
    (h) The list of British Approved Names.

(2) Where the product is not described in a monograph, the British Approved Name (BAN).

(3) If neither of the above apply, then the international non-proprietary name (INN).

(4) If none of the above apply, then the accepted scientific name or other name accurately describing the product.

This hierarchy of definitions means that wherever possible the product is labelled with a name which is clear to all users. These names are usually referred to as 'generic' names.

Appropriate quantitative particulars

This means the quantity of each active ingredient, expressed in terms of weight, volume, capacity or as a percentage.

Proprietary medicinal product

This means a ready-prepared medicinal product marketed in the UK with a particular name and in a special pack – in other words a branded or proprietary medicine.

Expiry date

Since January 1990, all licensed medicinal products have been required to carry an expiry date in clear language (Medicines (Labelling) Amendment Regulations 1985, SI 1985 No. 1558).

The product 'expires' at the end of the month stated, or after the date stated, e.g. 'June 1992' means the product is not to be used *after* June 1992.

Small containers

Ampoules and other containers of 10 ml capacity or less are not required to have all of the standard particulars on the ampoule itself. The package must bear the full standard particulars. The small container itself must have the following:

● name of product
● appropriate quantitative particulars
● quantity
● expiry date
● batch number
● any particulars required by the product licence.

Blister packs

Where the container of a medicinal product is a blister pack which is itself enclosed in a fully labelled package, the label on the blister pack need only include:

(1) name of product
(2) expiry date
(3) the name of the holder of the marketing authorization of the product
(4) the manufacturer's batch reference.

What is a container?

The container is the receptacle which actually contains the tablets, capsules, syrup, etc.

What is the package?

The package is the box, packet, etc. in which the container is enclosed.

GSL Medicines

The MAR Regulations 1994 contain extra requirements for some common GSL products:

(1) products which contain aloxiprin, aspirin or paracetamol must be labelled with 'If symptoms persist, consult your doctor' and the recommended dosage
(2) products containing aloxiprin must be labelled with 'contains an aspirin derivative'
(3) products containing aspirin must be labelled with 'contains aspirin'. This is not necessary for external products or where 'aspirin' is included in the product name.

(4) products containing paracetamol must be labelled with 'contains para-
     cetamol', unless 'paracetamol' is included in the product name
(5) the words 'do not exceed the stated dose' must appear adjacent to the
     directions or dosage on paracetamol products
(6) the phrases above in (2)–(4) may be combined where appropriate
(7) the phrases in (2)–(5) must be printed in a rectangle, in a prominent posi-
     tion.

Pharmacy only medicines

A further set of requirements applies to P, which must be labelled as follows:

(1) All Pharmacy Only medicines must be labelled with the capital letter 'P' in a
     rectangle. This requirement also applies to sales by wholesale.
(2) Products which contain aspirin, aloxiprin or paracetamol must be labelled
     as described above.
(3) Some substances are exempted from POM control when present in a
     product below a specified level. The products must generally be labelled
     'Warning. Do not exceed the stated dose'. Products for external use are dealt
     with in a different way, as are products where the substance is an anti-
     histamine or similar substance.
(4) Products for the treatment of asthma or bronchial spasm, and those which
     contain ephedrine or its salts, must be labelled 'Warning. Asthmatics
     should consult their doctor before using this product'.
(5) Anti-histamine products, except those for external use, must be labelled
     'Warning. May cause drowsiness. If affected do not drive or operate
     machinery. Avoid alcoholic drink'.
(6) Liquid or gel products for external use, including embrocations, liniments,
     lotions or antiseptics must carry the words 'For external use only'.
(7) Human medicines containing hexachlorophane must either be labelled 'Not
     to be used for babies' or carry a warning that the product is not to be
     administered to a child under the age of two except on medical advice.

The warning phrases must be in a rectangle which does not contain any other
matter.

Prescription Only Medicines

The containers and packages of POM must be labelled with the letters 'POM' in a
rectangle. The label must also carry the appropriate warnings listed above for
external medicines and for medicines containing hexachlorophane. These
requirements apply when the products are sold by wholesale, which includes
sale to doctors or dentists.

When sold by wholesale, POMs do not need to be labelled 'Keep out of reach
of children' but this is necessary for retail sale.

Radiopharmaceuticals
(1) The container and the package shall be labelled in accordance with the 1985
     Edition (as amended in 1990) of the Regulations for the Safe Transport of

Radioactive Materials recommended by the International Atomic Energy Agency.

(2)   The labelling on the shielding shall explain in full the codings used on the vial and shall indicate, where necessary, for a given time and date, the amount of radioactivity per dose or per vial and the number of capsules, or for liquids, the number of millilitres in the container.

(3)   The vial shall be labelled to show:

    (a)   the name or code of the medicinal product, including the name or chemical symbol of the radionuclide
    (b)   the international symbol for radioactivity
    (c)   the name of the manufacturer; and
    (d)   the amount of radioactivity as specified in paragraph 2 above.

Labelling for dispensed medicinal products

A dispensed medicinal product is a medicinal product prepared or dispensed in accordance with a prescription given by a practitioner.

What the label of a dispensed medicine must contain

The container shall be labelled with

(1)   the name of the patient
(2)   the name and address of the person who sells or supplies the product
(3)   the date of dispensing
(4)   the following details if requested by the practitioner:

    (a)   the name of the medicinal product or its common name
    (b)   the directions for use
    (c)   the precautions relating to its use

(5)   the words 'keep out of reach of children' or similar
(6)   the words 'for external use only' if the product:

    (a)   is a P or POM medicine which is a liquid or gel,
    (b)   consists of an embrocation, liniment, lotion, antiseptic or other preparation and
    (c)   is for external use.

Where the pharmacist believes that any of the particulars in (4) as requested by the practitioner are inappropriate, he may substitute those he believes to be appropriate. This may only be done after taking all reasonable steps, and failing, to consult with the prescriber.

Quantity dispensed

A RPSGB Council Statement in 1984 advised that labels of dispensed medicines should indicate the total quantity of the product dispensed in the container. The requirement applies to solid and liquid medicines, and to both internal and external preparations.

Counter prescribing and recipes

Where a product is dispensed in accordance with a specification furnished by the purchaser, or the pharmacist counter prescribes to a person present in the pharmacy, the product may be labelled as a dispensed medicine or with the standard particulars. This means that products ready labelled for retail sale do not require the addition of the patient's name, the date or the address of the pharmacy.

Standard labelling requirements for homoeopathic products

Containers and packages of homoeopathic products must be labelled in clear and legible form to show a reference to their homoeopathic nature, in particular by clear mention of the words 'homoeopathic medicinal product'. This is in addition to any other particulars required by regulations. See Chapter 14.

Pharmacists' own remedies

Products prepared in a pharmacy for retail sale from that pharmacy, and which are not advertised, are sometimes known as 'nostrums'. They must be labelled with the following:

- name of product
- pharmaceutical form on the package
- appropriate qualitative details
- quantity
- directions for use
- special handling and storage requirements
- expiry date
- name and address of seller
- 'keep out of reach of children'
- where appropriate, the warnings for 'P' medicines.

Child resistant containers

The retail sale of certain products must be in child resistant containers (CRCs). The original regulations, the Medicines (Child Safety) Regulations 1975, SI 1975 No. 2000, only covered aspirin and paracetamol for children. They were amended by the Medicines (Child Safety) Amendment Regulations 1976, SI 1976 No. 1643, which made CRCs a requirement for aspirin and paracetamol used for adults.

A 'child resistant container' is:

- an opaque or dark-tinted reclosable container complying with BS 6652 (SI 1987 No. 877)

- *or* opaque or dark-tinted unit packages in the form of bubbles, blisters or other sealed units.

The products covered by the Regulations are: aspirin products in unit-dose form (except effervescent tablets containing less than 25% weight in weight) for human use; paracetamol products for human use.

When packed for administration to children the medicinal products must be white, although flavours are allowed. Each container may not contain more than 25 unit doses.

Exemptions

The Medicines (Child Safety) Regulations 1975, SI 1975 No. 2000 do not apply when the sale or supply is:

(1) on prescription
(2) made by a doctor or dentist for a patient
(3) from a pharmacy by a pharmacist responding to a request from a patient to use his judgment as to treatment
(4) by a doctor or dentist to a colleague for a patient
(5) in the course of business of a hospital for use in accordance with the directions of a doctor
(6) for export or not for retail sale
(7) of products not for human use.

Dispensed medicines in CRCs

There is no law requiring the use of CRCs for dispensed medicines. However, in 1981 the pharmaceutical and medical professions agreed that all solid-dose oral preparations should be dispensed in CRCs or in strip or blister packs. Exceptions are allowed for:

- original packs
- patients who experience difficulty in opening CRCs
- specific requests from patients.

The voluntary scheme became a professional requirement from 1 January 1989, and appears as a requirement in the RPSGB Code of Ethics. This was extended by a Council Statement in February 1994, which stated that from 1 January 1995 it was a professional requirement for CRCs to be used for all liquid medicines dispensed from bulk.

Ribbed or fluted bottles

According to the Medicines (Fluted Bottles) Regulations 1978, SI 1978 No. 40, certain medicinal products for external use must be supplied in ribbed or fluted bottles. The outer surface of the bottles must be fluted vertically with ribs or grooves recognisable by touch. The list of substances is contained in Appendix 6.

In these Regulations 'external use' means:

'... application to the skin, teeth, mucosa of the mouth, throat, nose, ear, eye, vagina or anal canal. It does not include throat sprays, nasal drops, nasal sprays, nasal inhalations, teething preparations or dental gels.'

Exceptions
The Regulations do not apply to:

- bottles over 1.14 litres
- containers for export
- products sold or supplied solely for scientific education, research or analysis
- eye or ear drops in a plastic bottle
- where the product licence specifies otherwise
- where there are exceptions in the Schedule.

Offences

It is an offence for any person in the course of business carried on by him to sell, supply or possess for sale any medicine which does not comply with the requirements. It is also an offence to have any leaflet which does not comply.

Medicinal products must be sold in containers. Containers, packages and leaflets must properly describe the product and must not mislead as to the nature or quality of the product.

Contravention is punishable by a fine of up to £2000 and up to two years' imprisonment.

Patient Information Leaflets

Council Directive 92/27/EEC on the labelling of medicinal products for human use and on package leaflets was adopted by the European Commission on 31 March 1992. It was fully implemented into UK legislation via the following statutory instruments.

- The Medicines (Leaflets) Amendment Regulations 1992 SI No. 3274.
- The Medicines (Marketing Authorisations etc) Regulations 1994 SI No. 3144.
- Section 86 of the Medicines Act 1968 is amended by the Medicines Act 1968 (Amendment) Regulations 1994 SI No. 101:

'(4) No person shall, in the course of a business carried on by him, supply a product to which Chapters II to V of the Directive apply, unless —

a) a leaflet enclosed in, or supplied with, the container or package of the product, or

b) the container or package itself, contains the particulars which a leaflet relating to the product is required by regulations under subsection (1) of this section to contain, and does so in the manner required by such regulations.'

Regulation 7 of the MAR Regs 1994 imposes an obligation on the holder of a UK marketing authorization to comply with 'all obligations which relate to him by virtue of the relevant Community provisions, including in particular ... obligations relating to package leaflets'. Schedule 3 para 11 states that it is an offence for the holder of a marketing authorization to sell or supply a product without a package leaflet which complies with the requirements of Council directive 92/27/EEC.

Paragraph 12 states that any other person who, in the course of a business carried on by him, sells or supplies a product without a package leaflet is also guilty of an offence.

The offence is punishable by a fine or imprisonment or both.

The content of these patient information leaflets (PIL) is set out in the Medicines (Leaflets) Amendment Regulations 1992, which substantially amended the principal Regulations which are the Medicines Leaflets Regulations 1977.

Regulations 3 and 8 set out the content of such leaflets, which is detailed in Schedule 2 of the 1992 Regs. The contents of the PIL must be approved by MCA.

Leaflets for 'relevant medicinal products' are to be drawn up in accordance with the Summary of Product Characteristics (SPC).

Leaflets may be printed in more than one language provided one is English and the same particulars appear in each language (regulation 5(4)).

The licensing authority may direct in the marketing authorisation that certain therapeutic indications shall not appear on leaflets (new regulation 4(7) as inserted by regulation (5(8)).

Symbols, pictograms or other information may appear on such leaflets if there is no promotional element (new regulation 4(8) as inserted by regulation 5(8)).

The Regulations provide for certain information to be shown where the name of a relevant medicinal product is given, where that information does not form part of that name (new regulation 4(9) as inserted by regulation 5(9), article 7.1(a) of the Directive).

Standard requirements for Patient Information Leaflets

(1) For identification of the medicinal product:

    (a) The name of the product followed, where the product contains only one active ingredient and its name is an invented name, by the common name.

    (b) A statement of the active ingredients and excipients expressed qualitatively and a statement of the active ingredients expressed quantitatively, using their common names, in the case of each presentation of the product.

    (c) The pharmaceutical form and the contents by weight, by volume or by number of doses of the product, in the case of each presentation of the product.

    (d) The pharmaco-therapeutic group, or type of activity in terms easily comprehensible for the patient.

    (e) The name and address of the holder of the product licence and of the manufacturer.

(2) The therapeutic indications.

(3) A list of information which is necessary before taking the medicinal product as follows:

   (a) Contra-indications.
   (b) Appropriate precautions for use.
   (c) Forms of interaction with other medicinal products, with alcohol, tobacco and food and any other form of interaction which may affect the action of the medicinal product.
   (d) Special warnings which:

      (i)   take into account the particular condition of certain categories of users;
      (ii)   mention, if appropriate, potential effects on the ability to drive vehicles or operate machinery;
      (iii) give details of those excipients, knowledge of which is important for the safe and effective use of the medicinal product.

(4) The necessary and usual instructions for proper use of the medicinal product which shall include:

   (a) The dosage
   (b) The method and if necessary route of administration.
   (c) The frequency of administration, specifying if necessary the time at which the medicinal product may or must be administered

and where the nature of the product makes it appropriate, shall also include:

   (d) The duration of treatment where it should be limited
   (e) The action to be taken in the case of an overdose
   (f) The course of action to take when one or more doses have not been taken
   (g) Indication, if necessary, of the risk of withdrawal effects.

(5) A description of the undesirable effects which can occur with normal use of the medicinal product and if necessary the action to be taken in such case, together with an express invitation to the patient to communicate any undesirable effect which is not mentioned in the leaflet to his doctor or pharmacist.

(6) A reference to the expiry date indicated on the label with:

   (a) A warning against using the product after this date
   (b) Where appropriate, special storage requirements
   (c) If necessary, a warning against certain visible signs of deterioration.

(7) The date upon which the leaflet was last revised.

Guidelines

Article 12 of the Directive makes provision for the publication of guidelines to be used in conjunction with the Directive. The Guideline on Excipients in the label and package leaflet of medicinal products for human use became effective on 1 September 1997. This guideline is currently under review and the updated version is due to become effective in the near future. The Guideline on the readability of the label and package leaflet of medicinal products for human use became effective on 1 January 1999.

Hospital practice

Where medicines are given to patients in hospitals as individual doses, e.g. on a ward, the leaflet need not be included in the packaging, but must be provided to the patient on request.

Chapter 16

Other Health Professions and Medicines

In addition to practising their own profession, other health professionals are often the subject of specific exemptions in the MA enabling them to handle medicines. Details of the exemptions are set out in the POM Order as amended. An Order may specify any or all of the following as 'appropriate practitioners' under the Medicines Act – PAMs, pharmacists, dental auxiliaries, ophthalmic opticians, osteopaths, chiropractors, nurses, midwives, health visitors, or any other health professionals the S of S specifies. In addition health care professionals may also be enabled to supply and administer specific medicines through a Patient Group Protocol.

Doctors

Doctors, along with dentists and vets, are generally exempted from the licensing requirements of the MA. Section 9, together with Schedule 1 of the MAR Regs 1994, allows doctors to:

(1) import medicines for patients
(2) manufacture, assemble, sell or supply medicines to patients
(3) procure the manufacture, assembly, sale or supply for patients
(4) do any of the above at the request of another doctor, for the other doctor's patients.

The sale or supply to patients is allowed by section 55 despite the provisions generally restricting supply to pharmacies. However the NHS Terms of Service stop GPs from charging for treatment given to their NHS patients. Dispensing doctors are allowed to supply and charge their dispensing patients for blacklisted medicines, i.e. those in the Selected List Scheme.

Nurses

Section 11 of the MA allows nurses to assemble medicinal products in the course of their profession, without an ML. They are also permitted to prescribe in certain circumstances (see below).

Midwives

Similarly, midwives may assemble medicinal products without an ML.

The restrictions on the sale or supply of products do not apply:

(1) To the sale or supply in the course of the professional practice of a midwife of products on a list.
(2) When the product is delivered or administered by a midwife on being supplied in pursuance of arrangements made by the S of S.

The list of products which a midwife may sell or supply is:

- all GSL and P products
- chloral hydrate
- ergometrine maleate (not parenterals)
- pentazocine hydrochloride
- triclofos sodium.

Administration

There is a list of POMs which midwives may administer parenterally in the course of their professional practice:

- ergometrine maleate
- naloxone hydrochloride
- oxytocin
- pentazocine lactate
- pethidine
- pethidine hydrochloride
- phytomenadione.

The following three drugs may be administered only while attending a woman in childbirth:

- lignocaine
- lignocaine hydrochloride
- promazine hydrochloride.

Ophthalmic opticians

Opticians may sell or supply a range of medicines in the course of their professional practice *and* in an emergency.
The products are:

(1) Eye drops or eye ointments of:

  (a) chloramphenicol (up to 0.5% drops, up to 1% ointment)
  (b) sulphacetamide sodium (up to 30%).

(2) Medicines which are POMs only because they contain any of the following:

- atropine sulphate
- bethanecol chloride

- carbachol
- cyclopentolate hydrochloride
- homatropine hydrobromide
- naphazoline hydrochloride
- naphazoline nitrate
- physostigmine salicylate
- physostigmine sulphate
- pilocarpine hydrochloride
- pilocarpine nitrate
- tropicamide.

Supply to opticians

Pharmacists may supply these medicines to a registered ophthalmic optician on receipt of a signed order.

Products only for use in practice

Opticians may purchase certain products for use in their practice, but not for sale or supply. The products are POMs which are classed as POM because they contain any of the following:

- amethocaine hydrochloride
- framycetin sulphate
- lignocaine hydrochloride
- oxybuprocaine hydrochloride
- proxymetacaine hydrochloride
- thymoxamine hydrochloride.

Chiropodists

State registered chiropodists who hold a certificate of competence from the Chiropodists Board are allowed to sell certain medicinal products. The sale or supply must be made in the course of their professional practice. The product must have been made up for sale or supply in a container elsewhere than at the place at which it is sold or supplied, i.e. chiropodists cannot supply from their own bulk stocks. Chiropodists are also allowed to expose or offer for sale medicines on the list.

Chiropodists may sell:

(1) The following P medicines for external use:

- potassium permanganate crystals or solution
- heparinoid and hyaluronidase ointment.

(2) P for external use containing any of the following as active ingredients, and up to the strengths listed:

- borotannic complex 9%
- buclosamide 10%

- chlorquinaldol 3%
- clotrimazole 1%
- crotamiton 10%
- diamthazole hydrochloride 5%
- econazole nitrate 1%
- fenticlor 1%
- glutaraldehyde 10%
- hydrargphen 0.4%
- mepyramine maleate 2%
- miconazole nitrate 2%
- phenoxypropan-2-ol 2%
- podophyllum resin 20%
- polynoxylin 10%
- pyrogallol 70%
- salicylic acid 70%
- thiomersal 0.1%.

(3)

- co-dydramol 10/500 tablets where the quantity sold or supplied at any one time does not exceed 3 days treatment (maximum 24 tablets)
- amorolfine hydrochloride cream up to 0.25%
- amorolfine hydrochloride lacquer up to 5%
- topical hydrocortisone up to 1%
- ibuprofen other than POM preps, and only for three days treatment at a maximum daily dose of 1200 mg and a maximum pack size of 3600 mg.

Administration of parenteral analgesics

Chiropodists who hold a 'certificate of competence in the use of analgesics' approved by the Chiropodists Board are allowed to administer parenteral analgesics in the course of their practice. The list of analgesics is:

- bupivacaine hydrochloride
- hydrochloride with adrenaline (maximum strength of adrenaline 1 in 200 000, i.e. 1 mg in 200 ml).
- lignocaine hydrochloride
- lignocaine hydrochloride with adrenaline (maximum strength of adrenaline 1 in 200 000, i.e. 1 mg in 200 ml).
- mepivaine hydrochloride
- prilocaine hydrochloride.

Ambulance paramedics

Arrangements have been made to enable specially trained paramedics to administer certain POM to patients in their care, without the requirement to be acting in accordance with the directions of a doctor.

The POM Order 1997 allows 'persons who hold a certificate of proficiency in ambulance paramedic skills issued by, or with the approval of the Secretary of State' to administer specified parenteral medicines on their own initiative 'only for the immediate necessary treatment of sick and injured persons'.

In the case of POM medicines containing heparin sodium the administration is only to be for the purpose of cannula flushing.

The list of medicines is:

- diazepam 5 mg per ml emulsion for injection
- succinylated modified fluid gelatin 4 per cent intravenous infusion.

and POM containing one or more of the following substances, but no other active ingredient:

- adrenaline acid tartrate
- anhydrous glucose
- benzyl penicillin
- compound sodium lactate IV infusion (Hartman's Solution)
- ergometrine maleate
- ergometrine maleate 500 mg/ml with oxytocin 5 iu/ml
- frusemide
- glucose
- heparin sodium
- lignocaine hydrochloride
- meloclopramide
- morphine sulphate
- nalbuphine hydrochloride
- naloxone hydrochloride
- polygeline
- sodium bicarbonate
- sodium chloride
- streptokinase.

Diazepam and morphine are controlled by the Misuse of Drugs Regulations. A 'group authority' has been issued by the Home Office (under powers contained in Regulations 9(4)(a) and 10(4)(c) of the Misuse of Drugs Regulations 1985) which allows lawful possession by ambulance paramedics, and supply by ambulance stations for the purpose of administration as described above.

Ambulance paramedics may administer the above medicines, in the specified circumstances, whether or not they are officially on duty.

Any ambulanceman may also administer:

(1) Any non-parenteral POMs (as may anyone).
(2) Those POMs in Article 7 of the POM Order (for the purpose of saving life in an emergency).
(3) Any POM in accordance with the directions of a doctor.

Nurse prescribing

Ministers are empowered to determine the 'appropriate practitioners' for the purpose of the sale and supply of POM medicines. Nurses are now one of the 'appropriate practitioners' referred to in the Medicines Act and the POM Regulations. As such they are able to prescribe within the limits set by the legislation.

What is the definition of 'a nurse prescriber'?

A community nurse or practice nurse who is identified as a nurse prescriber on the UKCC register, writing a prescription for an item in the Nurse Prescribers' Formulary using form FP10(CN) or FP10(PN), within a nurse prescribing demonstration scheme or within a Health Authority or Trust that has implemented nurse prescribing.

It is important to remember that two sets of rules apply to nurses who prescribe: the general rules and the NHS rules which limit prescribing in the NHS.

General rules

The Medicinal Products: Prescription by Nurses etc. Act 1992 was an enabling measure which amended both the Medicines Act 1968 and the NHS Act 1977 so that secondary legislation could then set out the details of nurse prescribing. The 1992 Act came into effect in 1994.

Section 58 of the Medicines Act 1968 lists the practitioners who can authorize the supply of POM medicines. Section 1 of the 1992 Act adds nurses to that list, and section 63 of the HSC Act 2001 adds 'other persons'.

Section 58 reads:

'The appropriate ministers may by order specify descriptions or classes of medicinal products for the purpose of this section; and in relation to any description or class so specified, the order shall state which of the following, that is to say —

a) doctors
b) dentists
c) veterinary surgeons and practitioners
d) registered nurses, midwives and health visitors who are of such description and comply with such conditions as may be specified in the order, are to be appropriate practitioners for the purposes of this section
e) other persons who are of such a description and comply with such conditions as may be specified in the order.'

Ministers are given power to specify the subcategories of nurses, etc. who may prescribe. This may be done by specifying the training and qualifications which are necessary. Statutory Instrument 1994 No. 2402 sets out the necessary training and qualifications for nurses to prescribe. It states that nurses who are able to prescribe must:

- be registered on parts 1–12 of the UKCC register
- have a district nurse qualification and be employed by a Health Authority, Trust or fundholding practice

- be registered on Part 11 as a health visitor and be employed by a Health Authority, Trust or fundholding practice
- be named on the professional register and marked as qualified to prescribe.

Amendments to this Statutory Instrument have been made to allow eligible nurses employed in Primary Care Act pilots to prescribe.

Article 2(b) of the POM Order designates appropriate nurse practitioners as appropriate practitioners for the sale and supply of certain medicinal products, which are set out in Schedule 3 of the Order. The Medicines Act 1968 already allows any person to prescribe medicines. The restrictions are placed on the dispensing of the prescriptions by pharmacists. Thus no changes to the Medicines Act were necessary in respect of P and GSL medicines.

Parenteral administration

Section 58(2) allows doctors, dentists and vets to delegate the parenteral administration of POM medicines to anyone. Section 1 of the 1992 Act allows Regulations to prohibit this delegation by nurses.

Which nurses can prescribe

Three conditions must be fulfilled:

- registration
- qualification
- employment.

A nurse prescriber must hold a district nurse or health visitor registration, and must have completed the recognized training for prescribing. In addition, in order to prescribe the nurse must be employed as a District Nurse or as a Health Visitor by a HA or a Trust, or be a practice nurse. The law enables all nurses who meet the criteria to prescribe any of the products in the Nurse formulary, whether on NHS forms or as private prescriptions.

Registration

Nurse prescribers must be either:

(1) (a) registered on Part 1 or 12 of the Register maintained by the United Kingdom Central Council for Nursing, Midwifery and Health Visiting under Section 10 of the Nurses, Midwives and Health Visitors Act 1979, *and*

   (b) have a district nursing qualification additionally recorded in the professional register under rule 11 of the Nurses, Midwives and Health Visitors Rules 1983 *or*

(2) registered as a health visitor on Part 11 of the Register maintained by the United Kingdom Central Council for Nursing, Midwifery and Health Visiting under section 10 of the Nurses, Midwives and Health Visitors Act 1979.

Note that the district nursing qualification is now known as Specialist Practitioner: district nursing in the home, and the health visitor qualification as Specialist Practitioner Public Health Nursing – Health Visitor.

Qualification

In each case the nurse's name must be held in the professional register with an annotation signifying that the nurse is qualified to order drugs, medicines and appliances for patients having successfully completed a Nurse Prescriber's Training Course approved by the English National Board.

Dispensing nurse prescriptions in the NHS

Section 41 of the NHS Act 1977 sets out the duties of FHSAs to arrange for the provision of pharmaceutical services in response to orders from doctors and dentists.

> 'It is the duty of every Health Authority, in accordance with regulations, to arrange as respects their area for the provision to persons who are in that area of –
>
> d) such drugs and medicines and such listed appliances as may be determined by the S of S for the purposes of this paragraph which are ordered for those persons by a prescribed description of person in accordance with such conditions, if any as may be prescribed, in pursuance of functions in the health service, the Scottish health service, the Northern Ireland health service or the armed forces of the Crown.

What can be prescribed by nurses?

Nurse prescribers may only prescribe from the items listed in the Nurse Prescribers' Formulary (listed at the back of the BNF). This has not been laid down as a Statutory Instrument, and can be amended as required. A few amendments were made to this from 1st December 1998. This list is a 'white' list, i.e. any item prescribed by a nurse which does not appear on this list will be disallowed by the PPA.

Patient Group Directions

The general position

In general the effect of section 58(2)(b) of the Medicines Act is that POM medicines may only be supplied to patients by doctors or pharmacists in accordance with a prescription which complies with the requirements of section 15(2) of the POM Order. This requirement may be varied by order. Patient Group Directions (PGDs) are effected by amendments to the POM Order and to the Medicines (P&GS-EX) Order 1980. Both original orders widen the restrictions imposed in the Medicines Act so as to allow medicines to be supplied in certain circumstances without there being a prescription in the normal form. The amending legislation is mainly in four statutory instruments:

- the Prescription Only Medicines (Human Use) Amendment Order 2000, SI No. 1917
- the National Health Service (Pharmaceutical Services) Amendment Regulations 2000, SI No. 121
- the Medicines (Pharmacy and General Sale – Exemption) Amendment Order 2000 No. 1919
- the Primary Care Trusts (Functions) (England) Regulations 2000 No. 695.

Section 52 of the Medicines Act is unaffected by these provisions. Section 52 restricts the retail sale of P and POM medicines, in the course of business, to pharmacies.

Protocol

The Patient Group Direction allows certain named health professionals on their own account or on behalf of 'NHS bodies' to sell, supply or administer named medicines within the terms of a protocol. There is a special exemption for persons lawfully conducting a retail pharmacy business.

Administration of injections

Since Article 9 of POM order allows any person to administer a non-parenteral POM to human beings, the effect in practice of PGD is also to allow pharmacists and other health professionals to give injections in accordance with a PGD.

Patient group direction

A 'patient group direction' is defined in the POM Order as 'a written direction relating to the supply and administration of a description or class of prescription only medicine and which is signed by a doctor or dentist, and by a pharmacist and relates to supply and administration, or administration, to persons generally'. It applies to groups of patients who may not be individually identified before presenting for treatment.

Patient group directions are drawn up locally by doctors, pharmacists and other health professionals, signed by a doctor or dentist, as appropriate and approved by an appropriate healthcare body.

Limited to NHS

The use of patient group directions is confined to NHS bodies and to NHS funded services provided through the private, charitable or voluntary sector. This is because there is no appropriate independent body to approve directions in the private sector. Patient group directions must be authorized by the NHS Trust, Health Authority or Primary Care Trust as appropriate. The process by which patient group directions must be authorised by the NHS Trust, Health Authority or Primary Care Trust, as appropriate, is contained in guidance.

Not CDs

The supply or administration of controlled drugs is excluded from the scope of patient group directions.

Persons able to supply under PGD

- nurse
- midwife
- health visitor
- pharmacist
- optometrist
- chiropodist
- radiographer
- orthoptist
- physiotherapist
- medical laboratory technicians
- ambulance paramedics.

Particulars required for a lawful patient group direction

- name of the business to which the direction applies
- coming into force and expiry dates
- description of the medicine to which the direction applies
- signature of a doctor or dentist as appropriate
- signature by an appropriate health organization
- clinical condition or situation to which the direction applies
- clinical criteria under which the patient is eligible for treatment
- exclusions from treatment under the direction
- circumstances in which further advice should be sought from a doctor or dentist
- details of applicable or maximum dosage, quantity, pharmaceutical form and strength, route of administration, frequency and duration of administration
- relevant warnings
- details of any necessary follow-up action
- arrangements for referral for medical advice
- record-keeping arrangements.

Particulars concerning medicines must be consistent with the Summary of Product Characteristics for the relevant product.

Supply may be made by pharmacies or by health service bodies or by certain health professionals. In addition the conditions set out below must be met:

- The PGD must relate to the supply or administration of a description or class of POM.
- The PGD must be in effect at the time of supply or at the time of administration.
- The PGD contains the relevant information.
- The PGD is signed by an 'authorizing person'.
- The individual who supplies or administers the medicine is designated in writing for the purpose, and is one of the authorized classes.

- The medicine supplied or administered has a valid product licence, marketing authorization or homoeopathic certificate of registration.

The new legislation allows:

- A pharmacy to supply or administer a POM without a normal prescription, but instead under the authority of a PGD (s. 12C). Previously any person could administer a non-parenteral POM under the direction of a doctor, so the effect of the new legislation is to allow the administration of a parenteral POM. Under the PGD the administration must be by a pharmacist or by another person in one of the specified classes.
- A HA, a Trust, a PCT (and a SHA and the CSA) itself to supply a POM for the purpose of being administered to a particular person in accordance with written directions (s. 12A). This extends the exemption previously confined to hospitals which allows supply without a formal prescription. Hospitals can only make such supplies in the course of their business, and as a result of the 2000/1917 amendment of s. 12, only for specific patients. Now, where the hospital is an NHS one it will, as a Trust, be able to make supplies in other circumstances.
- A person (not a doctor or a pharmacy business) who has made an arrangement with a HA, a Trust, a PCT (and a SHA and the CSA) to supply for the purpose of being administered to a particular person in accordance with written directions (s. 12A).
- A HA, a Trust, a PCT (and a SHA and the CSA) itself to supply a POM for the purpose of being administered to a particular person in accordance with a PGD (s. 12A).
- A HA, a Trust, a PCT (and a SHA and the CSA) itself to administer a POM to a particular person in accordance with a PGD provided the individual who administers the POM is a pharmacist or other person in Part III of the schedule (s. 12A).
- A person who is a pharmacist or other person in Part III of the schedule, who has made an arrangement with a HA, a Trust, a PCT (and a SHA and the CSA) to administer a POM to a particular person in accordance with a PGD (s. 12A).
- A person who is a pharmacist or other person in Part III of the schedule to supply or administer a POM under a PGD in order to assist in the provision of NHS primary care services (s. 12B).

Chapter 17

Poisons and Other Controls

There are a number of controls on the sale, storage, labelling and other dealings with those poisons which are not medicines.

The Poisons Act 1972 sets up a mechanism to designate substances as poisons, and to lay down rules on how they are to be treated.

The Poisons Board

Section 1 of the Poisons Act creates an advisory committee (in reality a continuation of one established by earlier legislation, the Pharmacy and Poisons Act 1933).

The Board consists of at least 16 members. Five of them must be appointed by the RPSGB, and one of these must be engaged in the manufacture of pharmaceuticals. Members hold office for three years. The chairman is appointed by the S of S.

The Poisons List

The main task of the Board is to recommend to the Secretary of State which substances should be listed as poisons. Section 2 of the Act creates a Poisons List, which is set out from time to time in a Poisons List Order. The list consists of two parts.

Part I is a list of poisons which can only be retailed from a pharmacy.

Part II is a list of poisons which can be sold from either a pharmacy or by a 'listed seller'.

Listed sellers

A 'listed seller' is a person allowed by the local county or borough council to sell Part II poisons. The local authority can refuse permission if it believes the person is unfit. Names may also be removed from the list for non-payment of the retention fee. A court may remove a name from the list following a conviction which would make the person unfit to sell poisons.

The local authority list must include particulars of the premises, and the names of the persons listed. The permission is specific to the person. Up to two deputies may be named. The list is open to public inspection without charge.

The local authority is entitled to charge reasonable fees for inclusion, and for retention.

Listed sellers may not use any title, emblem or description which might suggest an entitlement to sell poisons other than those in Part II.

Enforcement

Enforcement is shared between the RPSGB and the local authorities, with the RPSGB dealing with pharmacies. Both appoint inspectors, but the local authorities may appoint one of the RPSGB inspectors to work on their behalf. RPSGB inspectors must be pharmacists.

Penalties

A person who fails to comply with the law relating to poisons is liable on conviction to a fine of up to £1000. Offences involving the misuse of titles, or the obstruction of an inspector may incur a fine of £100.

When the offences are related to the sale or supply of a poison, the employer remains liable even though an employee acted without his authority (section 8)

Substances on the List

Only substances which appear on the Poisons List are legally poisons. Other substances, despite their toxicity, are not legally poisons.

Some poisons may only be sold by listed sellers when the poison is in a specified form. Some poisons may only be sold to certain categories of purchaser.

The Poisons Rules

The detail of the law is found in the Poisons Rules, which categorize poisons into a number of Schedules. There are different rules governing each of the Schedules. The current law is found in the Poisons Rules 1982, SI 1982 No. 218, as amended (mainly) by the Poisons Rules Amendment Order 1985 SI 1985 No. 1077. The Rules also contain a number of general provisions which apply to all poisons.

General requirements

Generally, poisons in Part I must be sold:

(1) by a pharmacist or person lawfully conducting an RPB
(2) at the pharmacy
(3) by or under the supervision of the pharmacist.

Poisons in Part II must be sold:

(1) from a pharmacy, *or*
(2) by a listed seller from his premises.

Listed sellers may not sell any Part II poisons which they have altered or processed in such a way as to expose the poison.

Schedule 1

Extra conditions are specified for the sale, storage and record-keeping of poisons in Schedule 1.

Supervision

All Schedule 1 poisons, even those on Part II of the List, must be sold under the supervision of the pharmacist when sold from a pharmacy. When sold from 'listed premises' the sale must be effected by the listed seller or one of his deputies.

Storage

Schedule 1 poisons must be stored separately from other items. They must be in: a cupboard or drawer used solely for poisons; or a part of the premises separated from the rest so as to exclude the public; or on a shelf used only for storing poisons, and which has no food below it.

Schedule 1 poisons which are used in agriculture, horticulture or forestry must be kept separate from food products. If stored in a drawer or cupboard no other products may be kept with them.

When poisons are transported in vehicles adequate steps must be taken to avoid contamination of any food carried in the same vehicle.

Knowledge of the purchaser

Purchasers of Schedule 1 poisons must be known to the seller, or to a responsible person on his staff, as being 'of good character'. In the case of listed sellers, the responsible person is the person in charge of the premises or of the department.

Where the purchaser is not known, they must present a certificate stating that they are of good character. This must be in the prescribed form, and given by a householder. If the householder is not known to the seller then the certificate must be endorsed by a police officer in charge of a police station. The endorsement certifies that the householder is known to the police as a person of good character. It does not itself certify the purchaser.

Records

Sellers of Schedule 1 poisons are required to keep a Poisons Book and enter in it:

(1) date of sale
(2) name and address of purchaser
(3) name and address of person giving the certificate
(4) date of the certificate
(5) name and quantity of poison
(6) purpose for which the poison is stated to be required.

The format is laid down in Schedule 2 to the Poisons Rules.

The entry must either be signed by the purchaser, or purchasers who require a poison for trade or professional purposes may present a signed order instead of signing the Poisons Book.

A Poisons Book must be retained for two years after the last entry.

Signed order

A signed order must contain the following:

(1) name and address of purchaser
(2) trade, business or profession
(3) purpose for which the poison is required
(4) total quantity to be bought.

The seller must be reasonably satisfied that the signature is genuine, and that the person does indeed carry on the trade or profession stated.

The seller must retain the certificate, giving it a reference number for identification.

In an emergency a Schedule 1 poison may be supplied on an undertaking to supply a signed order in 24 hours.

Relaxations

The requirements relating to knowledge of the purchaser, and entries in the Poisons Book do not apply to the sale of poisons:

(1) for export
(2) by wholesale.

There are specific relaxations for the sale of nicotine dusts (less than 4%), and rat poisons containing barium carbonate or zinc phosphide.

Schedule 1 poisons subject to extra controls

The following Schedule 1 poisons are listed also in Schedule 12 and are subject to extra controls:

- sodium and potassium arsenites
- strychnine
- fluoroacetic acid, its salts or fluoracetamide
- thallium salts
- zinc Phosphide.

They may only be sold or supplied:

(a) by wholesale
(b) for export
(c) for education, research or analysis.

These poisons may also be sold or supplied in the circumstances outlined below.

Strychnine is subject to additional controls made under the Control of Pesticides Regulations 1986. They mean that purchasers of strychnine must have TWO written permits, both issued by MAFF:

(1)   Form LP10 (Rev 82), which is issued under Poisons Rules. This authorizes the purchase for killing moles. This form is valid for three months. The permit must be retained by the pharmacy for two years.

(2)   Form STRYCH3, which is issued under the Control of Pesticides Regulations, to persons who have satisfied MAFF that they are trained and competent in the use of strychnine. This form is a duplicate form. The pharmacy must keep the yellow copy for two years, and the other copy is returned to the purchaser.

The quantity of strychnine which may be sold is limited to 50 g in Britain, and to 25 g in Northern Ireland.

Strychnine must only be sold in the manufacturers' original unopened containers of 1 or 2 g. No more than 8 g may be sold to 'providers of a commercial service'.

Fluoroacetic acid, its salts or fluoroacetamide may be sold to a person with a certificate authorizing the use as a rodenticide. The certificate must state the quantity, and identify the place where it is to be used.

It may only be used in ships, sewers, drains and dock warehouses. Certificates are issued by local authorities or port health authorities, or by MAFF.

Thallium salts may be sold to:

(1)   Local authorities or port health authorities.
(2)   Government departments.
(3)   Persons with a written authority issued by MAFF authorizing the use of thallium sulphate for killing rats, mice or moles for pest control.
(4)   Manufacturers who regularly use them in the manufacture of articles in the business (except thallium sulphate).
(5)   Any person, when it is an ingredient in any article not intended for consumption by persons or animals (except thallium sulphate).

Zinc phosphide may be sold:

(1)   To a local authority.
(2)   To a government department.
(3)   To a person for his trade or business.

Calcium, potassium and sodium cyanides may only be sold under the so-called section 4 exemptions. Sales are not allowed for private purposes.

Section 4 exemptions

The main effect of section 4 of the Poisons Act is that in some circumstances poisons may be sold by persons who are neither listed sellers nor pharmacists.

The following activities are exempted from the provisions of the Poisons Act, except as provided specifically in the Poisons Rules:

(1)   Wholesale dealing.

(2) Export.
(3) Sale to doctor, dentist, vet for professional purposes.
(4) Sale for use in hospital or similar public institution.
(5) Sale by wholesale:

    (a) to government department
    (b) for education or research
    (c) to enable employers to meet any statutory obligation with respect to medical treatment of employees
    (d) to a person requiring the substance for trade or business.

Sales for resale

Where a wholesaler sells a Part I poison, he must either reasonably believe that he is selling to an RPB, or alternatively obtain a statement from the purchaser that he does not intend to sell the poison by retail (Rule 11). There have been instances where wholesalers have unwittingly (and unlawfully) supplied drug stores operated by a customer who also operated a pharmacy.

The CHIP Regulations 1994

All poisons must be labelled and packaged in accordance with the Chemicals (Hazard Information and Packaging) Regulations 1994, SI 1994 No. 3247 made under the Health and Safety at Work etc. Act 1974. They came into force on 31 January 1995, replacing an earlier, less extensive set of Regulations made in 1993. The 1994 Regulations also replace the Classification, Packaging and Labelling of Dangerous Substances Regulations 1984.

The Regulations require the manufacturer or distributor of a 'chemical' to classify it according to its danger. If it fits into one of the three broad classifications of danger given in the Regulations then it must be specially labelled, and information must be given when it is supplied.

Classification

'Chemical' includes solids, liquids and gases, and includes pure chemical substances such as ethanol as well as preparations of chemicals such as cleaning fluid. They are classified as follows:

(1) Chemicals which are dangerous because of their physical or chemical properties: explosive, oxidizing, extremely flammable, highly flammable, flammable.
(2) Chemicals which are: toxic, very toxic, harmful, corrosive, irritant, carcinogenic, mutagenic, toxic for reproduction, sensitizing.
(3) Chemicals which are dangerous for the environment.

Information

When classified chemicals are supplied in connection with work they must be accompanied by a 'safety data sheet'. Should any new safety information become available, the data sheet must be revised, and copies of the revised data sheet must be given to anyone who obtained the chemical during the previous 12 months. There is thus an implicit requirement to keep records of sales of chemicals for use in connection with work.

The information on the safety data sheet must be given under 16 standard headings.

Labelling

The Regulations set out details of labelling, which include:

- the name and address of the supplier
- the name of the chemical
- the type of danger
- warnings about use
- EU number
- a warning pictogram in black on orange background.

Packaging

Chemicals must be packaged safely. Toxic, very toxic and corrosive chemicals which are sold to the public must be in containers with child-resistant closures. This requirement applies regardless of the quantity sold. It also applies to solid products. Tactile danger warnings must be on containers sold to the public of chemicals which are harmful, highly flammable, extremely flammable, toxic, very toxic or corrosive.

Exemptions

Certain categories of products are exempt from the CHIP Regulations because they are already controlled under more appropriate legislation, e.g. radioactive substances. 'Medicinal products' are exempt from these Regulations, being subject to other rigorous control (see Chapter 15).

Enforcement

The RPSGB is the enforcement authority for pharmacies.

The Environmental Protection Act 1990

This Act imposes a duty of care on 'waste producers' to dispose of 'controlled waste' legally. Waste producers are persons in business, but not householders where their own household waste is concerned. Controlled waste is any household, commercial or industrial waste. Regulations define various types of waste, and lay down further rules for handling. The Collection and Disposal of Waste Regulations 1988, SI 1988 No. 819, which are made under the Control of Pollution Act 1974, define drugs and pharmaceutical products as 'clinical waste'. The Control of Pollution (Special Waste) Regulations 1988, SI No. 1709 include all POMs as 'special waste'.

Medicines and other pharmaceutical waste must be disposed of through licensed 'waste disposal authorities'. Each consignment must be documented.

Packaging waste

The Producer Responsibility Obligations (Packaging Waste) Regulations 1997 SI No. 648 implement the European Directive 94/62/EEC on the recycling of waste. The Regulations are made under the Environment Act 1995.

The Regulations place a 'producer responsibility' on businesses involved in the packaging chain to recover and recycle certain percentages of packaging waste. The obligation applies to businesses with a turnover of more than £5 million per year and which handle more than 50 tonnes of packaging per year. Packaging which contained 'special waste' including medicines is partially exempted from the regulations.

Smaller businesses are subject to a requirement to keep records of the tonnage of waste handled each year, and of any steps taken to promote the recovery of this packaging.

Other products subject to statutory control

The Food Safety Act 1990

The Food Premises (Registration) Regulations 1991 require all premises which sell food to be registered with the Local Authority. It is an offence to use unregistered premises for a food business. Food includes packed baby foods, confectionery, etc.

The Offensive Weapons Act 1996

Section 6 of the Act came into force on 1 January 1997. It prohibits the sale of knives and similar objects to people under 16 years old. The prohibited items include 'any knife, knife blade or razor blade' and 'any other article which has a blade or which is sharply pointed and which is made or adapted for causing injury to the person'. Items in pharmacies which might fall within these wide definitions include the obvious ones, plus items such as corn knives, metal nail files, scissors and the like.

Chapter 18

Controlled Drugs

The Misuse of Drugs Act 1971 controls activities concerned with certain dangerous and harmful drugs. It covers the import, export, production, supply and possession of 'controlled drugs' (CDs).

The Act achieves control by means of extensive and detailed Regulations. It prohibits all activities with CDs except where the Regulations provide exceptions.

The Misuse of Drugs Act 1971 extends to Northern Ireland, although there are separate Regulations for Northern Ireland.

Basic provisions of the Misuse of Drugs Act 1971

The Act prohibits the possession, supply, manufacture, import or export of controlled drugs except as allowed in the Regulations, or by a licence from the Secretary of State.

(1) Sections 7, 10 and 22 enable and require the Home Secretary to make Regulations affecting the way health professionals and others deal with controlled drugs.
(2) Section 12 enables the Home Secretary to give directions to a doctor, dentist or pharmacist who has been convicted of an offence under the Act (or a related offence under the Customs and Excise Management Act). The directions can prohibit the person concerned from dealing in CDs or in authorising their administration.
(3) Section 13 enables similar directions to be given where a doctor contravenes the Misuse of Drugs (Supply to Addicts) Regulations 1997 SI No. 1001.
(4) Section 13 also allows for directions to be given after a tribunal has found a doctor or dentist to have prescribed CDs in an irresponsible manner.
(5) Section 23 empowers the police or other authorized persons to enter business premises to inspect stock of CDs and related documents.

Controlled drugs

The drugs subject to control are listed in Schedule 2 of the Act. The Schedule is divided into three classes depending on the degree of danger the drugs present. The three classes: Class A, Class B, and Class C are used when determining penalties for offences under the Act (section 25). Class A are the most harmful drugs and attract the severest penalties.

The list of CDs may be altered by an Order in Council approved by an affirmative resolution of both Houses of Parliament. The Advisory Council on the Misuse of Drugs must be consulted before any change.

The original list contained in the Act has been changed by the following Orders: SIs 1973/771, 1975/421, 1977/1243, 1979/299, 1985/1995, 1986/2230, 1989/1340, 1990/2589, 1995/1966, 1996/1300 and 1998/750.

International convention

Many of the changes to both the Act and the Regulations are made because of the UK's obligations under the United Nations Single Convention on Narcotic Drugs 1961 and the United Nations Convention on Pschotropic Substances 1971. These conventions seek to regulate the world wide traffic in drugs of abuse. The Government is advised on any communication relating to the conventions by the Advisory Council.

The Advisory Council on Misuse of Drugs (ACMD)

The Advisory Council was established by the Act in 1972. Its purpose is to advise the relevant Ministers on various matters concerned with drug misuse.

The relevant Ministers are:

(1) In England: the Home Secretary, Secretary of State for Health and Secretary of State for Education.
(2) In Scotland, Wales and Northern Ireland: Ministers responsible for Health and Ministers responsible for Education.

Composition of the Advisory Council

There are at least 20 members, who are appointed by the Secretary of State after consultation with appropriate organisations. Members are required to have wide and recent experience of each of the following:

- practice of medicine
- practice of dentistry
- practice of veterinary medicine
- practice of pharmacy
- the pharmaceutical industry
- chemistry
- the social problems connected with the misuse of drugs (Schedule 1 of the Act).

Duties of the Advisory Council

The ACMD is required to keep under review the situation in the UK with respect to drugs which are being, or appear likely to be, misused (section 1). If it considers that misuse could cause harmful effects which might then constitute a social problem it must advise on the action to be taken. It must advise on measures:

- to restrict the availability of such drugs or to supervise the arrangements for their supply
- to enable persons affected by the misuse of such drugs to obtain proper advice
- to secure the provision of proper facilities and services for the treatment, rehabilitation and aftercare of such persons
- to promote cooperation between the various professional and community services which it believes have a part to play in dealing with the social problems of drug misuse
- to educate the public (particularly the young) in the dangers of drug misuse, and to publicize those dangers
- to promote research into, or obtain information about, any matter relevant to drug misuse prevention or the social problems of drug misuse.

The Secretary of State is empowered to conduct such research, or to assist it (section 32). Additionally the ACMD must advise on any matter relating to drug dependence or drug misuse if asked to do so by a relevant Minister. The ACMD must be consulted before any Regulations are made under the Misuse of Drugs Act. The ACMD discharges these duties by holding meetings either of the full Council or of committees established by it, and by issuing reports.

Regulations concerned with misuse of drugs

Three sets of Regulations have been made under the Act:

(1) The Misuse of Drugs Regulations 1985, SI No. 2066, amended by the Misuse of Drugs (Amendment) Regulations 1986/2330, 1988/916, 1989/1460, 1990/2630, 1995/2048, 1995/3244, 1996/1597, 1998/882, 1999/1404.
(2) The Misuse of Drugs (Notification of and Supply to Addicts) Regulations 1997 SI No. 1001.
(3) The Misuse of Drugs (Safe Custody) Regulations 1973 as amended by the Misuse of Drugs (Safe Custody)(Amendment) Regulations in 1974, 1975, 1984/1146, 1985/2067 and 1986/2332 and 1999/1403.

The Misuse of Drugs Regulations 1985

The Misuse of Drugs Regulations 1985 provide exceptions to the blanket restrictions of the Act so that certain classes of people can produce, supply, prescribe or administer CDs in the practice of their profession.

The Regulations contain Schedules of drugs. It is these Schedules which are of most importance to practice, as they affect the degree of control to be applied to various drugs and medicines when they are used for lawful purposes.

Controlled drugs are listed in five schedules, according to the degree of control required.

Schedule 1

This Schedule contains drugs subject to the strictest controls. The drugs have little or no medical value, but cause social problems through misuse. A licence from the Home Secretary is necessary to possess, produce, supply, offer to supply, administer or cause to be administered these drugs. They include: cannabis, LSD, mescaline, raw opium and coca leaf.

Schedule 2

This Schedule contains most of the drugs with medical use, including the opiates (such as heroin, morphine and methadone) and the stimulants such as amphetamines. The drugs in this schedule are subject to the full controls relating to prescriptions, safe custody and record keeping. Licences are needed for import or export. They may be manufactured or compounded by a pharmacist, doctor, dentist or vet, or by a person who holds a licence.

Schedule 3

This Schedule includes the barbiturates, diethylpropion, meprobamate, penta-zocine and phentermine. Transactions do not need to be entered in the CD Register, although invoices must be retained. The requirements concerning destruction do not apply. Safe custody rules apply to temazepam, diethylpropion, buprenorphine and flunitrazepam. Other drugs in Schedule 3 are exempt from safe custody requirements.

Schedule 4

This Schedule is split into two parts. Part I contains anabolic steroids. Drugs in Part I require a Home Office licence for import or export unless the substance is in the form of a medicinal product for personal use. Possession of listed steroids is an offence unless they are formulated as medicines. Part II contains most of the benzodiazepines.

Drugs in Schedule 4 are generally exempt from restrictions on import and export. There are no restrictions on their possession as medicinal products. Records need not be kept by retailers. There are no safe custody requirements.

Schedule 5

This Schedule contains dilute preparations of drugs in Schedule 2, which are not likely to produce dependence or to cause harm if they are misused. Examples are tablets and oral mixtures containing small amounts of codeine or morphine. Controls are minimal, consisting mainly of a requirement to keep invoices for two years. For this reason this schedule is sometimes referred to as 'CD Inv'.

Exempt products

Certain products, used for scientific or diagnostic purposes, and which contain an extremely small amount and proportion of controlled drugs are exempted from the prohibitions on production, supply and possession.

The Misuse of Drugs (Amendment) Regulations 1999 SI No. 1404 sets out the definition. An exempt product is a preparation or other product consisting of one or more components parts, any of which contains a controlled drug, where:

'(a) the preparation or other product is not designed for administration of the controlled drug to a human being or animal

(b) the controlled drug in any component part is packaged in such a form, or in combination with other active or inert substances in such a manner, that it cannot be recovered by readily applicable means or in a yield which constitutes a risk to health; and

(c) no one component part of the product or preparation contains more than one milligram of the controlled drug or one microgram in the case of lysergide or any other N-alkyl derivative of lysergamide.'

Import

The import of a CD is prohibited except in accordance with a licence granted by the Home Office or where the drug is exempted by Regulations. The regulations exempt Schedule 4 and 5 drugs from import controls. In addition, patients arriving in the UK with no more than a 15 day supply of a prescribed drug may do so without a licence.

Production

Production is generally prohibited by section 4 of the Act. 'Production' means producing the drug by manufacture, cultivation or by any other method.

The Regulations provide that the following persons may lawfully produce, manufacture or compound a CD:

(a)   a practitioner acting in his capacity as such
(b)   a pharmacist acting in his capacity as such
(c)   a person lawfully conducting a retail pharmacy business at his registered pharmacy (reg. 8)
(d)   a person authorised in writing by the Secretary of State may produce drugs in Schedules 3 and 4. The authority specifies the premises, and may specify other conditions
(e)   persons holding a licence issued by the Secretary of State.

Cannabis plants

The cultivation of any plant of the genus *Cannabis* is illegal without a Home Office licence. The maximum penalty for conviction in the Crown Court is 14 years plus a possible fine. Merely positioning a plant in the window to secure the best light, with the objective of growing the plant, is sufficient (*Tudhope* v. *Robertson* 1980). It is a defence for the accused to show that he neither knew of nor suspected nor had reason to suspect that the plant was a controlled drug.

Supply

Section 4 of the Act prohibits the supply of (or the offer to supply) controlled drugs, except where Regulations permit. 'Supply' includes distribution. A person who is authorized by the Regulations to supply a CD may only do so:

- to a person authorized to possess *and*
- subject to any provisions of the Medicines Act 1968 (e.g. the requirements of the POM Regulations).

Various categories of persons are allowed by the Regulations to supply or distribute CDs in Schedules 2, 3, 4, and 5.

Health professionals
- A practitioner
- a pharmacist
- a person lawfully conducting a retail pharmacy business
- a person or acting person in charge of a publicly maintained hospital or nursing home, except where there is a pharmacist
- sister or acting sister in charge of ward or department of hospital or nursing home.

Analysts, laboratories, etc.
- A person in charge of a laboratory
- a public analyst
- a sampling officer
- a sampling officer (Medicines Act)
- a person employed in connection with an NHS drug testing scheme
- RPSGB inspector.

Person in charge of a hospital or nursing home
The Regulations allow the person in charge of a publicly maintained hospital or nursing home to possess and supply CDs in Schedules 2–5, if no pharmacist is responsible for dispensing. The person in charge of a private hospital, nursing home or hospice without a pharmacist needs a Home Office licence to supply Schedule 2 CDs.

'Publicly maintained' means wholly or mainly maintained:

- by a public authority out of public funds or
- by a charity or
- by voluntary subscriptions.

Thus 'publicly maintained' includes NHS Trusts, but excludes private nursing homes and hospitals which are operated for profit.

Sister in charge of ward or department
The sister or acting sister in charge of ward or department may only supply drugs for administration to a patient in that ward or department in accordance

with the directions of a doctor. The authority only applies to drugs supplied by the person responsible for dispensing at the hospital or nursing home.

A person in charge of a laboratory

The laboratory must be recognized as one whose activities include the conduct of scientific education or research, and which is attached to a university, university college or hospital which is publicly maintained. The S of S may approve any other institution for the purpose.

Ships and oilrigs

Special arrangements are made for the unusual situations encountered on ships and oilrigs. The following persons are authorised to supply any drugs in Schedules 2–5 to anyone on the ship or rig as set out below: 'the owner or master of a ship which does not carry a doctor among the seamen employed in it ... the installation manager of an offshore installation'.

The CDs may be supplied as follows:

- in order to comply with certain statutory requirements
- to return drugs to the person who lawfully supplied them
- to supply drugs to a constable for destruction.

The statutory obligations are found in:

(a) the Merchant Shipping Acts
(b) the Mineral Workings (Offshore Installations) Act 1971
(c) the Health and Safety at Work etc. Act 1974.

Any person holding a licence under section 16(1) of the Wildlife and Countryside Act 1981 may supply or offer for sale any drug in Schedule 3 for the purposes for which the licence was granted.

It is not a supply to inject a person with that person's own CD. Thus where Charlie injects Snow with heroin at Snow's request, Charlie has not unlawfully supplied it – at least not by injecting it (*R. v. Harris* 1968).

Possession

Various categories of persons are allowed by the Regulations to possess CDs.

Health professionals
- A practitioner
- a pharmacist
- a person lawfully conducting a retail pharmacy business
- the person or acting person in charge of a hospital or nursing home
- the sister or acting sister of a ward, theatre of other department of a hospital or nursing home.

Analysts, laboratories, etc.
- A person engaged in a forensic laboratory
- a person in charge of a laboratory
- a public analyst appointed under section 27 of the Food Safety Act 1990
- a sampling officer under Schedule 3 to the Medicines Act 1968
- a person in connection with the NHS Drug Testing Scheme.

Carriers
- A carrier
- a person engaged in the business of the Post Office
- a person engaged in conveying the drug to a person who may lawfully have it in his possession.

Various officials
- A constable in the course of his duty
- a Customs and Excise officer
- an RPSGB Inspector, under sections 108 and 109 of the Medicines Act.

Persons authorized by the Home Office
- A person authorized under a Home Office group authority (Schedules 2 and 3)
- a person holding a Home Office written authorization (Schedules 3–5 only).

Ships and oilrigs
The master of a foreign ship in a port in Great Britain may possess any Schedule 2 or 3 drug so far as necessary for the equipment of the ship.

Any person may possess Schedule 2 or 3 in order to comply with statutory requirements.

Possession as a patient

A person may possess a CD for his own use or for administration to another, in accordance with the directions of a doctor. This authority is negated where a patient lied in order to obtain the prescribed drug, or failed to notify the doctor that he was already being supplied with that drug by another doctor. These provisions are intended to prevent drug misusers and dealers from obtaining several prescriptions from different practitioners.

Doctors treating themselves

Doctors and dentists are allowed to possess and supply CDs when they are 'acting in their capacity as practitioners'. It has been held by the courts (*R. v. Dunbar* [1982] 1 AER 188) that a doctor *bona fide* treating himself is 'acting in his capacity as a doctor' for these purposes.

Confiscated illicit CDs

Illicitly obtained drugs are sometimes handed over to teachers, social workers, etc. by those who no longer require them. The Act states that in certain circumstances the person who receives them will not himself be committing an offence. The circumstances are that:

(1) he knew or suspected the substance to be a controlled drug
(2) he took possession for the purpose of: preventing another person from committing an offence or continuing to commit an offence in connection with that drug *or* delivering it into the custody of a person lawfully entitled to take custody of it
(3) as soon as possible after taking possession he took all steps reasonably open to him to either: destroy the drug *or* deliver it into the custody of a person lawfully entitled to take custody.

Midwives

Special arrangements are made for midwives, who routinely use pethidine in their professional practice.

A midwife may possess and administer any controlled drug which she may lawfully administer under the provisions of the Medicines Act. The POM Order 1997 contains a list of drugs which a midwife may give by parenteral administration. This list includes pethidine, and pethidine hydrochloride. The MDA Regulations impose further conditions:

● she is a registered midwife
● the local supervising authority has been notified of her intention to practise
● the authority is given only so far as is necessary to her professional practice
● excess stocks must be surrendered to the appropriate medical officer
● the drugs must have been obtained on a midwife's supply order signed by the appropriate medical officer.

A 'midwife's supply order' means an order in writing specifying the name and occupation of the midwife obtaining the drug, the purpose for which it is required and the total quantity to be obtained. It must be signed by a doctor who is for the time being authorised in writing for the purpose of the Regulations by the local supervising authority for the region or area in which the drug is or was to be obtained.

Requirements for writing prescriptions

Regulation 15 lays out the requirements for prescriptions for CDs other than those in Schedules 4 or 5.

Prescriptions for Schedule 2 and 3 CDs must meet the following requirements:

(a) in ink or otherwise indelible
(b) must be signed by the prescriber with his usual signature
(c) must be dated by the prescriber
(d) specify the address of the prescriber (except for FP10 and variants)
(e) state 'for dental treatment only' if issued by a dentist

(f) if issued by a vet, state that the CD is prescribed for an animal or herd under his care

(g) where instalment dispensing is intended the script must contain a direction specifying the interval between instalments, and the amount to be given on each occasion

(h) certain details must be in the prescriber's own handwriting:

- name and address of the patient
- the dose to be taken
- the pharmaceutical form and (where appropriate) the strength of the preparation of the CD
- the total quantity (in both words and figures) *or*
- the number (in words and figures) of dosage units of the preparation where the prescription is not for a preparation, then the total quantity (in words and figures) of the CD.

Although most of the prescription must be handwritten by the prescriber, the date may be inserted by a rubber stamp. The requirement in the Regulations is that the prescription be 'dated' by the prescriber. The Home Office takes the view that computer-generated dates are not acceptable as these could have been added by someone other than the prescriber.

The requirement to specify the 'form' is interpreted by the Home Office as requiring the pharmaceutical form, e.g. tablets to be specified even if only one form of the product is available. It should also be specified where the brand name gives an indication of the form, e.g. MST.

The prescription requirements above do not apply where the script is for phenobarbitone, phenobarbitone sodium, or a preparation of either of those, or for temazepam. Phenobarbitone prescriptions are exempted from the handwriting requirements. There are no special CD requirements for temazepam prescriptions, which have to comply with the POM regulations.

There are no specific requirements for Schedule 4 and 5 CDs other than the POM regulations.

Handwriting exemptions

The Home Office is allowed to waive the requirement that the body of a prescription for CDs must be in writing. In practice it does so only for specific named doctors, who either are working in drug dependency units or are physically unable to write. The prescription must be signed by the doctor and he must date the prescription. The current view of the Home Office and the RPSGB is that a computer-dated script is not legal, but one dated by the prescriber with a rubber stamp or a typewriter is legal.

If the date is generated by the computer without intervention by the prescriber it is arguable that the prescriber has not dated the script. But conversely if the computer program requires the doctor operating the computer to type in the date, which is printed out in the appropriate space, it arguably *is* dated by the prescriber.

'Signed' means signed by the prescriber with his usual signature. This may be only a set of initials, or presumably a symbol such as a cross.

What the pharmacist must do

A pharmacist may only dispense a script for a Schedule 2 and 3 CD if:

(a) the script complies with the requirements set out above
(b) the prescriber's address is in the UK
(c) the pharmacist knows the prescriber's signature, and he has no reason to suppose it is a forgery *or*
(d) the pharmacist has taken 'reasonably sufficient' steps to satisfy himself that it is genuine
(e) it is not before the date specified on the script
(f) it is not later than 13 weeks after the date on the script
(g) the script is marked, at the time of supply, with the date on which the drug is supplied.

With instalment prescriptions the first supply must be made not later than 13 weeks after the date in the script. The script must be marked with the date of each dispensing. It must be retained for two years after the last instalment is supplied.

Emergency supply

Supplies may be made to a practitioner in an emergency. He must represent that he urgently requires a CD for professional purposes. The supplier must:

● be satisfied that the statement is true
● be satisfied that because of some emergency the practitioner is unable to furnish a requisition before the supply is made
● obtain an undertaking from the practitioner to furnish a requisition in 24 hours.

It is an offence for the practitioner not to produce the requisition as promised.

Supplies within the hospital or nursing home

The assumption is that the normal supply is by pharmacists or doctors, who are authorised to supply drugs in Schedules 2–5. The Regulations recognize that some institutions do not have a pharmacist available and provision is made for other persons to possess and supply.

Supplies within the hospital or nursing home are governed by Regulation 14(6) of the Misuse of Drugs Regulations 1985:

'Where a person responsible for the dispensing and supply of medicines at any hospital or nursing home supplies a CD to the sister or acting sister for the time being in charge of any ward, theatre, or other department he shall:

1) Obtain a requisition in writing, signed by the recipient, which specifies the total quantity of the drug to be supplied, *and*

2) Mark the requisition in such manner as to show that it has been complied with, *and*

3) Retain the requisition in the dispensary for two years.'

A copy of the requisition or a note of it shall be retained by the recipient for two years.

Hospital prescriptions

The general requirements for writing CD prescriptions apply to all hospital and nursing home situations, with an exception. The requirement to put on the name and address of the patient is relaxed where the prescription is written in the patient's bed card or case sheet.

Prescription requirements do not apply when medicines are administered to patients from ward stocks. This procedure is considered to be 'administration in accordance with the directions of a doctor'.

Storage

Schedule 2 drugs (except quinalbarbitone) and the Schedule 3 drugs buprenorphine, diethylpropion and temazepam must be kept in a CD cupboard in nursing homes and private hospitals.

How are supplies made commercially?

Supplies may be made by pharmacies, practitioners or wholesalers. Wholesalers handling CDs require Home Office authority. A separate licence is required for each Schedule 2 CD. The Misuse of Drugs Act defines a 'wholesale dealer' as someone who 'carries on the business of selling drugs to persons who buy to sell again'. Retail pharmacies who undertake a small amount of wholesaling to other health professionals and hospitals, etc. are not usually required by the Home Office to be separately licensed. Where the amount of wholesaling is substantial, as is the case with some NHS hospital pharmacies which are registered with RPSGB then the Home Office will require a licence to be held.

Requisitions

A wholesaler does not need a requisition in order to supply a pharmacy. The list of persons from whom a requisition is required is in Regulation 14(4).

A requisition is required where a supply is made to:

- a practitioner
- the person in charge of a hospital or nursing home
- the person in charge of a laboratory
- the owner of a ship, or the master of a ship which has no doctor on the crew
- the installation manager of an offshore installation
- the master of a foreign ship in a port in Great Britain.

Hospital requisitions

A requisition is required before a supplier can make a supply to a hospital or nursing home. In this case 'supplier' means any person other than a doctor, dentist or vet.

The requisition must:

- be signed by the recipient
- state the name and address of the recipient
- state the occupation of the recipient
- state the purpose for which the drug is required
- specify the total quantity of drug to be supplied.

The supplier must be reasonably satisfied that the signature is authentic and that the person is engaged in the profession or occupation specified.

Residential homes

Residential homes cannot themselves possess or supply CDs. CDs may be prescribed for individual patients resident in the homes. Residential homes are not subject to the safe custody requirements.

Messengers

When a person supplies a CD on requisition, he may not give that CD to a person who claims to be a messenger unless:

- he has a written statement, which the supplier reasonably believes is genuine, from the person giving the requisition, stating that he is empowered to collect the drug
- the messenger is otherwise authorized by the Regulations.

Export

The export of a CD is prohibited except in accordance with a licence granted by the Home Office or where the drug is exempted by Regulations. The regulations exempt CDs in Schedules 4 and 5.

Doctors who wish to take emergency supplies of CDs out of the country require a licence from the Home Office, which is usually granted only when there is a real need, such as a hazardous expedition. Special arrangements are made where doctors wish to accompany pilgrims to Lourdes. Form MD50A is available from the Home Office and should be used to make the application.

Import licences may be required for the country being visited.

Patients requiring CDs when abroad

An 'Open General Licence' (OGL) was introduced by the Home Office in 1987. It provides a general authority for the export of small quantities of CDs which are in medicinal products, for medical reasons. It applies to:

- a traveller carrying CDs for administration to himself
- a member of his household who is unable to administer the medicine himself
- a doctor accompanying a patient who requires treatment during a journey to or from the UK.

The CDs, and the maximum quantities which may be exported are set out in a Schedule. An explanatory leaflet is available. The CD must be under the direct personal supervision of the person importing or exporting it. Maximum quantities are based on an average 15 days' supply. Personal export of more than this amount requires a Home Office licence. No records are required to be kept of CDs imported or exported under this licence. The licence is made under section 3(2)(b) of the Misuse of Drugs Act.

Records

The Regulations contain a number of requirements relating to the keeping of records for CDs.

CD register

Particulars of Schedule 1 and 2 drugs purchased or supplied must be entered in a register. The register must be a bound book. The regulations specifically prohibit a loose-leaf or record-card system. Either a different register, or a separate part of the same register must be used for each class of drugs. Basically a class consists of a different drug together with its stereo-isomers, its salts and any preparations containing them. The words of Regulation 19(1)b are:

> 'he shall use a separate register or separate part of the register for entries made in respect of each class of drugs, and each of the drugs specified in paragraphs 1 and 3 of Schedule 1 and paragraphs 1, 3 and 6 of Schedule 2 together with its salts and any preparation or other product containing it or any of its salts shall be treated as a separate class, so however that any stereo-isomeric form of a drug or its salts shall be classed with that drug.'

The commercially available registers, which consist of a number of bound sections held in loose-leaf binder, therefore comply with the regulations, as each section constitutes a separate register. It is permissible to use separate parts of a register for different drugs or strengths within the class. A register must not be used for any other purpose. It must be kept at the premises to which it relates. Only one register for each class must be in use at one time. Where the premises consist of several departments the Home Office may approve the keeping of separate registers in each department. Registers must be preserved for two years from the date of the last entry.

Entries in the register

All entries must be made in chronological order. Entries must be made on the day of the transaction or on the next day. Entries must not be cancelled, obliterated or altered. Corrections should be made by dated notes on the page. All entries and corrections must be in ink, or otherwise indelible.

Who must keep a register

Any person authorised to supply Schedule 1 or 2 drugs must keep a register except that a sister or acting sister in charge of a ward, theatre or register is not required to keep a register. The person who dispenses the drugs to the ward, whether a pharmacist or a person in charge of the hospital must keep a register.

Preservation of prescriptions, etc.

Requistions, orders or prescriptions for CDs in Schedules 1–3 must be retained for two years. NHS prescriptions are used for payment purposes and are not required to be retained.

Invoices

Pharmacists must keep the invoices or copies when they receive and supply drugs and medicines in Schedules 3 and 5. There are similar rules for producers, wholesalers, hospitals and laboratories for the drugs they may handle. The invoices must bear the date of the transaction, and the identity of the parties involved. The invoices must be kept for two years.

Requests for information

Certain people are authorised by the Secretary of State to request details about stocks, supplies and receipts of CDs. They may also inspect the stock, registers, requisitions and invoices. Confidential personal records, e.g. patient medication records need not be produced.

The authorized persons are:

- inspectors of the RPSGB
- Home Office Drugs Branch Inspectors
- authorized Medical and Dental Officers of the Health Departments of England, Scotland and Wales.

The people required to produce the information are:

- producers
- persons authorised to import and export CDs
- wholesalers
- pharmacists
- practitioners
- persons in charge of hospitals or nursing homes
- persons in charge of laboratories
- persons authorized to supply Schedule 3 and 4 drugs.

Destruction of CDs

(1) By patients. Patients may destroy any CDs in their possession, which are left over from their treatment. No records are required.

(2) By pharmacists. Pharmacists may destroy controlled drugs which are returned by a patient or patient's representative. There is no need to make any records or have the destruction witnessed. Medicines used for animal treatment may be similarly dealt with by vets as well as pharmacists. Other than above, pharmacists may only destroy CDs in the presence of a witness authorised by the Secretary of State.

The persons authorized include:

- Police officers
- Inspectors of the Home Office Drugs Branch
- RPSGB Inspectors
- Regional Pharmaceutical Officers
- Senior Administrative Officer employed on duties in connection with the administration of any NHS hospital
- Medical Officers of the Regional Medical Service of the Department of Health
- Chief Dental Officer of DoH, or a Senior Dental Officer to whom the authority has been delegated
- Supervisors of midwives
- Regional Medical Officers of SHHD
- Chief Administrative Pharmaceutical Officers (for their Health Board's area only
- Deputy Chief Dental Officer of SHHD
- Regional Dental Officers of SHHD
- Regional Medical Officers of the Welsh Office
- The Pharmaceutical Advisor for Wales
- Health authority pharmaceutical advisors
- NHS Trust Chief Executives
- Senior trust officers reporting directly to CEO, with responsibility for health and safety and security.

Where drugs are destroyed in this way a record must be made of the date of destruction and the quantity destroyed. The record must be signed by the authorized witness.

(3) Ships and offshore oilrigs. Excess Schedule 2 drugs in the possession of a master or owner of a ship, or the installation manager of an offshore installation may not be destroyed. They should be handed to a constable or to a pharmacist or licensed dealer.

Schedules 3–5

Schedule 3–5 CDs may be destroyed without an authorized witness. It is not necessary to keep records of the destruction.

Re-use of controlled drugs

The legal position of re-use or 'recycling' of CDs is the subject of some debate. The question usually relates to the use by Patient B of medicine originally prescribed for, and supplied to Patient A and which is no longer required by Patient A. This may happen in a hospice for instance.

The advice of the Home Office is that such re-use is legal, even where the pharmacist has been given the medicine in question 'for destruction'. The Home Office argues that the regulations do not *require* the pharmacist to destroy the medicines, they merely empower him to do so. Provided the correct records are kept the medicines may be used by him in the same way as if he had obtained them from his wholesaler.

The RPSGB advise that controlled drugs returned to the pharmacy by a patient should not be returned to stock. The RPSGB Code of Ethics states that 'Medicines returned to a pharmacy from a patient's home or a nursing or residential home must not be supplied to any other patient'.

Safe custody

The Misuse of Drugs (Safe Custody) Regulations 1973 (as amended) require Schedules 1–3 CDs (with some exceptions) to be kept in a locked receptacle. Where CDs are kept in a 'retail pharmacy' or in a nursing home or private hospital the receptacle must be a safe, cabinet or room which meets certain standards.

The general requirement

A person in possession of CDs must store them in a locked receptacle to which only he (and persons authorized by him) has the key. The courts have held that a car does not constitute a locked receptacle for this regulation.

Exceptions to the general requirement

This requirement does not apply to:

- a carrier in the course of his business
- a person engaged in the business of the Post Office
- a person who has been supplied with the CD on prescription, for his own use or for the treatment of another person or an animal.

In addition, a CD can remain out of the cabinet as long as it is under the pharmacist's direct personal supervision.

The safe custody requirements apply to all controlled drugs in Schedules 1 and 2 (except quinalbarbitone), and to diethylpropion, temazepam and buprenorphine.

Locked safe, cabinet or room

The Regulations specify that when CDs are kept on any premises occupied by a person lawfully conducting a retail pharmacy business they must be stored in a locked safe, cabinet or room which complies with the structural standards laid down in the Regulations. It is with these standards that the 'CD cabinet' complies.

The requirement also applies when CDs are kept in:

(a) any premises occupied by a pharmacist engaged in supplying drugs to the public at a NHS health centre
(b) any nursing home within Part II of the Registered Homes Act 1984.

Hospitals

Regulation 3 does not apply to hospitals unless the pharmacy department is registered as a RPB with the RPSGB. Hospital wards are required to keep CDs in a locked receptacle.

Standards

The standards specify that cabinets must be made of steel sheet or welded mesh. It must be designed with a close-fitting door fitted with a dead-bolt, and a five-lever lock or equivalent. The cabinet must be rigidly attached to a wall or floor with at least two rag-bolts which pass through an internal anchor plate.

Nothing shall be displayed outside a safe or cabinet to indicate that drugs are kept inside it.

There are detailed standards for secure rooms which contain CDs. The room is an alternative to the use of a cabinet or safe.

Where the CDs are kept in a 'retail pharmacy' the local police can issue a certificate stating that a room, safe or cabinet provides an adequate degree of security even though it does not comply with the specific standards laid down. This procedure enables the use of 'money' safes which may be constructed in a different way. The certificate lasts for a year after the inspection visit, and may be renewed.

Addicts

The Misuse of Drugs (Notification of and Supply to Addicts) Regulations 1973, SI 1973/799 deals with the treatment of addicts by doctors.

What is an 'addict'?

A person is to be regarded as an addict 'if, and only if, he has as a result of repeated administration become so dependent upon the drug that he has an overpowering desire for the administration of it to be continued.'

Which drugs are affected

The Regulations apply to the following drugs: cocaine, dextromoramide, diamorphine, dipipanone, hydrocodone, hydromorphone, levorphanol, methadone, morphine, opium, oxycodone, pethidine, phenazocine and piritramide. Also included is any salt, ester or ether or stereo-isomer (except dextrorphan) of the above drugs.

Supply to addicts

If a doctor considers, or has reasonable grounds to suspect that a person is addicted to any drug listed in the Supply to Addicts Regulations then he may not prescribe cocaine, diamorphine or dipipanone (or their salts or preparations) to that person unless:

(a)　he is treating an organic disease or injury *or*
(b)　he holds a Home Office licence.

Notification

Until May 1997, doctors were required to pass on details of addicts to the Home Office. The 1997 Regulations set up a Regional Drug Misuse Database to which doctors are expected to report treatment demands.

NHS prescriptions for addicts

Two types of NHS prescription forms are provided in E & W for doctors to use when prescribing for addicts. The forms enable addicts to receive supplies of drugs in daily instalments.

FP10(HP)Ad

This form is used by doctors in drug addiction clinics. There are no regulations specifically covering this form, but the form itself bears the information that it may only be used for prescribing the following drugs: cocaine, diamorphine hydrochloride, dextromoramide, dipipanone, methadone hydrochloride, morphine and pethidine hydrochloride.

The prescription must state the amount to be dispensed on each instalment and the interval between instalments. Other drugs and appliances may be ordered on the same form, but the supply may be made on one occasion only.

FP10(MDA)

Use of this form is governed by the NHS (GMS) Regulations 1992.

The form is issued by HAs to any GP on request. The form may be used for the instalment prescribing of any Schedule 2 Controlled Drug being used in the treatment of addiction in the patient. Only Home Office licensed doctors may prescribe diamorphine, cocaine or dipipanone (or their salts) to addicts for their addiction.

Some preparations of Schedule 2 drugs appear in Schedule 5 (e.g. tablets of dihydrocodeine) and the Home Office interpretation is that those preparations are consequently not in Schedule 2. It appears that Schedule 2 consists of a list of drugs, and Schedule 5 a list of preparations of some of the drugs in Schedule 2. An alternative interpretation would be that the word 'drug' in the Instalment Prescribing Regulations refers to entries in Schedule 2, and that an additional entry in Schedule 5 is irrelevant. There has been no case law on the issue to date.

The prescription must state the amount per instalment and the interval between instalments. The Regulations restrict the supply to a maximum of 14 days per form.

The form may not be used for any purpose except instalment prescribing for addicts. It may, however, be used to order a single supply of a quantity of water for injection.

Failure to comply with the conditions for use of the form would make a doctor liable to disciplinary committee action. A pharmacist would seem to be in a slightly different position. The question remains open whether a form which does not meet the conditions of use may still be dispensed by the pharmacist without breach of his Terms of Service.

Controls on specific drugs

In recent years the Misuse of Drugs Act and its regulations have been used to impose new controls on certain products which are subject to abuse and illicit use.

Temazepam

The Misuse of Drugs (Amendment) Regulations 1996, SI No. 1597 deal with Temazepam products. Although must benzodiazepines remain in Schedule 4, Temazepam has been moved to Schedule 3. However it is not subject to the normal prescription writing and records keeping rules which apply to Schedule 2 and 3 drugs:

- prescriptions do not need to be in the prescriber's own handwriting
- the debate does not need to be written by the prescriber
- no CD register entry is required.

All temazepam products, including liquids are subject to safe custody requirements.

Steroids

The Misuse of Drugs Act 1971 (Modification) Order 1996, SI No. 1300 adds anabolic and androgenic steroids, polypeptide growth hormones and the adrenoceptor stimulant Clenbuterol to the compounds in Class C of the MDA.

The Misuse of Drugs (Amendment) Regulations 1996, SI No. 1597 splits Schedule 4 into two parts. Part I contains the steroids, etc. and Part II contains mainly benzodiazepines.

Steroids are subject to the usual Schedule 4 requirements. In addition they require a Home Office licence for import or export unless the substance is in the form of a medicinal product for personal use. Possession of listed steroids is an offence unless they are formulated as a medicine.

Drug Trafficking Offences Act 1986

Section 34 of this Act added a new S9A to the MDA 1971, making it an offence for anyone to knowingly sell or supply items to drug addicts which could help them prepare or administer illicit controlled drugs. The section states:

It is an offence for a person to supply or offer to supply any article which may be used or adapted for use in the administration of a controlled drug to himself or another, believing that the article is to be so used, or to supply or offer to supply any article which may be used to prepare a controlled drug for administration to himself or another, believing that the article is to be so used in circumstances where the administration is unlawful.

Any administration of a controlled drug which is not in accordance with the instructions of a practitioner will be unlawful.

Syringes and needles are exempt from this, by virtue of section 9A(2). The sale of citric acid has recently been sanctioned in Scotland.

Chapter 19

Confidentiality and Records

Confidentiality

The confidentiality of information held by pharmacists is a matter both of law and of ethics.

The Data Protection Act 1998

The Data Protection Act 1998 controls the use of 'personal data', which is data relating to an identifiable living person. The Act came into effect in March 2000 and there is a transition period up to October 2001, by which time all systems must comply. The DPA 1998 implements an EC Directive, 95/46/EC which requires Member States 'to protect the fundamental rights and freedoms of natural persons, in particular their right to privacy with respect the processing of personal data'.

Personal data covers both facts and opinions about the individual. It also includes information regarding the intentions of the data controller towards the individual, although in some limited circumstances exemptions will apply.

'Data' is information which is being processed by equipment operating automatically in response to instructions given for that purpose, is recorded with the above intention, is recorded as part of a structured filing system, or forms part of accessible record, e.g. a health record.

The DPA 1998 applies both to computerized data and to paper records and filing systems. All computer records come within the terms of the DPA 1998 if they can be used to identify the individual the record refers to, no matter how they are filed. Manual records will be covered if specific information relating to particular individuals is readily accessible.

Data controller

The data controller is the person responsible for determining how any personal data are processed. The data controller is responsible for ensuring that the terms of the DPA 1998 are followed.

The data processor

The data processor is any person (other than an employee of the data controller) who processes the data.

Processing

Processing includes obtaining, recording or holding information and the organization, alteration, retrieval, accessing, disclosure or erasure of the data, whether in a manual or electronic form.

Data Protection Commissioner

The DPA 1998 is administered by a 'Data Protection Commissioner', created by the Act to maintain a register of data users (those who hold or process the information).

Registration

It is an offence to hold or process personal data unless registered with the Commissioner. The use of computers for labelling medicines, or for stock control does not require registration. However, the keeping of patient medication records on computer must be registered. The data controller must notify the Commissioner of:

- the name and address of the data controller (and a representative if one is nominated)
- the description of the data being processed
- the purposes of the processing
- other parties who may have access to the data.

Offences

Failure to comply with the notification requirements of the Act may result in a maximum fine of £5000 in the Magistrates Courts and unlimited fines in Crown Courts.

The Principles

Section 2 of the Act requires data users to comply with a set of 'Principles' which are found in Schedule 1 of the Act. These state that personal data shall be:

- fairly and lawfully processed
- processed for limited purposes
- adequate, relevant and not excessive
- accurate
- not kept longer than necessary
- processed in accordance with the data subject's rights
- secure
- not transferred to countries without adequate protection.

These principles apply to the handling of all data. The general effect is that data may not be processed at all unless either the subject has given permission, or a series of other conditions are met.

The Act imposes extra requirements for 'sensitive personal data'.

Sensitive personal data

Sensitive personal data are personal data consisting of information as to:

(a) the racial or ethnic origin of the data subject
(b) his political opinions
(c) his religious beliefs or other beliefs of a similar nature
(d) whether he is a member of a trade union (within the meaning of the Trade Union and Labour Relations (Consolidation) Act 1992)
(e) his physical or mental health or condition
(f) his sexual life
(g) the commission or alleged commission by him of any offence, or
(h) any proceedings for any offence committed or alleged to have been committed by him, the disposal of such proceedings or the sentence of any court in such proceedings.

Where sensitive personal data are health data, including health records, the relevant extra conditions which apply are either that:

'(1) The data subject has given his explicit consent to the processing of the personal data *or*

8. – (1) The processing is necessary for medical purposes and is undertaken by –

(a) a health professional, or
(b) a person who in the circumstances owes a duty of confidentiality which is equivalent to that which would arise if that person were a health professional.'

Medical purposes

'Medical purposes' includes the purposes of preventative medicine, medical diagnosis, medical research, the provision of care and treatment and the management of health care services. Generally, sensitive personal data requires that the subject give explicit consent, but this is not required when the data are processed for a health professional and are for medical purposes.

What is a health record?

A 'health record' is a record which consists of information relating to the physical or mental health or condition of an individual which has been made by or on behalf of a health professional in connection with the care of that individual.

The individual must be identifiable from that information, or from that together with other details held by the record holder. It is clear, therefore, that many of the records being held by pharmacies, surgeries, NHS Trusts, and other health care institutions will constitute 'health records' and will therefore fall within the scope of the 1998 Act's subject access provisions. The definition of a 'health record' could apply to material held on an X-ray, an MRI scan or a blood pressure monitor print-out, for example.

Individual's rights

The DPA 1998 gives seven main rights to the data subject.

Right of access

Section 7 of the Data Protection Act 1998 gives a right of access to all information held about a person. A copy may be obtained by applying in writing to the data user. A period of 40 days is allowed for the copy to be supplied. A fee of up to £10 may be charged.

Unauthorized disclosure may entitle the person to compensation.

There are various exemptions to the right of access, e.g. where data are held for taxation purposes.

Right to prevent processing likely to cause damage or distress
An individual can serve written notice prohibiting a controller from processing data that can cause substantial damage or distress. The controller has 21 days to either comply or to give reasons why the request is unreasonable.

Right to prevent processing for direct marketing
Individuals can prevent their data being used for marketing purposes.

The Act also gives individuals rights to compensation when they have suffered damage as a result of a contravention of the Act; and rights to rectification of incorrect records. Individuals can also ensure that decisions which affect them are not based solely on automated processing. They can ask the Commissioner to assess compliance with the Act.

Use of personal data for research or analysis
Personal data may be used for research without explicit permission where:

- the data are used exclusively for that purpose
- the analysis does not identify individuals
- the analysis is not in support of decisions relating to particular individuals
- no damage or distress is caused to any individual.

The Access to Medical Records Act 1988

The Access to Medical Records Act 1988 gives a patient a right to view the clinical information contained in his or her own medical history when released by the GP as a medical report for insurance or employment purposes. A medical report is a 'report relating to the physical or mental health of the individual prepared by a medical practitioner who is or has been responsible for the clinical care of the patient'.

The GP may charge a 'reasonable fee' if a copy is provided. The rights given under this Act relate solely to records prepared by a GP. There is no direct effect on pharmacists, and the information is included to give a complete picture.

Use of anonymized data for research

The Court of Appeal has held in 1999 that the disclosure by pharmacists of anonymized prescription data does not amount to a breach of confidentiality. The case was a Judicial Review brought by Source Informatics to challenge guidelines produced by the Department of Health to prohibit such sales. Source Informatics is a UK subsidiary of an American company concerned for commercial reasons to obtain information as to doctors' prescribing habits. It then sells this information on to pharmaceutical companies so that they may more effectively market their products.

Control of patient information under the Health and Social Care Act 2001

The Health and Social Care Act 2001 enables the S of S to regulate the sharing of medical information to improve patient care, or in the public interest.

Under section 60, the S of S may make regulations which require or regulate the processing of patient information in prescribed circumstances. This will, for instance, make it possible for patients to receive more information about their clinical care and for confidential patient information to be lawfully processed without informed consent to support prescribed activities such as cancer registries.

Safeguards
The HSC 2001 Act builds in a number of safeguards over the use of this power, to protect patients' interests.

Firstly, regulations can only provide for the processing of patient information for medical purposes where there is a benefit to patient care or where this is in the public interest. Medical purposes means –

'a) preventative medicine, medical diagnosis, medical research, the provision of care and treatment and the management of health and social care services
b) informing individuals about their physical or mental health or condition, the diagnosis of their condition or their care and treatment'

Secondly, regulations can only require the processing of confidential patient information, where there is no reasonably practicable alternative. The S of S can only make following consultation with those likely to be affected and with the new Patient Information Advisory Group.

Thirdly, any such regulations can only be made under the affirmative resolution procedure, requiring the consent of both Houses of Parliament.

Fourthly, all the controls of the Data Protection Act remain in place.

Patient Information Advisory Group
A Patient Information Advisory Group will be set up to advise the S of S on Regulations and on wider matters in relation to the processing of patient information. The advice provided by the Advisory Group on proposed regulations must be published.

Minors – the Gillick case

The RPSGB advises that when the patient is a child, the pharmacist may have to decide whether to release information to parents or guardians without the consent of the child but in the child's best interests. Much will depend on the maturity of the child concerned and his or her relationship with parents or guardians.

Such decisions are particularly difficult when the issue concerns contraception. The courts have laid out some helpful guidance in this area, following a case brought by Victoria Gillick.

Mrs Gillick sought to have the courts rule that DHSS guidance to doctors was unlawful and wrong. The guidance had stated that in exceptional circumstances doctors could give contraceptive advice and prescriptions to girls under 16 without the consent of the parents.

The House of Lords gave judgment in 1985 (*Gillick* v. *West Norfolk and Wisbech Area Health Authority and the DHSS*). They held that parental rights exist for the benefit of the child, not the parent. Although the courts will hesitate to enforce parental rights against the wishes of the child (and the more so the older she is) it is recognized that the best judges of what is in the child's best interests are the parents. However there will be cases in which a doctor is a better judge of what is in a girl's best medical interests, and whether or not the girl's parents should know of the advice should be a matter for the doctor's judgment.

A girl under 16 can consent to contraceptive advice and treatment, and the doctor can proceed without her parent's knowledge or consent if satisfied:

(1) She understands the advice.
(2) She cannot be persuaded to inform her parents, or to allow the doctor to do so.
(3) She is likely to have sexual intercourse with or without contraceptive treatment.
(4) Unless she has contraceptive advice or treatment her health (physical or mental) will suffer.
(5) Her best interests require that she receive contraceptive advice and treatment without the knowledge or consent of her parents:

The phrases used in the judgment are particularly relevant to doctors. Similar conditions will apply to the supply of over the counter products by pharmacists. It may be more difficult for pharmacists to satisfy the criteria, especially number (4).

The Caldicott Review 1997

This Review was commissioned by the Chief Medical Officer of England because of the increasing concern about the ways in which patient information is used in the NHS in England and Wales and the need to ensure that confidentiality is not undermined.

The Review set out a list of principles which should be followed by everyone concerned with patient information:

- justify the purpose(s)
- do not use patient-identifiable information unless it is absolutely necessary
- use the minimum necessary patient-identifiable information
- access to patient-identifiable information should be on a strict need-to-know basis

- everyone with access to patient-identifiable information should be aware of their responsibilities
- understand and comply with the law.

Caldicott guardian

Recommendation 3 of the Review was that a senior person, preferably a health professional, should be nominated in each health organization to act as a guardian, responsible for safeguarding the confidentiality of patient information. This person has become known as the 'Caldicott guardian'.

National Confidentiality and Security Advisory Body

This body was set up following the Caldicott Review on patient confidentiality. It has the following functions:

- set standards to govern the confidentiality and security of patient information
- promote awareness of issues surrounding patient records, including access and security
- produce guidance and support to Caldicott guardians
- advise Ministers, the NHS Executive, the Department of Health and the NHS Information Authority on a range of confidentiality and security issues.

Confidentiality and the RPSGB Code of Ethics

The RPSGB Code of Ethics deals with confidentiality. Section C of Part II repeats the general requirements of the data protection legislation. It specifies that pharmacy computer and manual systems which include patient-specific information should incorporate access control systems to minimize the risk of unauthorized or unnecessary access to data.

The Service Specifications in Part III include a section on patient medication records.

Information for research

The legal position regarding anonymized information is not clear-cut, but the RPSGB Code of Ethics states that the collation of data from patient records is allowed, on condition that it is presented anonymously, for the purpose of research or as information to interested commercial sources. Anonymous information is exempted from the provisions of the Data Protection Act.

Records

Pharmacies keep various records which include personal details of patients. Some records are kept because of a legal requirement, e.g. CD register, some by a contractual requirement, e.g. patient medication records (PMRs) for the elderly, and some for professional reasons only, e.g. PMRs for children.

The following are likely to be encountered:

- CD register
- NHS PMRs (written)
- NHS PMRs (on computer)

- private PMRs (written)
- private PMRs (on computer)
- prescription book.

Various legal issues arise in relation to the different types of record.

CD register

The legal requirements are dealt with in Chapter 16. For convenience the list of persons having access to the register is repeated here:

- Home Office (HO) inspectors
- RPSGB inspectors
- DoH medical officers
- SHHD regional medical officers
- DoH Chief Dental Officer or SDO
- SHHD Deputy Chief Dental Officer
- SHHD regional dental officers
- Welsh Office dental offices
- Welsh Office medical officers.

NHS patient medication records

The arrangements made by an HA include the provision of 'additional professional services'. These services may be provided by a pharmacist if he wishes. If he wishes to receive remuneration for providing them he must apply to the HA, on a form, confirming that a minimum number of records are kept. If the services are provided as additional professional services then their provision is a service governed by Regulations.

Payment is only made in respect of the records for certain categories of patients, even if records are also kept for other categories. Under the NHS Regulations records may be kept for:

(1) Any person agd 60 or over (a person who claims exemption under Regulation 6(1)(c) of the NHS (Charges for Drugs and Appliances) Regulations 1989).
(2) A confused patient. This is defined as a patient who, in the opinion of the pharmacist supplying the drug, is likely to have difficulty understanding the nature and dosage of the drug supplied and the times at which it is to be taken.

Additionally the patient must be on long term medication. This is defined as being circumstances where the nature of the drug is such that, in the opinion of the pharmacist supplying it, the same or a similar drug is likely to be prescribed for that person regularly on future occasions.

The DT contains some rules about payment. Payment is only made if a minimum number of records are maintained. There must be records for a minimum of 100 patients. For a pharmacy receiving Essential Small Pharmacy Scheme support the minimum number is 50.

Each record should cover all the drugs supplied to one patient. One or more of the drugs supplied should be long term as described above.

The record system should be suitable for the purpose and provide appropriate levels of security.

The records must contain the following information:

- name and address of patient
- name, quantity and dosage of drug supplied
- date of supply.

Fees are only paid where the pharmacist employed to operate the scheme has a certificate of completion of an approved training course.

Guidance issued by the DoH to HAs asks them to monitor the provision of additional professional services by pharmacists. In order to do this officers of the HA need access to the records. They are required to check that the pharmacy is keeping the requisite number of records for payment. They are also to check that the records contain the required information.

The NHS (Pharmaceutical Services) Regulations 1992 (as amended) require the pharmacist to 'make available to the HA all records kept as additional professional services'.

Prescription book

The following details must be recorded about the sale or supply of POMs:

(1) date of sale or supply
(2) name and quantity of medicine (where it is not apparent from the name, the strength and pharmaceutical form must also be included)
(3) date of the prescription
(4) name and address of prescriber
(5) name and address of patient (or owner of animal).

Repeat prescriptions
It is sufficient to record the date of supply, together with a reference to the original entry.

Keeping the prescription book
The book used to record POM supplies must be kept for two years after the last entry.

Keeping the prescriptions
The prescriptions must be retained for two years after they were dispensed.

Legislation will be introduced in 1997 which will allow pharmacists to keep POM records on computer or microfiche.

Computer records
The Medicines (Sale or Supply) (Miscellaneous Provisions) Amendment Regulations 1997, SI No. 1831 amended the law to permit records of private prescriptions and emergency supplies to be held on computer. The same details are required as for paper records. The computer records must be kept for two years. The RPSGB has advised that the computer records should contain an accurate audit trail of entries.

Chapter 20

The European Union

The law of the European Union (EU), commonly referred to (confusingly) as European Community law is automatically part of UK law, and consequently it is necessary for pharmacists to have some knowledge of the EU, and of the way it works.

The European Economic Community (EEC) was established by the Treaty of Rome in 1957. The original members were Belgium, France, Germany, Italy, Luxembourg and the Netherlands. The UK joined in 1972, along with Denmark and Ireland. They were then joined by Greece, Spain and Portugal.

In 1994 the EFTA (European Free Trade Area) countries of Austria, Finland, Iceland, Norway and Sweden joined to form the European Economic Area.

The original Treaty was modified in 1992 by the 'Maastricht' Treaty on European union.

Law-making institutions

The Treaty of Rome established several institutions to deal with the law-making process of the Community.

The Council of Ministers

This is the decision-making body of the EU. It is composed of Ministers from each of the member governments, normally the Foreign Ministers but it may be any appropriate Minister. One Minister attends from each state. Most decisions are taken on a majority basis. The Presidency rotates between the states at six-month intervals.

The Committee of Permanent Representatives (known by the French acronym COREPER) consists of senior civil servants from each state, and it acts as the administrative arm of the Council. The members are the heads of the permanent delegations in Brussels. Disputes are often sorted out here.

The European Council is the name given to the regular meetings of heads of governments, which discuss broad policy.

The Commission

The Commission is charged with seeing that the Treaties are implemented. There are 20 Commissioners with a large supporting staff. Commissioners are appointed for a five-year term, serve the EU as a whole, and can only be removed from office by the European Court of Justice or by the European Parliament (which can only dismiss the entire Commission on a two-thirds majority vote). Each Commissioner is responsible for an area of policy. The staff are organized into Directorates-General. The Commission is:

(1) a policy-planning body
(2) a mediator between governments
(3) the executive arm of the Community
(4) the prosecutor of those who breach the treaty rules.

The European Parliament

The Parliament is composed of directly elected representatives of the citizens of the member states. It has little direct power of legislation, although its powers were enlarged at Maastricht, but gives an opinion on Commission proposals. Its power lies in control of the Commission's budget.

The European Court of Justice (ECJ)

The ECJ is based in Luxembourg. It is responsible for ensuring that Community legislation is correctly interpreted and applied. Cases may be brought by a member state, an institution of the EU, or an individual. The ECJ responds to requests from national courts for an interpretation of Community law. It has the power to impose fines. Member states in breach of Community law are required to comply with the orders of the ECJ. Judges are appointed from each country.

There is a Court of First Instance which has jurisdiction relating to anti-dumping law, competition policy and employment disputes of the Commission staff.

Economic and Social Committee

This influential committee, known as 'Ecosoc' advises the Commission and the Council on economic matters. It is made up of representatives of the employers, workers and other interest groups in the member states. The representatives are proposed by the governments, and appointments are made by the Council.

Community law

There are four categories of Community law.

Regulations are laws issued by the EU which have effect throughout the EU as they stand. There is no need for Community law to be 'transposed' into national law.

Directives are binding on the member states. They lay down the result to be achieved but leave to the national authorities the task of enacting the necessary national legislation.

Recommendations are merely advisory statements.

Decisions are binding on the individuals or institutions to whom they are addressed.

Directives affecting pharmacy

Community law overrides national laws of the member states.

A number of Directives have been issued concerning medicines. They are based on Articles 100 and 100A of the Treaty of Rome. The majority of the medicines Directives are concerned with the licensing process, laying down the procedures to be adopted, the types of data to be required and giving definitions.

Directive 65/65/EEC
The main Directive is Directive 65/65/EEC which sets out the most important aspects of the marketing of medicines. These include the common principles which should be adhered to by each member state with regard to the conditions for granting a marketing authorization, manufacture and quality control procedures, labelling and information leaflets, and detailed guidance on data requirements.

The Directive requires that a marketing authorization is granted on grounds of safety, efficacy and quality, the same grounds as are laid down in the MA 1968.

Directive 65/65/EEC applies to 'medicinal products' which are defined as:

'any substance or combination of substances presented for treating or preventing disease in human beings or animals. Any substance or combina-tion of substances which may be administered to human beings with a view to making a medical diagnosis or to restoring, correcting or modifying physio-logical functions in human beings or animals'.

This directive, together with a number of others, was amended by the 'Future Systems' package of legislation which was designed to complete the single market in pharmaceuticals.

Regulation 2309/93 and Directive 93/39/EEC amend Directives 65/65/EEC, 75/318/EEC and 75/319/EEC. Directive 93/41/EEC repeals Directive 87/22/EEC.

The new systems are put in place in the UK by the Medicines for Human Use (Marketing Authorisations, etc.) Regulations 1994, SI 1994 No. 3144.

Directive 89/341/EEC
A main requirement of Directive 89/341/EEC is the requirement for ready-prepared medicines to be supplied with a 'patient information leaflet'.

The Transparency Directive
Directive 89/105/EEC is known as the 'Transparency Directive'. It requires member states which impose controls on the prices of medicinal products, or on the profits of the pharmaceutical industry, to publish their criteria, and the reasons for the decisions. The intention is to ensure that all procedures are operated in accordance with the Treaty, i.e. that they are fair and are not discriminatory.

Article 1 states:

'Member States shall ensure that any national measure, whether laid down by law, regulation or administrative action, to control the prices of medicinal products for human use or to restrict the range of medicinal products covered by their national health insurance systems complies with the requirements of this Directive'.

Later articles lay down a timetable of 90 days for the authorities to make a decision about a product.

The Directive applies to the Selected List scheme, the ACBS approval scheme and, by virtue of Article 5, to the Pharmaceutical Price Regulation Scheme.

Free movement of pharmacists

Three Directives of the Council of the European Union are concerned with pharmacy qualifications.

(1) Directive 85/432/EEC (known as the 'Training Directive') which is concerned with ensuring a common minimum standard of training for pharmacists in the EU.
(2) Directive 85/433/EEC (known as the 'Recognition Directive') is concerned with the mutual recognition of qualifications, and gives certain rights to practise pharmacy.
(3) Directive 85/584/EEC took account of the accession of Spain and Portugal to the EC.

These Directives have been implemented in Great Britain by an Order in Council, *viz.* the Pharmaceutical Qualifications (EEC Recognition) Order 1987, SI 1987 No. 2202.

The Order mainly amends the Pharmacy Act 1954, but also amends the MA 1968, the NHS Act 1977, and the NHS (Scotland) Act 1978. The main amendment to the Pharmacy Act 1954 inserts a new section 4A into the Act. This provides that EU nationals who hold one of the listed 'Qualifying European Diplomas in Pharmacy' are entitled to registration as a pharmacist in Great Britain. The diplomas are now listed in Schedule 1A to the Act.

The 'Greek derogation' – During negotiations on the Directive it was agreed that for a period, Greece was allowed to derogate from the requirement to recognize the qualifications of other Member States. The Directive allowed the individual state to decide whether it would in return refuse fully to recognize Greek qualifications. The UK government decided that for the period of the Greek derogation, the UK authorities would recognize qualifications obtained in Greece only for employees. Greek pharmacists are consequently prohibited from becoming the proprietor of a UK pharmacy.

Qualifying European Diploma

The new section 4A designates the RPSGB and the PSNI as 'competent authorities'. Together the two organizations cover the whole of the UK. The Free Movement Directives lay down a procedure by which nationals of one member state are entitled to registration as pharmacists in another member state. This procedure depends upon either the possession of a certificate or diploma (Qualifying European Diploma) where the training conforms with the Directive's requirements, or a certificate of training together with a period spent in practice. The competent authority can confirm the applicability of the relevant criteria.

Disqualifications
Section 4A also provides that the Statutory Committee of the RPSGB, when exercising its disciplinary powers, may take account of disqualifications to practise incurred in another member state.

Personal control of 'new' pharmacies
Article 3 of the 1987 Order amended section 70 of the MA 1968 so as to impose a condition that a pharmacy which has been registered for less than three years should not be under the personal control of a pharmacist who qualified in another Member state. This is the so-called 'Prag Amendment' (after the MEP who proposed it) which was intended to soften the expected impact of migrating pharmacists. At the time of the debate on the Directive several countries, including the UK, had no controls on entry to practise. In the UK at the time an application to dispense NHS prescriptions was automatically granted. This is no longer the case, although of course there are no restrictions of that nature on the establishment of a non-NHS pharmacy.

Linguistic ability
Article 4 of the Order amended the NHS Act 1977 to enable FHSAs to be satisfied that the linguistic competence of EU trained applicants for NHS contracts is adequate for the provision of services in the locality.

Article 5 inserted a similar provision into the NHS (Scotland) Act 1978.

Linguistic ability is now covered by Regulation 4(5) of the NHS (PS) Regulations 1992.

The Council of the RPSGB has made the following statement about competence in the English language.

'A pharmacist must have that knowledge of English which, in the interests of the pharmacist and the persons making use of the services offered by that pharmacist, is necessary for the provision of pharmaceutical services in Great Britain.

The superintendent of any body corporate conducting a retail pharmacy business must ensure that each employee pharmacist has that knowledge of English which, in the interests of that pharmacist and persons making use of his services, is necessary for the provision of pharmaceutical services, by that body corporate, in Great Britain.'

Titles
Pharmacists from other EU states are entitled to use the titles by which they are known in their own state, provided this does not cause confusion.

RPSGB byelaws
An Order of the Privy Council, dated 6 January 1988, amended the RPSGB byelaws to take account of the registration of overseas pharmacists. The byelaws

list the evidence which the Council of the RPSGB requires, and the fees to be paid. The evidence required is of:

- identity
- good character
- good physical and mental health
- the holding of a relevant EU diploma.

Many EU nationals hold diplomas which were granted before the states agreed the basic core knowledge of the course. They may be registered in the UK if they have lawfully practised pharmacy in another EU state for a period of at least three consecutive years during the last five years. The evidence for this is a certificate from the competent authorities of the member state. This process is referred to as the 'acquired rights' route.

Other professions

Similar Directives cover doctors, dentists, nurses, midwives and vets. A Directive issued in 1989 deals with the principle that a person fit to practise a professional activity in one state should in principle be allowed to practise in any other. Generally, professional qualifications achieved after a course of training equivalent to university are to be recognized. Where differences are substantial, a short test of ability may be imposed.

Chapter 21

The Pharmacy Profession

History

Chemists and druggists

The history of pharmacy as a profession distinct from the practice of medicine begins in 1794. Until then medicines had been dispensed by physicians and apothecaries as part of an ancillary service, but the compounding of prescriptions became more complex and expensive new avenues of supply were explored. Chemists and druggists had started to appear, with the primary purpose of dispensing the prescriptions of medical men.

An association

In response to the commercial threat posed by this new breed of merchant, the apothecaries formed a pharmaceutical association to restrain chemists and druggists from dispensing prescriptions and interfering with what was perceived as the legitimate business of apothecaries. The association was formed in 1794. When the association failed to stem the chemists and druggists, the apothecaries tried to enlist help at Westminster. In the original draft of the Apothecaries Act 1815 the apothecaries sought to prohibit the dispensing of medicines other than by apothecaries licensed under the provisions of the Act. After much intense lobbying by the chemists and druggists the proposal was abandoned. Section 28 of the Apothecaries Act expressly preserved 'the trade or business of a chemist and druggist in the buying, preparing, compounding, dispensing, and vending drugs, medicines, and medicinable compounds, wholesale and retail'. This was the first recognition of the pharmacy profession in an Act of Parliament.

Training

There was nevertheless a problem. Whereas the apothecaries could practise only after passing examinations required by the Apothecaries Act 1814, there was no equivalent requirement for chemists and druggists. Yet the measuring and compounding of medicines was a skilled and exact science. Compulsory pharmaceutical training was required in other European countries such as France, Germany and Sweden, and there was genuine concern that chemists and druggists in this country were neither licensed nor trained. On a number of occasions enterprising individuals tried to introduce an improved system, but few chemists and druggists supported ideas for reform.

The Hawes Bill

The introduction of a medical Bill by Mr Hawes provided the necessary catalyst for reform in 1841. The Hawes Bill sought to give supervision of chemists and druggists to medical practitioners, who would set up a system of education and licensing along European lines. In order to oppose the Bill leading chemists in London formed a Society, the Pharmaceutical Society, the object of the Society being to improve the education of pharmaceutical chemists.

Royal Charter

The Hawes Bill failed, but the legislative attempt achieved its purpose. Following discussions with London University, the College of Physicians and the College of Surgeons, the Pharmaceutical Society established an educational programme and founded its own Board of Examiners. The Pharmaceutical Society's membership grew from 668 members (not including associates and apprentices) in 1841 to 1640 in 1843 when a Royal Charter was granted. The Royal Charter declared that existing chemists and druggists could be admitted as members, but assistants, apprentices and students would be admitted only after being examined and certified as qualified for admission. After a few years, the Pharmaceutical Society obtained the introduction of a Bill in order to place the education and certification of pharmaceutical chemists on a statutory footing. The Society of Apothecaries did not oppose the Bill.

Statutory regulation

The Pharmacy Act 1852 confirmed the Royal Charter, empowering examiners appointed by the Pharmaceutical Society to grant or refuse certificates of competent skill and knowledge to exercise the business of pharmaceutical chemist. It became a criminal offence fraudulently to exhibit a certificate purporting to be a certificate of membership.

In the 150 years which have followed, the Pharmaceutical Society has grown from strength to strength. The Royal Charter was superseded by a second Charter in 1953. The Pharmacy Act 1852 was repealed and replaced by the Pharmacy Act 1954, and together these provisions govern the education and organization of the modern profession. Members of the Pharmaceutical Society were divided into pharmaceutical chemists, and chemists and druggists, but the latter class was abolished in 1953. In 1988 the Queen permitted the Society to be known as the Royal Pharmaceutical Society of Great Britain (RPSGB). In 1999 the RPSGB had more than 43 000 persons on the Register of Pharmaceutical Chemists. The number of pharmacy premises had risen to 12 311.

Contemporary challenges

The RPSGB is currently responding to a number of different challenges, in particular:

(i)		the challenges set by government in the development of pharmacy and the way in which the profession is to be regulated
(ii)	the regulatory challenges presented by Internet pharmacy, and its impact on Community pharmacy in general.

The Royal Pharmaceutical Society of Great Britain

Objects

The main objects of the RPSGB are as follows:

(1)		To advance chemistry and pharmacy.
(2)		To promote pharmaceutical education and the application of pharmaceutical knowledge.
(3)		To maintain the honour and safeguard and promote the interests of members in the exercise of the profession of pharmacy.
(4)		To provide relief for distressed persons who are either members, former members, widows, orphans or other dependants of former members, or students.

These objects previously defined were confirmed by the 1953 Royal Charter and have been considered in detail by the courts on two occasions.

Not a trade association

In the first case, *Jenkin* v. *Pharmaceutical Society* (1921), the court decided that the RPSGB's objects were not intended to cover activities normally associated with a trading association. It followed that the RPSGB was unable:

(1)		To regulate the terms of employment (hours, wages and conditions) between employer and employee members of the RPSGB.
(2)		To expend its funds in the formation of an industrial council committee to further these purposes.
(3)		To insure its members against insurable risks.

A distinction had to be drawn between activities which promoted the interests of those engaged in the exercise of the profession of pharmacy as a whole and the promotion of the interest of an individual or individuals. The formation of an industrial council committee was an activity which fell into the latter category and therefore could not be said to promote the exercise of the profession of pharmacy within the meaning of the Charter. Although decided under the 1843 Royal Charter, the same decision would almost certainly be reached today.

The National Pharmaceutical Association

Shortly after this decision, the National Pharmaceutical Union was formed to represent pharmacists on the trading aspects of pharmacy. Now known as the National Pharmaceutical Association, the Association offers indemnity insurance through the Chemists' Defence Association which is operated under its auspices.

No power to restrain trade

In the second case, *Pharmaceutical Society* v. *Dickson* (1970), the RPSGB had sought to include in the Code of Ethics a rule which amongst other things, would have confined the trading activities of new pharmacies to pharmaceutical and 'traditional' goods. The sale of 'non-traditional' goods, such as jewellery, beachwear, handbags, Thermos flasks etc. was, in the Society's opinion, degrading the quality and status of the profession. As in *Jenkins*, the House of Lords held that the proposed restrictions went outside the expressed objects of the Society. In the absence of evidence to show that professional standards had been eroded by reason of the trade in 'non-traditional' goods, the proposed restraint could not be said to be necessary to maintain and safeguard the honour of the profession or to promote the interests of members in the exercise of the profession.

The Council

The Council of the RPSGB manages the affairs of the Society. There are 24 members, of whom 21 must be elected by the members. The remaining three members are appointed by the Privy Council.

Membership

Members of the RPSGB are defined as those whose names are registered as pharmaceutical chemists with the RPSGB.

Register of pharmaceutical chemists

Under section 1 of the Pharmacy Act 1954 the Council of the RPSGB is obliged to appoint a registrar. The registrar's principal duty under the Act is to maintain a register of pharmaceutical chemists. The register must contain the names and addresses of all persons who are entitled to have their names registered, and the registrar must publish a list known as the 'annual register of pharmaceutical chemists' every year. Registration is essential to a practising pharmacist. Only a registered pharmacist is entitled to buy and sell drugs and to compound and dispense medicines. Similarly, only a registered pharmacist can run an RPB. Every registered pharmaceutical chemist must pay an annual fee to the RPSGB.

A person is entitled to have his name included in the register if he satisfies the registrar that he is qualified, whether by examination or under bye laws made by the RPSGB, to receive a certificate of competence to practise.

Section 16 of the Pharmacy Act 1954, together with byelaws made under the Act, have the effect of prescribing a maximum number of attempts to pass the pharmacy registration examinations. Although the practice constituted a restraint of trade, it is justifiable in the interests of safeguarding the public and preserving the integrity of the profession – see *R. v. RPSGB ex parte Mahmood* (2000).

Certificate of registration

The Council of the RPSGB is obliged under section 5 of the Pharmacy Act 1954 to issue to a qualified pharmacist a certificate of registration. Under the MA 1968 a pharmacist is bound to 'conspicuously exhibit' his certificate of registration at each premises in respect of which he has personal control. It is a criminal offence fraudulently to exhibit a certificate purporting to be a certificate of membership of the RPSGB. It is further a criminal offence to forge a certificate or allow it to be used by any other person.

Removal of name from the register

The Council may direct the registrar to remove the name of a pharmaceutical chemist from the register if he has failed to pay the annual fee within two months of the date of demand. The Statutory Committee may also direct the removal of the name of a pharmaceutical chemist from the register if he has been guilty of a crime or professional misconduct.

Registration of premises

Under section 75 of the MA 1968 the registrar is obliged to keep a register in which he enters any premises in respect of which an application for registration is made. The registrar must be satisfied that at the time of the application the applicant is a person lawfully conducting an RPB or entitled to conduct an RPB lawfully from the premises. The meaning of these terms is explained earlier in Chapter 9.

Infringements

During 1999 the Ethics Infringements Committee and the Law Infringements Committee combined to form a new Infringements Committee. This Committee conducts investigations into allegations of misconduct and/or unlawful activity by a pharmacist, with a view to initiating criminal proceedings by the RPSGB in its own right as a prosecutor where a breach of the criminal law has occurred, or referring the matter to the Statutory Committee for further investigation. During 1999, 55 individual alleged breaches of the law or the Code of Conduct were considered by the Committee. The Committee recommended criminal prose-cution in seven of these cases.

Since the 25 September 2000 the RPSGB has been empowered to conduct covert surveillance under the Regulation of Investigatory Powers Act 2000. The RPSGB is included in a list of public authorities allowed to authorise directed surveillance as part of an investigation into the detection or prevention of crime. Directed surveillance is defined as covert surveillance which does not entail the presence of individuals or use of monitoring devices on residential premises or in private vehicles. The surveillance must be proportionate and be carried out for the purposes of a specific investigation.

Although covert surveillance was used only once in 1999, the inclusion of the RPSGB as an authorized public authority might encourage its use in the investigation of the most serious cases.

The Statutory Committee of the RPSGB

Introduction

The professional conduct of pharmaceutical chemists is supervised by a committee of the RPSGB known as the Statutory Committee. The Statutory Committee exercises its supervisory and disciplinary jurisdiction pursuant to section 7 of the Pharmacy Act 1954, and its procedures are governed by statutory instrument, i.e. the Pharmaceutical Society (Statutory Committee) Order of Council 1978, SI 1978 No. 20.

Composition

The Statutory Committee consists of five members appointed by the Council of the RPSGB and the chairman who must be legally qualified. The chairman is appointed by the Privy Council. Members of the Statutory Committee hold office for five years. The quorum for a meeting of the Statutory Committee is three, but the chairman must be present. The Council of the RPSGB also appoints a secretary who is usually present at all Statutory Committee meetings. In 1999 the Statutory Committee held 12 meetings over 38 days.

Reference to the Statutory Committee

If information concerning the criminal conviction or professional misconduct of a registered pharmacist or one of his employees comes to the attention of the RPSGB (either as a result of the activities of the inspectors or by complaint from a member of the public), the information may be passed to the secretary of the Statutory Committee. On receipt of the information the secretary must submit to the chairman a report which summarizes the information or complaint. The chairman may direct the secretary to write to the person affected by the complaint to invite that person to submit an answer or an explanation of the conduct in question.

After considering the totality of the information available to him, the chairman must direct himself as follows:

(1) If he considers that the case is outside the Statutory Committee's jurisdiction, or is otherwise frivolous, or that it should be disregarded due to lapse of time or some other circumstance, the chairman must decide that the case is not to proceed further.

(2) If he considers that the conviction or alleged professional misconduct is not of a serious nature, or for some other reason may be disposed of without an inquiry, he may, after consulting the other members of the Statutory

Committee, decide that the case is not to proceed further, but he may direct the secretary to send a reprimand to the person affected and caution him as to his future conduct.

(3) In any other case the chairman must direct the secretary to take the necessary steps to hold an inquiry by the Statutory Committee into the matter. In this event the secretary must instruct a solicitor to investigate the facts of the case. If the solicitor reports that there is insufficient evidence to prove the criminal conviction or alleged misconduct, the Statutory Committee must consider his report and decide whether to hold an inquiry.

Notice of inquiry

The secretary must send notice to the person affected that the Statutory Committee is to inquire into the circumstances of a criminal conviction or his alleged misconduct. The notice must be sent not less than 28 days before the date of the inquiry.

Procedure at the hearing

An inquiry is held in public, although the Statutory Committee may direct the public to be excluded if it appears that exclusion is in the interests of justice or there is some other compelling reason. The person affected and the 'complainant' (in effect, the RPSGB), may be represented by a solicitor or barrister at the hearing. If the person affected does not attend the inquiry, the Statutory Committee may proceed in his absence or adjourn the hearing. At the hearing the case is presented against the person affected, and witnesses are called to give evidence. The witnesses may be cross-examined. This will be followed by evidence from the person affected. The Statutory Committee has a wide discretion to receive evidence orally or in writing. However, the Statutory Committee is bound to disregard evidence from a person who is present but refuses to submit for cross-examination.

The decision

After hearing the evidence and submissions, the Statutory Committee retires to consider its decision. The Statutory Committee must decide:

(1) Whether the conviction or misconduct is proved.
(2) If so, whether the conviction or misconduct is such as to render the person with regard to whom it is proved unfit to be on the register.
(3) If so, whether one of the statutory directions should be made.
(4) Whether any reprimand or admonition should be addressed to the person affected.

The statutory directions are set out in section 8 of the Pharmacy Act 1954 and section 80 of the MA 1968. By section 8 of the Pharmacy Act 1954 the Statutory Committee may direct the removal of a registered pharmaceutical chemist, or person employed by him, from the register. Section 80 of the MA 1968 gives the same power to direct removal from the register of a limited company which carries on an RPB and any member of the company's board or any officer employed by the company. In either case a statutory direction does not take effect until three months after notice of the direction has been given or, where an appeal to the High Court is brought against the direction, until the appeal is determined or withdrawn.

The chairman must announce the decision in public, and the decision must be communicated to the person affected and the registrar, who must act on any statutory direction which has been given.

In 1999, 21 pharmacists received a direction from the Statutory Committee that their name should be removed from the register. Ten pharmacists and one company were reprimanded.

Application for restoration

A person whose name has been removed from the register as a result of criminal conviction or misconduct may apply to have his name restored to the register. The application must be supported by a statutory declaration made by the applicant and accompanied by at least two certificates of his identity and good character. In the past the application has been considered by the Statutory Committee in private, unless the chairman directed otherwise. However, the Statutory Committee can determine its own procedure, and in November 1990 the Statutory Committee changed its procedure. The chairman stated that the application will now always be held in public, unless there was some special reason for the application to be heard in private. Unless the Statutory Committee decides to grant the application without a hearing, the applicant is entitled to appear before the Statutory Committee and be represented by a solicitor or barrister. If the statutory direction had been given at the inquiry following a complaint, the complainant may be given an opportunity of being heard or submitting written evidence. The secretary must communicate the decision of the Statutory Committee to the applicant and to any objector, and also to the registrar who must act on any direction which has been given.

It is often difficult for a pharmacist who has been removed from the register to know when he should apply for restoration. Removal from the register is without limit, although in practice pharmacists have often sought guidance from the Law Department of the RPSGB as to when might be an appropriate time to apply for restoration. In order to assist pharmacists where a statutory direction has been given, in some cases the Statutory Committee has recently started to give an indication as to when it might be appropriate for the affected person to apply for restoration. However, the indication will be informal, and the Statutory Committee has stated that it will not consider itself bound as to its actions in the future in any way. Failure by the Statutory Committee to act in accordance with such an indication has yet to be judicially tested in the High Court. A strong argument can be made out that an affected person will have a legitimate expectation that he will be restored to the register in accordance with the indication if he remains of good conduct during the period of removal.

In 1999, of the 17 applications for restoration 13 were successful.

Appeals

A person or a limited company affected by a decision of the Statutory Committee to remove them from the register or not restore them to the register may, within three months from the date of the decision, appeal to the High Court. The RPSGB may appear on the hearing of an appeal as the respondent. On appeal the High Court may make any order as it thinks fit, including an order as to the costs of the appeal. The registrar is bound to make such alterations in the register as are necessary to give effect to the High Court's order on appeal. An affected person who has been reprimanded may also appeal to the High Court, but by way of judicial review. Again the appeal has to be lodged promptly and within a maximum time limit of three months from the date of decision.

It is difficult to appeal successfully against the Statutory Committee's decision. The function of the High Court is not to impose its own view in substitution for a view taken by the Statutory Committee unless it came to the conclusion that the Committee was plainly wrong or had misdirected itself in reaching its conclusion, see *Thobani* v. *Pharmaceutical Society of Great Britain* (1990) and *Singh* v. *General Medical Council* (2000).

The standards of professional conduct

Code of Ethics

Members of the RPSGB approved and adopted a revised Code of Ethics at the annual general meeting in May 2000. The new code seeks to distinguish between serious misconduct which would almost certainly result in complaint to the Statutory Committee and standards of professional etiquette and prudence which pharmacists should strive to attain but which might not attract censure if they fail. Further revisions of the Code of Ethics will be presented for adoption at the next annual general meeting in May 2001. The Code of Ethics and Professional Standards is reproduced on the RPSGB's website (www.rpsgb.org.uk).

Key responsibilities
The Code of Ethics identifies the key responsibilities of a pharmacist in the following terms:

> 'Pharmacists understand the nature and effect of medicines and medicinal ingredients, and how they may be used to prevent and treat illness, relieve symptoms or assist in the diagnosis of disease. Pharmacists in professional practice use their knowledge for the well-being and safety of patients and the public.
>
> - At all times pharmacists must act in the interests of patients and other members of the public, and seek to provide the best possible health care for the community in partnership with other health professions. Pharmacists must treat all those who seek pharmaceutical services with courtesy, respect and confidentiality. Pharmacists must respect patients' rights to participate in decisions about their care and must provide information in a way in which it can be understood.

- Pharmacists must ensure that their knowledge, skills and performance are of a high quality, up to date, evidence based and relevant to their field of practice.
- Pharmacists must ensure that they behave with integrity and probity, adhere to accepted standards of personal and professional conduct and do not engage in any behaviour or activity likely to bring the profession into disrepute or undermine public confidence in the profession.'

Principles
There are nine philosophical principles which stand at the core of the Code of Ethics. Apart from minor amendments these principles do not differ from the principles set out in the Code of Ethics approved by Council in 1984. The nine principles are as follows.

(1)   A pharmacist's prime concern must be for the welfare of both patients and public.
(2)   A pharmacist must uphold the honour and dignity of the profession and not engage in any activity which may bring the profession into disrepute.
(3)   A pharmacist must at all times have regard to the laws and regulations applicable to pharmaceutical practice and maintain a high standard of professional conduct. A pharmacist must avoid any act or omission which would impair confidence in the pharmaceutical profession. When a pharmaceutical service is provided, a pharmacist must ensure that it is efficient.
(4)   A pharmacist must respect the confidentiality of information acquired in the course of professional practice relating to patients and their families. Such information must not be disclosed to anyone without the consent of the patient or appropriate guardian unless the interests of the public or the patient require such disclosure.
(5)   A pharmacist must keep abreast of the progress of pharmaceutical knowledge in order to maintain a high standard of professional competence relative to his sphere of activity.
(6)   A pharmacist must neither agree to practise under any conditions of service which compromise his professional independence nor impose such conditions on other pharmacists.
(7)   Publicity for professional services is permitted provided that such publicity does not create an invidious distinction between pharmacists or pharmacies, is dignified and does not bring the profession into disrepute.
(8)   A pharmacist offering services directly to the public must do so in premises which reflect the professional character of pharmacy.
(9)   A pharmacist must at all times endeavour to cooperate with professional colleagues and members of other health professions so that patients and the public may benefit.

Obligations
The Council formed the view that it was necessary to elaborate on the nine principles so as to form a brief summary of the pharmacist's obligations in each

area. Any complaint of misconduct would be based upon an alleged breach of these obligations and, by inference, of the principle which governs them.

Guidance
In order to assist pharmacists in the practical discharge of their professional obligations, the Council has set out some guidance which is intended to reflect the standards which pharmacists should meet in their daily lives.

The Code is reproduced in Appendix 7.

A practical example
The operation of the Code of Ethics can be demonstrated by a consideration of a practical example which arises almost daily in a retail pharmacy. A customer wishes to purchase two bottles of codeine linctus cough mixture. The pharmacist recognizes the customer, and believes that she bought two bottles of the same mixture three days earlier. It would not be unlawful to make the sale. But what does the Code of Ethics say?

'Principle 1. A pharmacist's prime concern must be for the welfare of both the patients and public.

Obligation: paragraph 1.7. A pharmacist must exercise professional judgment to prevent the supply of unnecessary and/or excessive quantities of medicines and other products, particularly those which are liable to abuse or which are claimed to depress appetite, prevent absorption of food or reduce body fluid.

Guidance on Obligation 1.7. Many POMs and CDs have a potential for abuse or dependency. Care should be taken over their supply even when it is legally authorized by prescription or signed order. A pharmacist should be alert to the possibility of drug dependency in health care professionals and patients and should be prepared to make enquiries to ensure that such medicines are to be used responsibly.

Some over-the-counter medicines and non-medicinal products are liable to be abused, which in this context usually means (a) consumption over a lengthy period and/or (b) consumption of doses substantially higher than recommended. Requests for such products should be dealt with personally by the pharmacist and sales should be refused if it is apparent that the purchase is not for a genuine medicinal purpose or if the frequency of purchase suggests overuse. A pharmacist should not attempt on his own to control an abuser's habit, but should liaise with bodies such as drug abuse clinics in any local initiative to assist abusers.

An up-to-date list of products known to be abused nationally appears in the Medicines, Ethics and Practice Guide. The products which are abused are subject to change, and pharmacists should keep abreast of local and national trends. The professional requirements for the provision of needle and syringe exchange schemes are set out in Standard 17.

It is clear from this guidance that the pharmacist should not make the sale because the frequency of purchase suggests over-use. The pharmacist would err in his professional judgment if he made the sale because he would be supplying an excessive quantity of medicine which is liable to abuse. This error, particularly if it was repeated on more than one occasion, would render the pharmacist open to a finding of misconduct by the Statutory Committee.

Appendix to the Code

An appendix entitled 'Standards of good professional practice' is attached to the Code of Ethics. The appendix sets out standards which must be met by registered pharmacists. This obligation is imposed by Obligation 1.14 of the Code of Ethics, and failure to meet the standards could form the basis of a complaint of misconduct. Again, guidance has been set out to help in the interpretation of the standards.

There are 19 areas covered by the standards, as follows.

(1) Standards for premises – appearance, safety, condition and tidiness of premises, environment, size of dispensary, and hygiene.
(2) Standards for dispensary design and equipment – suitability of dispensary, work surface and shelves, floor covering, water supply, waste disposal, and dispensing equipment.
(3) Standards for procurement and sources for materials – responsibility for procurement, sources of supply, safe systems of work, and medical gases.
(4) Standards of manufacturing and quality assurance – good manufacturing practice, quality assurance and control, batch numbers, manufacturing formulae, and documentation, equipment and sources of supply for manufacturing.
(5) Standards for dispensing procedures – dispensing procedures, supervision of dispensing and sales, safety in dispensing procedures, forged prescriptions, dispensing containers, re-use of containers, re-use of medicines, labels, storage, recalls, and personal hygiene.
(6) Standards for professional indemnity.
(7) Standards for education, training and development – competency, self-assessment, legislative changes and new services.
(8) Standards for relationships with patients and the public.
(9) Standards for relationships with other health care professionals.
(10) Standards for administration and management.
(11) Standards for community pharmacists providing a repeat medication service.
(12) Standards for the sale of non-prescribed medicines – request for medicine by name, pharmacist's involvement, special purchasers or users, medicines requiring special care.
(13) Standards for pharmacists providing services to nursing and residential homes.
(14) Standards for pharmacists providing instalment dispensing services.
(15) Standards for the home delivery of medicines.
(16) Standards for pharmacists providing domiciliary oxygen services.
(17) Standards for pharmacists providing needle and syringe exchange schemes.

(18) Standards for the collection and disposal of pharmaceutical waste by community pharmacies.
(19) Standards for the provision of on-line pharmacy services: security/confidentiality, request for supply of medicines, information and advice, record keeping.

At the time of writing a proposed twentieth standard of good professional practice has been published, concerning standards for the dispensing of extemporaneous preparations. The standard will be added to the Standards for Good Professional Practice shortly.

Council statements

Subsequent to the revision of the Code of Ethics in May 2000, the Council has issued two Council statements which supplement the obligations set out in the Code. The first statement prohibits any involvement in petitions promoting self interest to the detriment of other existing pharmacy contractors. The second concerns the circumstances in which a dog may be present on pharmacy premises.

Professional Standards Fact Sheets

The RPSGB has also prepared a series of Professional Standards Fact Sheets addressing areas of practice which are frequently the subject of enquiry. At the time of writing sheets are available on the following subjects:

(1) controlled drugs and community pharmacy
(2) controlled drugs and hospital pharmacy
(3) the export of medicines
(4) the use of unlicensed medicines in pharmacy
(5) advertising
(6) prescription collection, home delivery and repeat medication services
(7) pharmacy and the internet
(8) labelling of MDS and compliance aids
(9) patient group directions
(10) dealing with dispensing errors.

The fact sheets are reproduced on the RPSGB's website. The RPSGB has also prepared guidance on counter prescribing for self-limiting minor illness and common conditions (see the *Pharmaceutical Journal*, 9 September 2000) and the supply of emergency hormonal contraception as a pharmacy medicine (see the *Pharmaceutical Journal*, 16 December 2000).

Breach of the Code

A breach of the Code of Ethics could form the basis of a complaint of misconduct but the Council, in considering whether or not action should follow, takes into consideration the circumstances of an individual case and does not regard itself as being limited to those matters which are mentioned in the Code. In law, the arbiter of what constitutes misconduct is the Statutory Committee. Misconduct does not necessarily involve some sort of moral censure; rather, misconduct may be defined as 'incorrect or erroneous conduct of any kind provided that it is of a serious nature', i.e. judged according to the rules written or unwritten of the pharmaceutical profession, see *R* v. *Statutory Committee of the Pharmaceutical Society of Great Britain, ex parte Sokoh,* 3 December 1986, unreported. Moreover, in that case the High Court held that it was possible that just one error may constitute misconduct, if the error was sufficiently serious.

The incorrect or erroneous conduct must, however, be regarded as so serious as to justify a finding of misconduct. Deliberate breach of the policy made by the Council will not automatically amount to misconduct – in such a case the Statutory Committee has to satisfy itself that the deliberate breach of policy was of such a quality as to constitute serious misconduct, see *R* v. *Statutory Committee of the Royal Pharmaceutical Society ex parte Boots the Chemists PLC,* 14th February 1997. In that case Boots deliberately flouted policy made by the Council in June 1993 to prohibit the introduction of collection and delivery services in areas where a community pharmacy already exists. The chairman of the Statutory Committee advised that Boots' conduct did not amount to misconduct in law. The High Court agreed and said that the legally unqualified majority of the committee should have followed the chairman's advice.

A Health Committee

Parliament has enacted the Pharmacists (Fitness to Practise) Act 1997 which establishes a new committee of the RPSGB, to be known as the Health Committee. The new committee is given power to impose conditions with which a pharmacist must comply if he continues to practise in circumstances where he is unwell. Investigations into a pharmacist's fitness to practise are initiated by the Council, which is required to inform the pharmacist involved and give him 28 days to respond. Following a hearing the Health Committee is empowered to dismiss the allegation of unfitness to practise or, if it considers it to be well founded, to impose conditions on practice or suspend registration. Pharmacists who have been suspended or made subject to conditions of practise are able to request a review of the order against them. The Act also set up an appeal procedure. Although the Act received Royal Assent on 19 March 1997, its provisions have not yet been brought into effect.

The future

At the time of writing the RPSGB has begun consulting its members on a major reform of the profession's disciplinary machinery and the introduction of a requirement on pharmacists to undertake appropriate continuing professional development if they wish to retain the right to practice.

The catalyst for reform was provided by the NHS Plan published in July 2000, which requires health self-regulatory bodies such as the RPSGB to change so that they:

● are smaller, with much greater patient and public representation in their membership

- have faster, more transparent procedures
- develop meaningful accountability to the public and the Health Service.

These principles were expanded upon in the government consultation papers issued in August 2000 for the new Nursing and Midwifery Council (NMC) and the new Health Professions Council (HPC). A specific requirement contained within the proposals for new legislation for these professions is that a professional majority of more than one on either the Councils, or their Committees, is unacceptable to government.

The consultation papers provide for the key functions for the new Councils to be:

- establishing and keeping the register ('registration')
- establishing and reviewing standards of proficiency, and the training required, for admission to the register ('education')
- establishing and reviewing standards of conduct and ethics ('standards setting')
- establishing and reviewing arrangements to protect the public from those who are unfit to practice ('discipline and health')
- establishing and reviewing requirements for re-admission and renewal of registration ('competence based practising rights').

In any event the RPSGB recognises that its powers and structures are outmoded and in need of reform, deriving principally from the Pharmacy Act 1954. The enactment of the Health Act 1999 enables professional regulatory bodies to amend their governing legislation by Order, and rising to the challenge in February 2001 the RPSGB distributed a paper to its members entitled 'Reform of disciplinary machinery and the introduction of competence based practising rights' containing radical proposals to this effect.

The paper proposes the delegation of disciplinary functions by Council to two Committees. An Investigating Committee would replace the Council's existing Infringements Committee, and a Disciplinary Committee would replace the Statutory Committee. In all cases it is proposed that members of the Committee will have security of tenure, to ensure that they are independent of influence. Lay members will be appointed after public advertisement and in consultation with the Privy Council.

The paper also addresses the need for the RPSGB's education division to explore ways to develop its continuing professional development pilot scheme in order to satisfy the government's broad requirements laid down in the NMC and HPC consultation documents.

It is proposed that the RPSGB will provide a framework for pharmacists to devise their own Personal Development Plans, to be maintained throughout their careers as pharmacists. The cycle is underpinned by the idea that pharmacists will now be required to identify their personal professional needs and improve their skills as practising pharmacists for the benefit of patients as well as for their own benefit. A Competence Audit Committee will set the framework for, determine the details of and monitor the operation of the continuing professional development requirements for eligibility to practice.

While the list is not exhaustive, elements in the programme are expected to include:

- continuing education
- critical incident analysis
- audit
- writing
- experiential learning
- learning from colleagues
- teaching
- problem solving.

Chapter 22

Liability in Negligence

Dispensing mistakes

A pharmacist, like any other professional person, can make a mistake and, like doctors, the consequences of a pharmacist's mistake can be most serious. The customer may suffer serious personal injuries as a result of the mistake.

It has been estimated that in the USA deaths due to medication errors exceed the number of fatal accidents on the roads. In the UK little research has been performed on dispensing errors in community pharmacy. Some research conducted in Glasgow in 1996 disclosed that dispensing errors occurred in 1% of prescriptions dispensed. Most of these errors related to dispensing the wrong medicine or strength of medicine (72%). Incorrect labelling accounted for 14% of errors.

The law concerning a pharmacist's civil liability for mistakes is considered in this section of the book. With the increase in professional negligence litigation, it is an area of law with which the contemporary community pharmacist needs to have some familiarity.

Breach of contract

Where a customer obtains medicinal products on the strength of an NHS prescription, even though he pays a prescription charge, the courts have held that the products are not supplied under a contract of sale, but rather by virtue of the pharmacist's statutory duty to supply the medicinal products (*Pfizer Corp* v. *Ministry of Health* (1965)). Accordingly, if the customer is to recover any damages for a mistake in the dispensing process, he has to establish a case in negligence against the pharmacist at common law.

Negligence

A customer who wishes to recover damages for personal injuries has to prove four things:

(1) That the defendant owed him a duty of care.
(2) That the defendant was in breach of that duty.
(3) That he has suffered damage as a result of that breach.
(4) That the damage was reasonably foreseeable in all the circumstances.

Duty of care

A duty to take reasonable care arises when the defendant can reasonably foresee that the claimant (the one who complains) is likely to be injured by his conduct. As Lord Atkin said in *Donoghue* v. *Stephenson* (1932) AC 562 at page 580:

'You must take reasonable care to avoid acts or omissions which you can reasonably foresee would be likely to injure your neighbour. Who, then, in law is my neighbour? The answer seems to be – persons who are so closely and directly affected by my act that I ought reasonably to have them in contemplation as being so affected when I am directing my mind to the acts or omissions which are called in question'.

Breach of duty

It is always a question of fact whether the defendant has failed to show reasonable care in the particular circumstances of a case. The law lays down the general rules which determine the standard of care which has to be attained, and it is for the court to apply that legal standard of care to its findings of fact so as to find whether the defendant has attained that standard. The legal standard is not the standard of the defendant himself, but that of a person of ordinary prudence or a person using ordinary skill. In cases where a person has a particular skill, such as a pharmacist, the person is required to show the skill normally possessed by persons undertaking work of a similar nature. Thus in the case of a pharmacist, the pharmacist must exercise the standard of skill which is usual in his profession; he must exercise the same degree of care which a reasonably competent pharmacist would exercise in performing the same task.

Occasionally situations arise where the claimant is not able to establish exactly how the accident occurred. Nevertheless, the mere fact of the happening of the accident in certain circumstances may justify the inference that the defendant has probably been negligent and his negligence caused the injury. The maxim, known as *res ipsa loquitur* (i.e. 'the thing speaks for itself'), is an evidentiary rule to the effect that the fact of the injury and the circumstances in which it was sustained, establish a prima facie case of negligence against the defendant, which he must then rebut in order to avoid a finding of liability.

Damage as a result of the breach

The claimant must show that the defendant's wrongdoing was a cause, though not necessarily the sole or dominant cause, of his injuries. In general, a defendant who commits a wrong takes his victim as he finds him. It is no answer to a claim for damages to say that the victim would have sustained no or less injury if he had not suffered from some pre-existing condition.

Foreseeable damage

There is a final hurdle which a claimant must surmount before he can recover damages for negligence. The type of injury which he has suffered must be reasonably foreseeable, in the sense that a reasonable man would have foreseen the type of injury as being likely to flow from the defendant's breach of duty.

Negligence causing death

All causes of action which accrue to the benefit of a claimant will survive for the benefit of his estate after his death under the provisions of the Law Reform (Miscellaneous Provisions) Act 1934. Additionally, where the breach of duty has caused death, the deceased's dependants may maintain an action and recover damages against the person liable in respect of the death under the Fatal Accidents Act 1976. The action must be brought by the deceased's personal representatives, and since only one action may be brought, claims must be included for all the dependants. In assessing damages under the Fatal Accidents Act, other than damages of £7500 for bereavement, the court seeks to compensate the dependants for the loss which they have sustained as a result of the death.

Choice of defendant

In some cases the claimant may be faced with a choice of defendants. A typical situation arises where the claimant was a passenger in a motor car, which was in collision with another. If there is evidence to show that both drivers are to blame, it is normal practice to commence legal proceedings against both drivers. The same principles will apply where a patient has suffered injury caused by the breach of duty of a doctor and a pharmacist. Both may be sued together in one action. The basic rule is that each of the two tortfeasors will be liable for the whole damage resulting from their tortious act. However, where tortfeasors are jointly liable, the tortfeasors can ask the court to assess their respective liability in respect of the accident. This is done by one of the tortfeasors commencing proceedings against the other for contribution under the Civil Liability (Contribution) Act 1978.

Defences

The obvious defence, raised in most negligence actions, is the basic denial that the defendant has been guilty of any negligence and the further denial that, in the event of the claimant establishing any breach of duty against him, the injury resulted from the accident. The following specific defences tend to arise in practice in cases where pharmacists are involved.

Contributory negligence

Where the injury suffered is partly the result of the fault of the claimant, the recoverable damages are reduced by the court to the extent it thinks fit, having regard to the plaintiff's responsibility for the injuries: the Law Reform (Contributory Negligence) Act 1945. The court determines the percentage of contributory negligence. It will not deal in minute percentages, so the normal practice is to disregard responsibility evaluated at less than 10%.

Novus actus interveniens

(A new act intervening.) Situations sometimes arise where the sequence of events following on from the defendant's act or omission is interrupted. Once it is established that, in the ordinary course of events, the defendant's act or omission would not have resulted in the damage but for the intervening act (whether of some third party or of the claimant), the chain of causation is broken. In such an event the defendant will not be liable.

Volenti non fit injuria

(That to which a man consents cannot be considered an injury.) To raise this defence it is necessary to show that the claimant agreed to run the risk involved; mere silence on the subject is not normally sufficient.

Limitation

In personal injury cases the claimant must normally commence his action within three years of the date when the cause of action accrued. The date when the cause of action accrued will be the date when the injury was sustained. There are, however, special cases. After sustaining personal injury a claimant may not have discovered the effects of the injury or the identity of the defendant until after the limitation period has expired. In this case a special period of limitation is prescribed. The period of limitation will be deemed to run for three years from the date when the claimant became possessed of full information about his case. The period begins to run when the claimant has knowledge of all of the following matters:

(1) That his injury was significant.
(2) That the injury was attributable in whole or in part to the acts or omissions complained of.
(3) The identity of the defendant.

However, it is right to add that a party who has sustained injuries will be imputed with knowledge which he might reasonably have been expected to acquire either by his own observation or inquiry or by expert advice, which it might have been reasonable for him to seek. Finally, a court may direct that the limitation provisions should be disregarded in a personal injury case if in the view of the court it would be equitable for action to proceed, having regard to the degree of prejudice suffered by the claimant on account of the rules of limitation as well as the prejudice the defendant would suffer if the limitation period were disregarded.

Application of the law to pharmacists

Amongst other duties it is clear that a pharmacist is obliged as a supplier of medicinal products to take reasonable care to:

(1) Ensure that the correct medicinal products are supplied.
(2) Warn customers of the potential dangers or adverse effects of the medicinal products.
(3) Ensure that customers are instructed as to the correct dosage.

Failure to take reasonable care in the discharge of any of these tasks will render the pharmacist liable to legal proceedings for breach of professional duty. The application of these principles is demonstrated by a consideration of the following reported cases.

Dispensing the wrong medicine

Collins v. Hertfordshire County Council (1947)

The pharmacist at a pre-NHS hospital was asked to dispense '100 ml of 1% cocaine with adrenaline, for injection'. The pharmacist did not question the order for an 'unheard-of dosage' of a dangerous drug. He made up the cocaine and adrenaline as an injection and supplied it to the operating theatre. During an operation the cocaine preparation was injected and the patient died. In fact the final-year student doctor who had ordered cocaine had herself misheard the consultant surgeon who had actually ordered procaine. The hospital's standing instructions on ordering dangerous drugs had not been complied with by either the doctor or the pharmacist. The hospital authority was held liable for the pharmacist's failure to question the order, and for the student doctor's mistake.

Prendergast v. Sam and Dee Ltd, Kozary and Miller (1989)

A pharmacist misread a doctor's writing on a prescription. The doctor had prescribed Amoxil but the pharmacist read it as Daonil. He dispensed Daonil, and the patient, who was not a diabetic, suffered hypoglycemia and irreversible brain damage.

The patient (Prendergast) sued the pharmacy company (Sam and Dee Ltd), the pharmacist (Kozary) and the doctor (Miller).

The court found all three defendants liable. The doctor's writing was adjudged to fall below the standard of legibility required of him in the exercise of his duty to the patient. The court also held that although the writing was bad, the word could have been read as Daonil, and that certain aspects of the prescription should have alerted the pharmacist.

On appeal the court specifically held that the chain of causation starting with the poor handwriting was not broken.

The court held that the pharmacist had a duty to give some thought to the prescription he was dispensing and he should not dispense mechanically. If there is any doubt the pharmacist must contact the doctor for clarification. In this case if the pharmacist had been paying attention he would have realised that there was something wrong with the prescription, since the dosage and the small number of tablets were unusual for Daonil. Additionally, the claimant had paid for the prescription, yet drugs for diabetes (such as Daonil) were free under the NHS.

The court apportioned damages between the defendants: 25% to the doctor, and 75% shared between the company and the pharmacist.

Dispensing the wrong dosage

Dwyer v. Roderick (1983)

This case is usually referred to as the Migril case. The facts can be summed up in three sentences.

(1) A doctor negligently directed the patient to take an overdose in the prescription.

(2) The pharmacist failed to spot the error.
(3) The pharmacist was held liable in negligence.

These facts illustrate the difficulties for pharmacists.

The owner of the pharmacy admitted negligence, and the court held that he was 45% liable for the damages of £100 000.

The judge emphasized that the pharmacist:

(1) Owed a duty to the patient to ensure that drugs were correctly prescribed.
(2) Should have spotted the error.
(3) Should have queried the prescription with the doctor.

As a result of this case the RPSGB issued this Council Statement:

'Pharmacists are reminded that patients who are prescribed Migril tablets should take no more than four tablets for any single migraine attack and no more than six in any one week. Because there have been occasional reports of severe toxic effects from overdosage, the Council advises pharmacists to ensure that patients are aware of the maximum dosage.'

Taking precautions

Community pharmacists would do well to take heed of the results of an Australian survey into the causes of dispensing errors. High prescription volumes, pharmacist fatigue, pharmacist overwork, interruptions to dispensing, and similar or confusing drug names were put forward as the principal contributing factors to dispensing errors.

In the UK some recent research has shown that the tendency of manufacturers to use similar packs for different medicines or strengths of medicines is a significant contributory cause of dispensing errors. Indeed, a survey of 33 hospitals revealed that the most frequent sources of error were different strengths of product in almost indistinguishable boxes, and different medicines with similar names made by the same manufacturer. Sometimes medicine packs are distinguishable when viewed individually but look similar when stacked together in a dispensary.

Accordingly, in order to reduce the chances of making a mistake, community pharmacists would be well advised not to put similar packs together, to express strengths uniformly (for example, either 60 mg in 2 ml or 30 mg/ml, but not both), and where possible to adopt uniform colours for different product strengths.

The future

As with medical negligence cases, the incidence of negligence claims against pharmacists will undoubtedly increase in future years. There are a number of situations which have not yet appeared in the reported cases. For example, a pharmacist will presumably be liable if he dispenses medicinal products which are obsolete or damaged in such a way as to be dangerous, or where he fails to supply product leaflets intended by the manufacturer to be passed to the user.

Recent research into the administration of carbamazepine (prescribed to epilepsy sufferers) has disclosed that dispensing errors occur, most often where the pharmacist confuses 200 mg and 400 mg modified release tablets. On occasions these errors led to profound medical, social and psychological consequences. The research concludes that inadvertent intoxication of epilepsy sufferers with carbamazepine is widespread as a result of dispensing errors, but that these errors could be avoided by changing the appearance of both the packaging and the tablets for different product strengths (see Research paper by Mack, Kuc, Grunewald, published in the *Pharmaceutical Journal*, 18 November 2000).

The RPSGB has given guidance in a fact sheet on how to deal with dispensing errors. See Chapter 21.

Insurers prefer to settle these cases quietly, rather than run the risks of an adverse result with unwanted media attention and significantly increased legal costs.

Liability as an occupier of premises

The Occupiers' Liability Act

A community pharmacist may also find himself liable as an occupier if an accident occurs on his premises. The provisions of the Occupiers' Liability Act 1957 regulate the duty which an occupier of premises owes to his visitors in respect of dangers due to the state of the premises, or to things done, or omitted to be done on them. Where an act or omission creates a dangerous condition which later causes harm to a visitor, the Act applies. Typical examples would be where a chair for customers waiting for prescriptions collapses because it was in need of repair, or where the floor covering had become raised, thus constituting a danger to all customers who might enter the pharmacy.

An occupier

In order to be an occupier of premises, exclusive occupation is not needed. The test is whether a person has some degree of control associated with, or arising from his presence in, and use of, or activity in the premises.

A visitor

A visitor includes all persons to whom the occupier has given an invitation or permission to enter the premises.

The duty

The duty of the occupier is to take such care as in all the circumstances of the case is reasonable to see that the visitor will be reasonably safe in using the premises for the purposes for which he is invited or permitted by the occupier to be there.

Warning and knowledge of danger

In determining whether an occupier of premises has discharged the common duty of care, regard will be had to all the circumstances. For example, where the occupier warns a visitor of danger, and despite the warning damage is caused to the visitor, the warning itself does not absolve the occupier from liability, unless in all the circumstances it was enough to enable the visitor to be reasonably safe.

Access for disabled people

The Disability Discrimination Act 1995 has particular relevance to a community pharmacy, since the provisions of the Act will apply to many patients visiting a pharmacy. The Act imposes a duty on a service provider, which includes a community pharmacist, to make 'reasonable adjustments' for disabled people to enable them to have better access to services.

With these considerations in mind, it is important for a community pharmacist to ensure that he does not have any practices or procedures which would make it difficult for a disabled person to make use of his services, that he provides auxiliary aids or services to enable disabled people to make use of his services, and that he provides a reasonable alternative method of making a service available where the physical features of the premises impede a disabled person in the use of the service.

Some community pharmacies operate from narrow retail units, where wheelchair access is often difficult if not impossible. Consideration must be given to constructing a ramp, or if this is not possible, to installing a bell at wheelchair height outside the pharmacy so that a disabled person could call for assistance. The layout of the pharmacy must also facilitate wheelchair access to the prescription dispensing area.

Before making any changes to the premises, a community pharmacist should contact the local disablement officer at the nearest Job Centre. In addition to advising on changes which could be made to comply with the provisions of the Act, the officer will know if there are any local funds available to assist with alterations made for this purpose.

The definition of a disabled person for the purposes of the Act is very wide. It embraces any person who has 'a physical or medical impairment which has substantial and long-term adverse affects on his or her ability to carry out day-to-day activities'.

Chapter 23

Business Premises

When setting up a pharmacy, a pharmacist has to decide whether to buy shop premises or rent shop premises from a landlord. The purpose of this part of the book is to assist a pharmacist in making this decision, by explaining the basic difference between the ownership and rental of business premises and by describing the principal rights and obligations of leasehold ownership.

Business premises, like residential dwellings, are either 'freehold' or 'leasehold'.

Freehold premises

The owner of freehold premises owns them absolutely. In other words, the owner has freedom to make such use of them as he wishes. He may lease the premises to a tenant, and he may raise a mortgage or loan against the equity in the property. The only qualification to this freedom will be in the form of easements or restrictive covenants.

Easements

An easement is a continuing right or privilege enjoyed by someone other than the freeholder over the freeholder's land. For example, where A and B own adjacent premises, B may enjoy a right of way over A's land.

Restrictive covenants

A restrictive covenant is a restriction attaching to the premises which prevents the owner from carrying out specified activities. Such covenants are of particular importance to the purchaser of business premises as one of the most common forms prevents the carrying out of specified trades or activities on the premises. For example, if A owns two shop premises in the same road and sells one of them to B, a covenant may be included whereby B undertakes not to pursue a similar trade to A in the newly purchased premises. When B subsequently sells to C, the burden of the covenant will continue to attach to the premises.

In the normal course of events such covenants will become apparent before purchase during the normal searches carried out by the purchaser's solicitors. Failure to detect and warn about easements or covenants may render the solicitor liable to the purchaser in damages for negligence.

Pre-contractual enquiries

There are significant pitfalls to be avoided when a community pharmacist buys an existing retail pharmacy business, particularly where there are unresolved applications for a new contract, minor relocation and/or doctor dispensing rights. Unexpected changes in the way in which general medical services or pharmaceutical services are provided can impact significantly on the profitability of a retail pharmacy business which is the subject of the purchase.

It is, therefore, imperative for the purchaser to discover the existence of any unresolved applications which might adversely effect the economic viability of the retail pharmacy business. This is not as easy as it sounds because a seller, whether a freehold seller or an assignor of leasehold premises, is under no legal obligation to disclose the existence of an unresolved application. There is no local register which can be consulted. Local health administrators may be prepared to reveal relevant information on request, but there is no duty on them to do so. Local health administrators are not obliged to do any more than make available for inspection a copy of the pharmaceutical list – see regulation 22(1)(a) of the National Health Service (Pharmaceutical Services) Regulations 1992.

In these circumstances it is absolutely vital for an intending purchaser and his solicitor to ask the right questions of the vendor/assignor. As well as asking both orally and in writing (by pre-contractual enquiries) about planning permission, the profitability of the retail pharmacy business and other matters of commercial interest which form the usual subjects of enquiry, an intending purchaser and his solicitor must ask the vendor/assignor whether there are any unresolved applications for a new pharmacy, minor relocation or doctor dispensing, whether any such applications have been made within the last five years, and whether the vendor/assignor has received notice (either formally or informally) that any such application is likely to be made. The intending purchaser must also probe the extent of the vendor/assignor's knowledge of any plans by a nearby doctors surgery to move premises. If the answer to any of these questions is 'yes', the vendor/assignor must explore full details of the application or plans and obtain details of any determination which was reached. Any incorrect answer may give rise to an action in damages as a breach of warranty and/or as a negligent misrepresentation under section 2 of the Misrepresentation Act 1967.

The importance of making careful pre-contractual enquiries was demonstrated in the case of *Banks* v. *Cox* (2000) where during the sale of a nursing home the purchaser asked the vendor whether there had been any material change in the nature or conduct of the business. The Court held that the vendor was guilty of fraudulent misrepresentation when he failed to bring to the purchaser's attention a change in social services policy which seriously affected the profitability of the business.

Leasehold premises

Instead of purchasing a freehold interest, a pharmacist may acquire a leasehold interest in business premises. A lease is, like a freehold, an interest in land. The leaseholder is in effect the owner of the leasehold premises for the duration of the lease. A business lease should be negotiated by a solicitor and contained in written form; however, more informal agreements do sometimes occur. Whether the lease is contained in a formal document or not, there are certain preconditions which must exist to create a lease, as opposed to a mere licence, which is no more than permission, revokable at will, to be present on the premises. For a lease to exist, the agreement must: be for a fixed term at a rent, and grant exclusive possession of the premises.

Fixed term

A lease does not have to be for a term of years, but must be expressed for a fixed, ascertainable duration. Usually the lease will be for a definite period of time terminating on a specific date. A periodic tenancy may also be created where the lease is renewable at short intervals, e.g. monthly, quarterly or yearly. As long as the intervals are expressly specified, a lease is capable of being created.

Exclusive possession

Exclusive possession means that the tenant has the sole right to occupy the premises. A possible qualification to this may be a clause in the lease which confers on the landlord a right to re-enter the premises from time to time in order to inspect them or to carry out repairs. A grant of anything less than exclusive possession is incapable of creating a tenancy.

Rent

The term 'rent' is more or less self-explanatory. Most leases will contain specific clauses dealing with the amount of rent payable and the dates upon which it should be paid. It is very unusual for rent to take a form other than money, but it is possible for it to take the form of the provision of services. If rent is not payable, it is highly unlikely that anything other than a mere licence has been created.

Formalities

In order to create a legal lease which exceeds three years in duration, it is necessary for the lease agreement to be contained in a deed (section 52 of the Law of Property Act 1925). The document creating the lease will set out the names of the parties and the period for which the lease is to run. A rent will be specified and each party will undertake in various clauses to abide by certain obligations. For example, the tenant may undertake to keep the premises in a good state of repair. There will usually be a clause by which the landlord is permitted to re-enter the premises should the tenant fail to pay the rent, or if he is in breach of certain of his obligations. If for some reason a lease has not been created by deed, it may be recognized by a court if it can be ascertained that the parties intended to create a lease, and that acts consistent with that intention have been carried out by the parties.

Terms of a business lease

A lease will, by its clauses, impose obligations on both parties. It will create rights for the benefit of one party in the event of a breach of an obligation by the other. A distinction exists between terms which are known as conditions, and those which are known as covenants.

Conditions

Conditions are terms which have to be fulfilled for the lease to come into existence, or for it to continue. For example, it may be a condition of the lease that the premises are to be used exclusively for the purposes of carrying on business as a pharmacy. Should the tenant cease to comply with this condition, the landlord will have the right to re-enter the premises whether or not that right is expressly reserved in the lease.

Covenants

A covenant is an agreement between the parties whereby one party promises to fulfil certain obligations. Examples include covenants:

- to pay rent
- to maintain the premises in a certain condition
- to insure the premises
- not to sub-let.

A breach of covenant may give rise to certain legal remedies such as damages or injunction. A breach on the part of the tenant will not automatically entitle the landlord to re-enter unless this has been expressly provided for.

If an enforceable lease has been entered into which does not contain covenants, a court will imply the usual covenants. These may include covenants on the part of the tenant:

- to pay rent
- to repair the premises at the end of the term
- to pay rates
- to deliver the premises up to the landlord at the end of the term.

The landlord will be obliged to grant quiet enjoyment of the premises to the tenant, and will be entitled to re-enter the premises for non-payment of rent.

Specific covenants

The covenants which commonly give rise to the greatest potential for difficulty or dispute during the currency of the lease are covenants:

- not to assign or sub-let
- not to change the use made of the premises
- not to alter or improve the premises
- to repair and to insure the premises.

Each of these merits some closer attention.

Covenants limiting the right to assign or sub-let

If the landlord wishes to restrict the tenant's right to sub-let or assign premises (i.e. to prevent the tenant from creating a sub-lease or vesting the benefit of a lease in a third party), he must do so by express words in the lease. Such a covenant will not be implied. If the words of the covenant are unconditional and prevent any sub-letting or assignment whatsoever, then the tenant is bound by the covenant absolutely.

However, it is common for a clause to be inserted whereby assigning or sub-letting is permitted subject to the landlord's consent. Where this is the case, section 19(1) of the Landlord and Tenant Act 1927 then inserts into the covenant a proviso that such consent will not be withheld unreasonably. The question of when it is reasonable for a landlord to refuse consent is discussed below, but the effect of an unreasonable refusal is the removal of the covenant, so that assignment or sub-letting can take place without consent. The usual course for the tenant to take when faced with an unreasonable refusal is to seek a declaration in the county court (under section 53 of the Landlord and Tenant Act 1954) that the landlord's refusal was unreasonable. The tenant bears the burden of proving unreasonableness.

Under the Landlord and Tenant Act 1988, section 1, a landlord who is asked to give his consent to assignment or sub-letting must give his consent or justify his refusal as reasonable. Failure to do so may render the landlord liable in damages or to an injunction.

A landlord can circumvent the application of section 19 of the Landlord and Tenant Act 1927 by either: including an express prohibition on any sub-letting or assigning; *or* by including a condition that if the tenant wishes to assign or sub-let, he must first offer to surrender the lease to the landlord. The landlord may then take possession of the premises if he does not wish to allow the assignment or sub-letting.

Unreasonable refusal   If the tenant is not satisfied that the landlord's refusal is reasonable, he must prove that it is unreasonable. The landlord is not obliged to provide reasons for his refusal. The landlord will not be held to have acted unreasonably if he has acted as a reasonable person might do. A refusal of consent will be unreasonable if the grounds for refusal do not relate to the personality or credit-worthiness of the proposed assignee or sub-tenant, or to the effect of the proposed assignment or sub-lease on the use or occupation of the premises (*Houlder Bros & Co.* v. *Gibbs* (1925)).

Motives   The landlord is entitled to be selfish in his reasons, except where the reason for his refusal is to achieve some purpose totally unconnected with the lease, or where there is such disproportion between the benefit to the landlord and the detriment to the tenant brought about by the refusal, that it would be unreasonable for the landlord to withhold his consent.

Where the assignee has an ulterior motive in obtaining the benefit of the lease, e.g. in using the nuisance value of the lease to force his way into a new development, refusal may be reasonable.

It is unreasonable for a landlord to refuse consent on the grounds of race or sex: Race Relations Act 1976, section 24; Sex Discrimination Act 1975, section 31.

Where the covenant provides that the landlord's consent is required for sub-letting or assigning, money may not be requested as a condition of consent being granted, but a reasonable amount may be requested to cover expenses.

In some cases, the covenant restricting assignment and sub-letting will clearly evidence the purpose for which the covenant was made. In such a case the words of the covenant will be strictly construed. An assignment or sub-letting will not be permitted where to do so would defeat the original purpose of the covenant.

It will usually be unreasonable for the landlord to refuse his consent on the grounds that he anticipates that the assignee or sub-tenant will breach a covenant restricting the use which can be made of the premises, as his right to enforce the covenant will remain unaffected.

Covenants concerning change of use

Many legal documents substitute the term 'user' for 'use'. The above heading will appear as 'Covenants concerning change of user'.

Many business leases contain a covenant preventing the tenant from changing the use made of the premises during the period of the tenancy. Such a covenant will either be absolute, or conditional upon the consent of the landlord.

Where the landlord's consent is required for a change of use, section 19(3) of the Landlord and Tenant Act 1927 prevents the granting of consent from being conditional upon the payment of money by the tenant. The landlord may, however, be entitled to compensation for any loss as a result of the change of use.

Unlike section 19(1) which imposes a requirement of reasonableness on the landlord's granting of consent, section 19(3) makes no such provision. Often the covenant may include words to the effect that the landlord may not refuse his consent unreasonably. In determining whether consent has been unreasonably withheld, similar considerations apply as to the requirement of reasonableness in consenting to sub-letting or assignment (see above). An example of unreasonable refusal can be found in the case of *Anglia Building Society* v. *Sheffield County Council* (1983) in which the refusal was held to be unreasonable where it was used merely as an attempt to secure an advantage for the landlord wholly unconnected with the lease, and wholly outside the intention of the parties.

The correct procedure for challenging the reasonableness of the landlord's decision is to seek a declaration in the county court under section 53 of the Landlord and Tenant Act 1954. If the refusal is declared unreasonable, the covenant becomes of no effect, and the tenant can change the use he makes of the premises as desired.

Landlord's remedies for tenant's breach of user covenant   Where the tenant breaches the change of user covenant, the landlord has a remedy in damages; and where the covenant contains a proviso for re-entry, the lease may be forfeited. The court may also grant an interlocutory injunction preventing the change of use pending a full trial of the issue.

It should be remembered that the change of use will be subject to any restrictive covenants attaching to the freehold of the premises, and to planning regulations. Any change of use should therefore always be carried out in consultation with the landlord.

Covenants against alterations or improvements

A lease may contain covenants not to carry out any alterations or improvements to the premises. These may be either absolute prohibitions, or qualified by the requirement of the landlord's consent. If the covenant is absolute, the tenant's hands are tied. Where the landlord's consent is required, section 19(2) of the Landlord and Tenant Act 1927 provides that any refusal must be reasonable if the alterations amount to improvements. The section also provides that the landlord: may require a sum of money for any diminution in the value of the premises, or of any neighbouring premises belonging to the landlord; *or* may require the tenant to reinstate the premises to its original state at the conclusion of the tenancy.

The court will decide whether an alteration amounts to an improvement from the tenant's point of view (*Lambert* v. *F.W. Woolworth and Co. Ltd* (1938)). It was also said in that case that many considerations, aesthetic, historic or even personal, may be relied upon as yielding reasonable grounds for refusing consent.

A tenant who breaches a covenant against alteration or improvement may be liable in damages and to forfeiture should the landlord succeed in proving that his consent was not unreasonably withheld. Therefore, as with activities encroaching on all types of covenants, the tenant should negotiate with the landlord, and as a last resort seek a declaration from the county court.

Repairing covenants

Covenants obliging either party to repair the premises will either be express or implied. In commercial leases such covenants will usually be expressed in the lease. Should no such covenants be contained in the lease, obligations may be implied by common law.

The only obligation imposed on the tenant at common law is to occupy the premises in a tenant-like manner, i.e. to take reasonable care of the premises and to make good any damage which is caused by the tenant or his employees or visitors. This does not extend to making good minor damage caused by fair wear and tear.

A landlord is obliged to maintain his own premises ancillary to the leased premises where maintenance of his premises is necessary for the enjoyment of the leased premises. For example, where the tenant has leased a shop on the ground floor of premises, the remainder of which is owned by the landlord, the landlord will be obliged to maintain the roof and common parts of the building unless the lease expressly provides otherwise.

The landlord may also be obliged to carry out such repairs as are necessary to give business efficacy to the agreement. For example, where the tenant has covenanted to maintain and repair the interior, the landlord may be required to ensure the good repair of the exterior.

Express covenants to repair Express covenants to repair are usually expressed as obligations to keep the premises in good, habitable or tenantable repair. The old case of *Proudfoot* v. *Hart* (1890) provides general guidance that this means:

'such repair as, having regard to the age, character and locality of the premises, would make it reasonably fit for the occupation of a reasonably minded tenant of the class who would be likely to take it at the time when the lease was granted.'

Covenants to repair do not create an obligation to renew or improve the premises. The line between repair and improvement is a difficult one to draw, but as a rule of thumb, the duty can be no higher than restoring the premises to the condition in which they were originally found. The question of what amounts to simple repair is a question to be decided in the specific circumstances. For example, repair will not normally include the duty to cure inherent defects in the premises, e.g., replacing defective guttering. However, in some circumstances the secondary damage can only be repaired by repairing the primary cause. The repair of the primary cause may be construed as an improvement, but may nevertheless be covered by the repairing covenant. The tenant is not obliged to repair a structural defect in the building which pre-dates the commencement of the lease (*Quick* v. *Taff Ely Borough Council* (1985)). If, however, a pre-existing defect causes secondary damage, e.g. a leaking roof causing damp penetration, secondary damage caused during the period of the lease will have to be repaired by the tenant.

Special care should be taken prior to the signing of the lease to ensure that the tenant is not to be held liable for the re-building of premises destroyed by fire or flood etc. It is common for the liability for rebuilding to be expressly attached to the landlord in the lease.

Landlord's remedies for breach of repairing covenant If a tenant is in breach of his covenant to repair, the landlord has the remedies of damages and forfeiture. The measure of damages is the difference between the value of the unrepaired premises, and the value of the premises had the repairs been executed. However, if it is the landlord's intention to demolish the premises at the end of the tenancy, there will be no justification for such an award of damages.

Forfeiture If a landlord seeks to obtain forfeiture of the premises consequent upon a breach of a repairing covenant, he must serve a notice under section 146 of the Law of Property Act 1925 containing details of the breach, requiring the breach to be remedied, and requiring the payment of compensation. In the case of premises leased for at least seven years with at least three years left to run, special procedures are provided by the Leasehold Property (Repairs) Act 1938. When the landlord serves a notice under section 46 of the Law of Property Act 1925, he must inform the tenant of his right to serve a counter-notice under the 1938 Act. If a counter-notice is served within 28 days, the landlord's action cannot proceed without the leave of the court. Leave will only be granted if one of the following five circumstances exists.

(1) The value of the landlord's interest in the premises has been, or is likely to be, substantially diminished if the repairs are not carried out.
(2) The repair is necessary to comply with an order of any authority or local byelaw.

(3) Where the tenant does not occupy the premises, the repair is necessary in the interests of another occupier.
(4) An immediate repair will avoid further deterioration leading to more expensive repairs.
(5) There are special circumstances making leave to proceed just and equitable.

The landlord does not have to prove the existence of one of these grounds outright, but merely has to show a prima facie ground.

Right of entry to repair   Under some leases the landlord may have a right to enter the premises to carry out repairs, and to recover the cost of repairs as a debt. The landlord cannot force the tenant to carry out the repairs (i.e. the contractual remedy of specific performance is not available), but must pursue his remedies of damages or forfeiture.

Tenant's remedies for breach of repairing covenant   The tenant of business premises may sue the landlord for damages if the landlord is in breach of a repairing covenant. In the past, damages have been awarded for discomfort, loss of enjoyment of the premises, and bouts of ill-health caused by the poor state of repair. There have also been some indications in the decided cases that the cost of alternative accommodation is recoverable. The landlord of business premises cannot be forced to repair, i.e. the remedy of specific performance is not available to the tenant.

Cost of repairs set off against rent   The case of *Lee Parker* v. *Izzet* (1971) decided that a tenant may deduct the cost of repairs from future rent. However, to avoid complications over whether the amounts spent on repair are reasonable, it is advisable for a tenant to obtain a county court declaration that the landlord is in breach of his covenant.

Insurance covenants

A commercial lease will make express provision for the insurance of the building. Often the tenant will be required to pay the insurance premiums and to refrain from acts which will suspend the cover.

Destruction of a building   A clause will usually be inserted to oblige the landlord to use insurance moneys to rebuild the premises should they be destroyed during the period of the lease. In the absence of such a covenant, the landlord will not be obliged to rebuild the premises.

Where a building has been destroyed and the landlord does not intend to rebuild, a dispute may arise as to which of the parties is entitled to the insurance moneys and in what proportions. Following the case of *Beacon Carpets Limited* v. *Kirkby* (1984) the most likely outcome is that the moneys will be divided between the parties in proportion to their interest in the building.

Rent

Commercial leases will invariably contain express terms setting out:

- the amount of rent to be paid
- the times at which it is to be paid
- the consequences of non-payment (usually forfeiture)

and often provision for a review of the amount of rent payable at a set date or dates during the tenancy.

It must be noted that the rent is payable for the land upon which the premises stand, and not for the premises themselves. Therefore, should the building be destroyed during the period of the lease, rent continues to be payable.

Rent on assignment or sub-letting

Until the Landlord and Tenant (Covenants) Act 1995, an original tenant used to be liable to the landlord for rent under the terms of the lease, even where he had assigned or sub-let the lease with the landlord's permission. The 1995 Act was passed to alleviate the considerable hardship which this rule imposed on original tenants, requiring them in effect to guarantee payment of rent for the duration of the term of the lease, even after their interest in the lease had been assigned to a third party.

The effect of the Act in easing the position of tenants is to some extent mitigated by allowing landlords to require tenants to enter into 'authorised guarantee agreements' which guarantee payments by the immediate person to whom the tenant may in future assign the lease, a transaction over which the tenant does, after all, have some control. The legal status of these guarantees, known as 'AGAs', is presently uncertain and any pharmacist who is asked to provide an authorised guarantee should obtain legal advice before doing so.

A landlord can assign his interest (the 'reversion') in the premises to a third party. If so, the rent becomes payable to the assignee, but only if the landlord has issued a notice to the tenant complying with section 151(1) of the Law of Property Act 1925.

Guarantors

If payment of rent is secured by guarantors under the terms of the lease, they will be fully liable for payment of unpaid rent should the tenant fall into arrear. The guarantors are then left to pursue the tenant for the sums in which they have been held liable. Where the tenant is a small private company it is common for landlords to require the directors or main shareholders (who are usually the same) to give guarantees in their personal capacity. This is to protect the landlord in the event of the company going into liquidation but means the directors/ shareholders carry considerable personal risk.

Rent review

A commercial lease will usually contain a clause stating that at a fixed date or dates during the lease the rent will be revised by an independent third party, usually a surveyor. The lease may provide that the landlord and tenant should agree on the appointment of a surveyor jointly, or it may provide that a third party, e.g. the President of the Royal Institution of Chartered Surveyors, should make the appointment.

The review clause will specify that the rent is to be revised according to the current market rent. The decision of the surveyor is usually expressed to be final, and a clause is often inserted whereby even if the surveyor determines that a reasonable market rent would be less than that already being paid, rent will nevertheless continue to be paid at the existing rate.

The surveyor is under a duty to carry out the rent review according to his professional standards. All relevant factors will be taken into account such as the rent being paid for similar premises in the same area, the condition of the premises and the effect of, for example, the existence of a covenant restricting change of user. For obvious reasons, it is vitally important that the tenant make himself aware of the rent review procedure at the outset.

Consequences of non-payment of rent

The usual remedy for non-payment of rent is forfeiture. All formal leases will inevitably include a clause providing for the surrender of the premises if the rent should cease to be paid for a specified period after the due date. The usual procedure is for the landlord to make a formal demand for unpaid rent before commencing forfeiture proceedings, although many leases will dispense with this requirement.

Once he has commenced forfeiture proceedings, if the landlord then does any act which indicates that he accepts the continuation of the tenancy, he loses the right to forfeiture. Accepting payment of arrears would constitute such an act. However, the landlord still has the right to receive rent for the continuing occupation. Such sums are known as 'mesne profits' (pronounced 'meen'), and are assessed at current market rates.

Relief against forfeiture   In High Court proceedings the tenant has a right to relief against forfeiture of the lease where he is no more than six months in arrears *and* if he pays all outstanding sums and costs into court before judgment is given.

Thereafter there is a mere equitable right to relief upon payment of all arrears and costs at any time up to six months from the date of the landlord's re-entry. As the right is only equitable, it will be granted only where the High Court considers it fair to do so in all the circumstances.

In county court proceedings, the tenant has the automatic right to relief against forfeiture if all arrears and costs are paid up to five days before the date set for the possession hearing.

Under section 138 of the County Courts Act 1984, the court has a discretion to order relief against forfeiture if all costs and arrears are paid within four weeks after the granting of the order for possession. By section 55 of the Administration of Justice Act 1985, the High Court may grant relief against forfeiture ordered by the County Court for up to six months following the date of the order.

Renewal of tenancies

The procedure for the renewal of business tenancies and compensation for improvements carried out by a tenant during the currency of the lease is governed by Part II of the Landlord and Tenant Act 1954, and by Part I of the Landlord and Tenant Act 1927. These statutes create mechanisms which come into play at the end of a tenancy, and which have as their object the resolution of matters between landlord and tenant by means of mutual agreement rather than resort to the courts.

The legislation creates a framework of procedural steps which must be complied with if a business tenancy is to be terminated, and provides for the continuation of the tenancy on its existing terms should these steps not have been taken. The legislation also creates a right to request a renewal of the tenancy for a period of up to fourteen years.

Tenancies covered by the legislation

Section 23 of the 1954 Act states that the Act covers:

> 'any tenancy where the property comprised in the tenancy is or includes premises which are occupied by the tenant and are so occupied for the purposes of a business carried on by him or for those and other purposes.'

These words are to a large extent self-evident. Formally agreed business leases in documentary form will invariably be covered if the business is not being carried out in breach of a user clause.

Under section 43(3)(a), the Act does not normally apply to tenancies granted for a period of less than six months where there is no provision for renewing the term. However, if in that case the tenant has been in occupation for over twelve months he is deemed to have an established business which will be protected by the Act. The only other notable exceptions are leases where the landlord is a government department, local authority, a statutory undertaking or a development corporation, or where the landlord has specified that the use of the premises will change on a specified date.

Contracting out of the 1954 Act

The parties to the lease may contract out of the 1954 Act, and thereby avoid the protection afforded by it, by making an application to the County Court, either before the commencement of the lease or at any time during the currency of the lease, under section 38. Contracting out can only be achieved through joint application: neither party can exclude the protection of the Act unilaterally.

The procedure for renewal

Section 24(1) of the 1954 Act provides that the lease will continue after its expiry upon the same terms as during the currency of the lease, until either party issues a notice to renew the tenancy.

The renewal procedure may be initiated by either the landlord or the tenant issuing a notice in the prescribed form. A tenant may make a request for a new tenancy under section 26. In order to issue such a notice, the tenant must have held the lease for at least one year and must request a starting date for a new tenancy between six and twelve months from the date of service of the notice. The notice must also refer to the property to be comprised in the new lease and to the terms and rent proposed. The landlord may serve a counter-notice to the request stating his grounds of opposition. He must do so within two months of the service of the tenant's notice.

The tenant cannot serve a notice under section 26:

(1) if the landlord has already served a notice under section 25 (see below); *or*
(2) if the tenant has already given notice to quit; *or*
(3) if he has given notice under section 27 that he will be surrendering the lease at the end of the fixed term.

Under section 25 the landlord may serve a notice to propose a new tenancy (usually with modified rent), or to state grounds of objection to a new tenancy under section 30. The landlord's notice cannot take effect until a specified date between six and twelve months from the date of service, and in any event, not before the expiry date of a fixed term lease. The notice must contain the proposed terms of the new lease, or if continuation is objected to, the grounds of objection must be set out. The tenant must serve a counter-notice within two months of the service of the landlord's notice stating whether he intends to give up possession.

In theory, the notice procedure is intended to stimulate negotiations between the landlord and tenant and to encourage settlement between the parties. Failure of either side to respond to a notice issued by the other within the prescribed two month period will result in an agreement being presumed in the terms of the notice. If no settlement has been achieved within four months of the issue of the notice, sections 29(3) and 24(1) require the parties to apply to the court for resolution of dispute. An application will either be for the grant of a new tenancy, or for possession.

During the negotiation period, the landlord may apply under section 24A of the Act for an interim rent to be determined by the court. The court will fix a rent which 'it would be reasonable for the tenant to pay'.

The landlord's grounds of opposition   Under section 30 the landlord has seven grounds of opposition to the grant of a renewed tenancy.

(1) Failure of the tenant to comply with repairing obligations under the lease resulting in the property being in a state of disrepair. The extent of the disrepair and the requirements of the repairing covenant will be the major factors the court will have to consider in exercising its discretion under this head.
(2) Persistent delay by the tenant in paying rent when it has become due.
(3) Other substantial breaches of covenant by the tenant, or 'any other reason connected with the tenant's use or management of the holding'. There is considerable room for judicial discretion under this head, but substantial and/or frequent breaches of covenant will have to be proved by the landlord.
(4) The offer by the landlord of suitable alternative premises on terms which are reasonable having regard to the terms of the current tenancy, and to all other relevant circumstances, e.g. the suitability of the proposed new premises for the tenant's business including the tenant's need to preserve goodwill.
(5) Where the current tenancy is a sub-letting of part of premises in which the landlord has an interest in the freehold reversion at the conclusion of the superior tenancy, and the landlord could get a much better return by letting the premises as a whole.

(6) Where on the termination of the tenancy the landlord intends to demolish or reconstruct the whole or a substantial part of the premises, and the proposed works can only be carried out by obtaining possession. In order for the landlord to succeed under this head he must be able to prove his intent at the date of the hearing. This is usually done by pointing to some actual steps which have been taken towards carrying out the intention. In order for the requirement of reconstruction to be proved, it must be proved that the demolition of at least part of the premises will be necessitated (*Cadle* v. *Jacmarch* (1957)).

The tenant has two defences, provided by section 31A, to the assertion that possession is required to execute the work:

(a) That a new lease could be granted, but containing a clause permitting the landlord to enter to execute the works. This will only succeed if it can be shown that the tenant's business will not be substantially interfered with or for a substantial time, and that the works can be carried out with the tenant remaining; *or*

(b) That the tenant could be granted a new lease in an economically severable part of the premises, and that the granting of such a lease would not prevent the landlord from carrying out the works.

(7) That the landlord intends to use the premises or part of them for his own business or residence at the end of the tenancy. This ground of objection requires the landlord to prove his intent, and to show that he is the one who will occupy the premises. It is not sufficient for him to intend to let it to others.

Where the landlord succeeds in proving one of the grounds for objection, he will be awarded possession after the expiry of a minimum period of three months.

Under section 31(2), if the court decides that one of the grounds (4), (5), or (6) above are not proved at the date of the hearing, but would be in twelve months time, the grant of a new tenancy may nevertheless be refused. In this event the tenant can apply to the court under section 31(2) for possession to be delayed for a year.

The grant of a new tenancy

Where no objection is raised by the landlord or where his objection fails, the tenant may be granted a new tenancy. Under section 32, the tenant has a prima facie right to a tenancy only of the premises to which the original lease applied. If this raises matters of dispute, they can be resolved by the court.

The court is in theory entitled to award a new tenancy of anything up to fourteen years' duration, but in practice tends only to grant leases of similar length to that which previously subsisted.

Rent under the new tenancy may be fixed by the court where the landlord and tenant fail to agree. It will be fixed at a level at which 'having regard to the terms of the tenancy, the holding might be expected to be let on the open market by a willing lessor ...' However, the court will not take into account the following:

(1) The tenant's previous occupation.
(2) Any goodwill attaching to the premises generated by the tenant's business.
(3) Improvements carried out by the tenant other than those required by covenant, provided: that the tenancy has always been protected by the Act, that the improvements were carried out within 21 years of the renewal *and* provided that the tenant did not surrender the premises at the end of the tenancy in which the improvements were carried out.
(4) The value attributable to a liquor licence on licensed premises.

Under section 35, the court has a very wide discretion to determine other terms of a new lease which the landlord and tenant have failed to agree, but there will be a strong presumption in favour of the terms of the original lease. This presumption can be rebutted if there is good reason, but such reasons would have to be very strong, e.g. certain terms will need to be included in order to give commercial efficacy to the agreement.

Tenant's compensation at the end of a tenancy

At the conclusion of a tenancy, whether by surrender or by court order, the tenant may be able to recover compensation for improvements made during the lease. Under section 37 of the 1954 Act the right to compensation arises where the tenant has been unsuccessful in obtaining a renewed tenancy due to a successful objection by the landlord on one of the grounds numbered (4), (5), and (6) in the list in the section above entitled 'The landlord's grounds of opposition' (i.e. the grounds in section 30), providing that the landlord has not offered suitable alternative accommodation.

The right to compensation is restricted by section 38 to tenants who have been in occupation for at least five years. However, if the tenant is a successor to a business which has been carried on on the premises for at least five years, the right will remain even if the successor has been in occupation for less than five years.

The parties may contract out of the compensation provisions at any time before the commencement or during the currency of the lease, as part of an application to the court to contract out of the protection afforded by the Act generally.

The amount of compensation payable is dependent upon the length of time the tenant has been in occupation. Section 37 provides that tenants who have been in occupation for more than 14 years will receive a sum of twice the rateable value of the premises times the 'multiplier' (which is currently three). Tenants who have been in occupation for less than 14 years will receive the rateable value times the multiplier.

Compensation for improvements

At the conclusion of a tenancy the tenant is able to claim compensation for loss of authorized improvements carried out by the tenant under section 1 of the Landlord and Tenant Act 1927.

The availability of compensation will not be affected by the reason for the termination of the tenancy, although the lease must have been formally terminated.

An application to the court for compensation must be made within three months of the service of the landlord's counter-notice if the tenant has terminated the tenancy by applying for a renewal; between six and three months before the termination of the tenancy if it is to terminate by effluxion of time; or within three months of a court order for forfeiture or re-entry.

In order to claim compensation the following requirements must *all* be met.

(1) The premises must have been used for business purposes.
(2) The improvements must have been executed by the tenant.
(3) The improvements must not have been executed pursuant to an obligation under the lease.
(4) The landlord must agree, or the court must have issued a certificate stating that the improvements add to the value of the premises without devaluing neighbouring property of the landlord.
(5) A formal claim for compensation must be made to the court.

Level of compensation

Section 1 of the 1927 Act provides that the level of compensation will be calculated either on the basis of the additional value to the premises by the improvements, or on the basis of the cost of carrying out the improvements at the end of the tenancy, minus an appropriate sum representing the cost of putting the improvements into a good state of repair. The court has a discretion to settle any differences arising and finally to settle the compensation sums.

Misrepresentation

Where the tenant can show that the court's refusal to grant a new tenancy was based on a misrepresentation by the landlord, 'the court may order the landlord to pay to the tenant such sum as appears sufficient as compensation for damage or loss sustained by the tenant as a result of the order or refusal' (section 55 of the 1954 Act). For example, where the landlord has successfully opposed an application for a renewed tenancy on the basis that he intends to use the premises for his own business, if he subsequently lets the premises to another party, the former tenant may apply for compensation to the court which ordered possession.

Compulsory acquisition

If the premises are acquired compulsorily, in assessing the compensation payable, the local authority is obliged, by section 47 of the Land Compensation Act 1973, to assess the potential loss that may be suffered by the tenant as a result of his loss of rights to renew the tenancy of the lease.

Chapter 24

Business Associations

When setting up in business there are several different ways in which a pharmacist may operate. He may set up either as a sole trader, in partnership with some other party, as a limited liability partnership, or as a corporate body. Each manner of operation has certain advantages and disadvantages. These are considered in this section of the book, with particular reference being made to the limited company.

The sole trader

The sole trader carries on business in either his own name or one created for the business. He bears the burden of full personal responsibility for the business and all its liabilities. Unlike a limited company, in which the company and its managing director are separate legal entities, the sole trader and his business are one and the same thing: the sole trader is liable for all the debts of the business, and his personal property is therefore put at risk.

Trading as a sole trader is therefore advisable only for those who do not expect to incur business debts or liabilities on any large scale. In setting up a pharmacy, a sizeable outlay will be made in the purchase of business premises and stock, and the potential personal liability will be considerable.

Partnership

Partnerships are comparatively common, and so require considerably more explanation. A partnership arises where two or more persons carry on a business in common with a view to making a profit. A partnership is called a firm, but the partnership has no legal entity of its own and the liability of the partners is personal.

The law relating to partnerships is to be found mostly in the Partnership Act 1890. This statute lays down the rules for determining the existence of a partnership, the relationship between partners and third parties, the relationship between partners, and the rules governing termination of partnerships.

All references to statutory sections below are to the Partnership Act unless otherwise indicated.

Partners and third parties

Every partner is an agent of the firm, and accordingly any acts done as a partner, including the incurring of extensive liabilities, will bind all the other partners.

The relationship between partners therefore has to be based upon a high degree of trust. The exception to this rule is where a partner pledges the credit of the firm for his own personal debts. In this event the firm will not be bound.

The partners' liabilities for the firm are joint and several. Thus each partner is potentially liable for the whole of the firm's liabilities, subject to the partners' rights of indemnity against each other. However, the right of indemnity may be of little use where only one of the partners in a firm has sufficient funds to pay a judgment debt to a creditor; he will have to pay the creditor and take his chance against the other partners.

By sections 10, 11, and 12 of the Act, partners are rendered liable for wrongful acts and omissions of other partners acting in the ordinary course of business or with the consent of the other partners, and for misapplication of money or property received for the firm or in the firm's custody. However, a partner is not liable for any liabilities incurred by the firm while he is not a partner. Furthermore, by section 14, any person who is not a partner of the firm, but who holds himself out as being a partner, is liable to the representee as if he were a partner.

Relations between partners

Formally created partnerships are usually governed by a partnership deed which will set out the rights and obligations of the partners in the firm. There is no express requirement for a partnership deed, but it lends certainty. By section 19 of the Act, partners may vary the terms of their partnership by mutual consent, or such variation may be implied from a course of dealing.

Fiduciary duty

The basic duty of a partner towards the others is one of good faith, i.e. to act honestly and for the benefit of the partnership as a whole. In modern times this is known as a fiduciary duty. There are three statutory aspects to this duty.

(1) Section 28 provides that 'partners are bound to render a true account of all things affecting the partnership to any partner or his legal representative'. This means that partners are bound to inform each other of all material facts in relation to partnership business.

(2) Section 29 provides that 'every partner must account to the firm for any benefit derived by him without the consent of the other partners from any transaction concerning the partnership, or from any use made by him of the partnership name or business connection'. An example of the operation of this section is where a partner makes a secret profit which he fails to disclose to the others. When it is discovered, the others may take out an action for account which may result in the secret profit being re-distributed amongst the partners.

(3) Section 30 provides that 'if a partner, without the consent of the other partners, carries on any business of the same nature as and competing with that of the firm, he must account for and pay over to the firm all profits made by him in that business'. This section is quite clear; the key question is whether the other business is in competition with the firm. If competition is established, liability is established.

Partnership property

Additionally, section 20 provides that all property originally brought into the partnership or acquired on account of the firm for the purposes and in the course of partnership business, constitutes partnership property and must be held and applied as such in accordance with the partnership agreement. Thus all partnership property is held jointly by all the partners for their mutual benefit.

Unless the contrary intention appears in the partnership agreement, the following provisions, created by the Act, apply.

Section 21 provides simply that unless it has been agreed otherwise, property bought with the firm's money is deemed to have been bought on behalf of the firm and will therefore be held for the benefit of all the partners.

Section 22 provides that all partnership property is to be treated as personal rather than real property. Thus if a partnership owns property or land, the interest of each of the partners is in their share of the potential proceeds of sale, and not in the land or property itself.

Section 24 provides that:

(1) Partners are entitled to take part in the management of the business, but are not entitled to remuneration for so doing. The idea is that each partner will receive his reward by a straightforward share of the profits, and possibly interest on his original capital investment.
(2) Partners are entitled to indemnity from the firm in respect of liabilities incurred in the proper conduct of the business or in its preservation. Partners are therefore entitled to reimbursement for expenses etc., incurred whilst carrying out partnership business.
(3) Partners are entitled to equal shares in the capital and profits of the firm, and are liable to contribute equally towards losses.
(4) Partners are entitled to interest on money advanced to the firm, but not on capital until the profits have been ascertained. In practice this provision makes little difference, as interest is frequently payable on capital, but it creates the automatic right to interest on money lent to the firm, subject to contrary agreement.

Taxation

A joint assessment to tax is made in the partnership name (Income and Corporation Taxes Act 1988). However, each partner may make a separate claim for allowances and deductions, his income from the partnership being deemed to be the share to which he is entitled in the partnership profits.

Termination of partnership

Where the partnership is for an indefinite duration, it may be dissolved by one partner giving notice to the others (section 32 of the Partnership Act 1890). A partnership may also be dissolved by the court on the application of a partner:

(1) Where one of the partners becomes permanently incapable of performing his part of the partnership contract.

(2) Where one of the partners has been guilty of conduct calculated to prejudice the carrying on of the business.
(3) Where the business of the partnership can only be carried on at a loss.
(4) Where circumstances arise which make it just and equitable that the partnership is dissolved.

A partnership may also be rescinded like any other contract for fraud or misrepresentation. In this eventuality section 41 gives the partner who has been the victim of the misrepresentation or fraud at the hands of another partner, the right to an indemnity for his loss and rights over partnership property to cover his loss.

On dissolution, the property of the partnership is applied first in the payment of the firm's debts and liabilities, then in the payment of what is due to each partner, first for advances and then for capital. Any surplus is divided among the partners in the proportion in which profits are divisible (according to the terms of the partnership agreement). Losses are paid out of profits if there are any, and if not, out of capital. If the residual capital is insufficient, losses are paid personally by the partners in the proportion in which they were entitled to profits.

Limited partnership

The limited partnership is a hybrid form where the firm has at least one general partner with unlimited liability, and one or more limited partners who contribute money or property to the partnership and are liable only to the extent of their contribution. This form of partnership is governed by the Limited Partnership Act 1907.

The main reason for instituting a limited partnership is to attract capital into the business. Hence the provisions in the Limited Partnership Act that the limited partner is prohibited on pain of unlimited liability from taking part in the management of the business and cannot bind the firm; his death or bankruptcy does not dissolve the partnership; his consent to the introduction of a new partner is not necessary; he has no power to dissolve the partnership; the charging of his share (i.e. the raising of money against it) is not a ground for dissolution; and he can take no part in the winding-up of partnership affairs unless the court directs. Furthermore the limited partner is unable to withdraw any part of his contribution during the continuance of the partnership. Precisely because the position of the limited partner is so precarious, i.e., he has no right to determine what use is made of his investment in the partnership, there are very few limited partnerships in existence. The modern simplification of the process of creating a limited company has almost entirely replaced the limited partnership.

Disadvantages of partnerships

The major disadvantage of partnership is the unlimited liability of members. The creation of a limited company avoids this problem and is far more attractive to those wishing to set up in a business which is going to incur any level of indebtedness, or in which extensive commercial risks will be taken. The many small businesses which make the transition to company status enjoy comparative security and have a prescribed structure within which to conduct the firm's affairs.

Limited liability partnership

From 6 April 2001 pharmacists have been able to utilize a new trading entity introduced by the Limited Liability Partnerships Act 2000. This new entity may be formed by two or more persons 'associated for carrying on a lawful business with a view to profit', and unlike a partnership, the entity will have a legal personality in its own right. The partners in a limited liability partnership may be individuals or companies, and since the entity will have its own legal identity the partners will not have any contractual liability to the partnership's creditors. It is unclear at the present time whether circumstances may arise where the corporate veil will be lifted in a case where an individual acts negligently.

The internal arrangements between the partners will closely resemble the position in a conventional partnership. Relations between the partners will be regulated by agreement, and where there is no agreement, the provisions in the Partnership Act 1890 will apply. However, the limited liability partnership will have to file an annual return, with audited accounts, and many of the provisions of the Companies Acts will apply. Partners will be taxed individually, and the creation of a limited liability partnership will be tax neutral. At the time of writing, a final version of the draft regulations giving further details about the proposed operation of a limited liability partnership is awaited.

There is no restriction on the type of business that can trade as a limited liability partnership. It is expected that the main users of limited liability partnerships will be firms of accountants and solicitors, but there is no reason why others, such as pharmacists, should not conduct their professional activities using this entity.

At the present time it is difficult to tell whether this new entity will prove popular with pharmacists as a vehicle for professional practice. It is quite possible that the more familiar limited company will continue to be a more attractive proposition when the competing advantages and disadvantages are taken into account.

The limited company

There are three types of limited company, the most significant of which for present purposes is the private limited company. The others are the public limited company and the company limited by guarantee.

Public limited companies (plcs) are usually quite large operations. They must have an allotted share capital of at least £50 000 (one quarter of which must be paid up), and the company may offer their shares or debentures (explained below) for sale to the public. Many public limited companies are quoted on the Stock Exchange, and their shares may be bought and sold through stockbrokers. Their basic structure, however, is similar to that of the private limited company (explained below).

Companies limited by guarantee are usually non-profit making companies formed for purposes ranging from the charitable, religious or educational, to the merely administrative, such as companies set up to manage a block of flats on behalf of the residents. This form of company is used chiefly as a method of incorporating groups of persons with common interest who do not have profit as the main motive.

Advantages of creating a limited company

There are a number of advantages in trading as a private limited company which can be summarized as follows.

(1) The liability of the members is limited to the value of their shares.
(2) The company has a legal personality of its own separate from its members.
(3) The name of the company is prevented from being used by other companies.
(4) There are certain advantages in borrowing money (see below).
(5) The interests and responsibilities of the persons engaged in the business are clearly defined, including the management responsibilities of the firm.
(6) The company has a continuing existence of its own independent of its members.
(7) In some circumstances there are taxation advantages.
(8) Whereas in the case of a sole trader maximum pensions contributions are limited on a sliding scale depending upon age to a percentage of income between 17.5% and 40%, there are greater possibilities for the directors of a company.
(9) The appointment, retirement or removal of directors is carried out in the prescribed manner.
(10) Employees may gain the opportunity of acquiring shares in the company, and outside investors may become shareholders.

The company's legal personality

An incorporated company has a separate legal personality which enables it to carry transactions and other functions in its own right. For example, the company may enter into contracts, purchase or lease property, sue or be sued in the company name.

A company is the beneficial owner of its own property, i.e. it does not hold it as trustee for its members, and they have no legal or equitable interest in it.

A company's transactions are carried out solely in the company name. A shareholder cannot enforce a contract made by his company; he is neither a party to the contract nor entitled to the benefit of it. Likewise, a shareholder cannot be sued on contracts made by his company, nor can a court compel a shareholder to vote at a company's general meeting in such a way as to ensure that the company fulfils its contractual obligations, or prohibit him from voting in any other way.

A member of a company cannot sue in respect of civil wrongs (known technically as 'torts') committed against the company, and cannot be sued for such wrongs committed by it. Even where it is proved that the company has committed a tort, the directors will only be liable where it can be shown that they actually participated in its commission.

Exceptions to the rule of separate legal identity

There are several exceptions to the rule that companies have a separate legal personality.

First, if a company continues trading without having at least two members for a period of more than six months, the person who is the remaining member during any period after the six months has elapsed, is liable jointly and severally with the company for its debts contracted during that period (section 24 of the Companies Act 1985). Liability does not arise until the period of six months has elapsed, and relates only to debts incurred after the expiration of that period. Liability can therefore be avoided by the single shareholder transferring some of his shares to a third party before the time expires. Furthermore, the remaining member will only be held personally liable for debts incurred at a time when he was a member of the company.

Secondly, if a person is involved in the management of a company while he is an undischarged bankrupt, or while a court order preventing him from being a company director remains in force, he will be personally liable for the debts of the company incurred while he is a director or is concerned in its management. A person who knowingly acts on the instructions of an undischarged bankrupt or of a person who is disqualified by court order from being a director, is also liable for company debts.

Thirdly, under the 1986 Insolvency Act, it is an offence for a person who has been a director of a company in the 12 months before it went into liquidation, to be a director of, or to be concerned directly or indirectly in the promotion, formation or management of another company with the same or similar name without leave of the court. A person committing this offence, or a person knowingly acting on the instructions of such a person, will be liable for the debts and liabilities of the company incurred during the period in which instructions were carried out for a person committing the offence.

Fourthly, if, when a company is wound up, it appears that it has been trading with intent to defraud its creditors or the creditors of another person, or for any other fraudulent purpose, the court may, on the application of the liquidator, order that any persons who are knowingly trading in that way are to be personally liable to such extent as the court thinks fit. A person who participates in fraudulent trading is guilty of a criminal offence, and a prosecution may be brought whether the company is being wound up or not.

Fifthly, if in the winding-up of a company which has gone into insolvent liquidation, it appears that a person who was a director at the time before the commencement of the winding-up knew or ought to have concluded that there was no reasonable prospect that the company would avoid such a liquidation, on the liquidator's application the court may order that person to contribute such amount to the assets of the company as it thinks fit. Such an order can be made where the director cannot be proved knowingly and fraudulently to have carried on the business, but where by the exercise of proper skill and care he must have concluded that liquidation could not be avoided.

Sixthly, in a minute number of cases the court may disregard the separate legal identity of a company where there is an overriding public interest in doing so, e.g. where in war time all the directors of a company are enemy aliens.

Seventhly, in a small number of cases the courts have disregarded the separate legal identity of a company where it had been formed solely for the evasion of a legal liability. For example, in *Gilford Motor Co* v. *Horne* (1933), a former company employee sought to evade the effect of a 'no competition' clause in his contract with his former employer by setting up a company in direct competition. The court decided that the company was a 'mere cloak or sham' employed solely to evade the effect of the clause, and an injunction was issued preventing the company from carrying on business in competition.

Eighthly, in some cases the courts have ignored the separate legal personality of a company where it appears that the company was acting as an agent for its shareholders, or that the company held its property as trustee for its shareholders. This is very rare and will usually occur only where the strict application of the principle of separate personality would work an injustice. This result may occur where, for example, the directors of a subsidiary company are also all directors of the parent holding company, and where the two companies carry on the same business and use the same accounting facilities. In such circumstances the court may discount the separate legal personality of the subsidiary and treat it merely as an agent of the holding company.

Limited liability

The concept of limited liability means that the liability of a company's shareholders is limited to the value of their shares (including any amount unpaid towards the value of the shares). In most private companies shares are fully paid up, so investors stand only to lose their investment plus any loan made to the company. Other potential liabilities may be personal guarantees for company borrowings or liabilities, e.g. bank overdrafts or guarantees of rent payments under business leases. In practice banks lending money to a small private company and landlords of business leases will inevitably require such personal guarantees so for these debts the concept of limited liability is a fiction.

If a company is unable to pay its debts, its creditors may petition the court to wind it up under the provisions of the Insolvency Act 1986. If the court orders the company to be wound up, a liquidator is appointed to realise the company's assets. If he fails to realize sufficient to meet liabilities through the sale of company assets, then the value of the shares in the company will be called up.

As a shareholder is not liable to pay the company's debts himself, a creditor of the company cannot sue him. A creditor can only obtain unpaid capital by petitioning the court to wind the company up, and awaiting such payment as can be met by the liquidator. The liquidator discharges the company's debts rateably, thereby ensuring that one creditor does not get preferred treatment merely by being the first to sue. (The protection afforded by limited liability is of course subject to the exceptions to the principle of separate legal identity discussed above.)

The protection of company names

Protection is given to company names by the Companies Act 1985. Under the Act the Registrar of Companies is not permitted to register a company in a name which is already in use. The Department of Trade and Industry is also empowered under the Act to require a company to change its name within a year of incorporation if it is the same as, or too similar to a name already on the register.

A certain amount of protection is afforded to partnership names under the Business Names Act 1985, but sole traders enjoy no such protection. However, if another business uses the name of a sole trader and members of the public can be shown to be unable to distinguish between the two concerns, the first user of the name may take out a 'passing off' action against the other for the damage done to his business. Such litigation is, however, costly and always carries substantial risk.

Financing the company – shares and loan capital

Shares

Most small companies have only one type of share known as ordinary shares. They are issued in order to provide permanent capital for the company, and will normally carry with them voting rights and an entitlement to a share of the company's profits or dividends.

The larger the company, usually the larger the number of shareholders. In companies where there are many shareholders, there may be different classes of shares. The most common form of shares other than ordinary shares are preference shares. The holder of preference shares is entitled to a dividend of a fixed amount before any dividend is paid to the holders of ordinary shares. The terms of issue of preference shares often provide that the holder is also entitled to a priority in the repayment of share capital in the event of a winding-up.

The preference shareholder is in a more secure position than the ordinary shareholder as he is entitled to fixed dividends, usually calculated as a percentage of the value of the shares. The ordinary shareholder however, has the opportunity of greater return as the level of dividend is not restricted to a fixed amount and will fluctuate in accordance with the company's profitability. Furthermore, in a winding-up, when preference shareholders have been repaid the nominal value of their shares, unless they have an express entitlement to a share in any surplus, the whole of the remaining assets of the company will be distributed among the ordinary shareholders in proportion to their holding.

Ordinary shareholders hold most of the power at general meetings, and it will be they who will control company affairs and appoint directors. Thus the ordinary shareholder has more rights in determining the way in which a company conducts itself, but the nature of the investment carries a greater risk.

Loan capital

Loan capital is an expression used to describe the long term indebtedness of the company secured by mortgages, debenture stock and loan stock. All companies have an implied power to borrow and to give security for loans made to them. Unless the company's Memorandum of Association (explained below) provides otherwise, the amount a company may borrow is unlimited.

One way in which a company may raise capital is to issue debentures. Debentures are similar to shares in that they have a nominal value. They are usually redeemable at a fixed future date, and their nominal value is the amount payable to the holder on redemption (unless by the terms of issue a premium is also payable on redemption). Debentures usually carry a fixed rate of interest on the amount invested in the company, and are usually secured by a fixed or floating charge over the company's assets. Thus in theory they represent a relatively safe form of investment. The debenture is therefore akin to an 'IOU' issued by a company to an investor, with pre-arranged terms concerning interest and repayment. As with preference shares, debentures enjoy priority in the repayment of interest and repayment of capital in the event of the company being wound up. However they do not carry voting rights, and holders do not participate in the running of the company.

Bank loans and overdrafts

Loans by banks are usually secured by a fixed or floating charge over company assets, and by personal guarantees given by directors. Even if assets are subject to a floating charge they may be dealt with freely, as the charge is not fixed to any asset or assets in particular until it becomes operational, i.e., until repayments are not made and the bank seeks to realize company assets to meet the debt. Loans subject to a fixed charge are secured against specific company assets, usually business premises and/or stock.

The creation and structure of a private limited company

The company name

When setting up a company, certain rules apply to the use of a company name.

(1) The new name must not be in the name of a company already on the register.
(2) Certain insensitive words cannot be used without the consent of the S of S or some other relevant body. For example, under section 78 of the MA 1968, the name 'chemist', 'druggist' or 'pharmacy' cannot be used unless it will apply to a registered pharmacy.
(3) The name must not give the impression of a connection with the government or local authority.
(4) The words 'limited', 'unlimited' or 'public limited company' must not be used except at the end of a name.
(5) The name must not be offensive.
(6) Unless exempted, the word 'limited' must be used at the end.

The S of S is empowered to direct a company to change its name where:

(1) The chosen name is too like a name already on the register.
(2) If within five years of incorporation he believes that false information was provided for the purpose of registration.
(3) If at the time the name by which it is registered gives so misleading an identification of the nature of its activities as to be likely to cause harm to the public.

It is imperative that once a company has been named, it continues to use exactly the same name, even down to the use of upper- and lower-case letters.

Formalities

To incorporate a company, various documents must be completed and lodged at Companies House.

(1) Memorandum of Association (discussed below).
(2) Articles of Association (discussed below).
(3) Statement of the particulars of the first director(s) and company secretary, together with their signed consents to acting in these capacities, and the address of the registered office.
(4) Statement of particulars of shares to be issued on incorporation signed by a director or by the secretary.
(5) Declaration of compliance with the Companies Act. This form may be made and signed either by a solicitor engaged in the formation, or by a director or by the secretary. The declaration must be made before a Commissioner for Oaths, Notary Public, Justice of the Peace, or solicitor having the powers conferred on a Commissioner for Oaths, and such person must also state where the declaration was made, sign and date the form.

The Memorandum and Articles of Association must be signed by at least two subscribers, who must write opposite their names the number of shares they agree to take. The names and addresses of the subscribers must be given and their signatures attested by one or more witness(es). The completed documents must then be lodged at the Companies Registry together with the appropriate capital duty at 1% of the capital subscribed for, and the official registration fee.

The Registrar examines the documents, and if they are correct a certificate of incorporation is issued. The issuing of the certificate may take several weeks, but once it is issued the company's subscribers may begin to act as a body corporate.

Memorandum and Articles of Association

The company's constitution is set out in two documents known as the Memorandum and Articles of Association. The Memorandum lays down the company's powers and its relationship with the outside world, and the Articles regulate dealings between the company and its members, directors and other officers.

The Memorandum of Association consists of clauses containing the following information.

(1) The name of the company.
(2) The location of the registered office, i.e. whether it is in England, England and Wales, Wales, or Scotland. It need not be more specific. Documents of companies whose registered office is to be situated in Scotland must be lodged at the Companies Registration Office in Edinburgh. These will be classified as Scottish companies. A company must at all times have a registered office at a particular address to which all communications and notices may be addressed.
(3) The objects of the company. It is invariably the longest clause and requires careful thought. The objects will set out the company's purpose and will set out the kind of activities in which the company seeks to be engaged. The clause will be sub-divided as follows.

    (a) The first sub-clause will set out the nature of the company's main business. It must be comprehensive and must detail all potential areas of business. If required, it can be amended at a later date by means of specific resolution.

    (b) The second sub-clause usually covers any other business which in the opinion of the directors may be advantageously or conveniently carried on in conjunction with the main business of the company.

    (c) The subsequent sub-clauses will cover general objects common to most businesses. These may include, for example, powers to lease, sell and purchase property; to purchase/lease equipment or machinery; to mortgage, charge or let out loans against company property; to issue and purchase shares; to issue debentures; to purchase shares in other companies; to sell the company; to draw bills of exchange and negotiable instruments; to distribute property amongst members; and to do all such things as may be necessary towards the attainment of the company's main objective. This list is by no means exhaustive, and will vary considerably between undertakings.

    Since the European Communities Act 1972, all transactions carried out by the directors in the company's name are binding as against the company even though they are apparently outside the scope of the Memorandum of Association. However, the shareholders may in this event take out an action for misfeasance against the directors.

(4) The limited liability of the members.
(5) The amount of share capital with which the company proposes to be registered and the nominal value of each of the shares into which the share capital is to be divided. The division of shares into different classes, the proportion of shares in each class and the rights conferred on the holders of each class of shares are sometimes stated, but this is very rarely done in practice as it is then more difficult to vary the rights at a later date. These matters are usually dealt with in the Articles so that any alteration can be effected by passing a special resolution.
(6) Further additional clauses may be included, usually of a kind found in the Articles of Association. The advantage of inserting additional matters in the Memorandum is that they can be protected against subsequent alteration,

whereas if they were in the Articles of Association, they could be altered by a special resolution passed by a general meeting of the company despite any provision to the contrary in the Memorandum or Articles.

(7) The Memorandum of Association concludes with an association clause by which two or more subscribers state that they are desirous of being formed into a company in pursuance of the Memorandum, and if the company has share capital, that they agree to take the number of shares set opposite their names.

The Articles of Association

The Articles of Association regulate the internal affairs of the company. These regulations govern the relationship between the company and its shareholders and the relationship of the shareholders between themselves. A table (known as 'Table A') of model articles is found in the Companies Act 1985. It is normal practice to adopt articles which include Table A and to make modifications.

The following is a non-exhaustive list of categories of provisions usually found in Articles of Association.

(a) Classes of shares   Where there is more than one type of share, the rights attaching to the owners of each class will be set out. For example, the priority of preference shareholders in the payment of dividends, the rules governing the apportionment of capital and the voting rights attaching to the holders of different classes will be set out. The Articles may also state the way in which these rights may be altered, or the classes of shares created.

(b) Share issue restriction   Sections 89–96 of the Companies Act 1985 accords existing shareholders the right of first refusal to any new shares issued. Existing shareholders must be offered the new shares in proportion to their current holding and must be notified in writing. These statutory rights may be altered or excluded by the Articles of Association. For example, directors may be given discretion over share issues. If this is the case, the directors' authority must be renewed every five years.

(c) Share transfer   The Articles will often give the directors the discretion not to register a transfer of shares. In a small business with only a few shareholders, the right of pre-emption is usually given to existing shareholders when one member decides to sell his shares. The Articles will contain detailed procedural provisions regulating this process.

(d) Company's purchase of its own shares   In a private limited company, the Articles may provide that a company has authority to purchase its own shares. However, advice should always be taken as to the taxation implications of such a course.

(e) Regulation 64 of Table A   This states that a company must have at least two directors, but is not restricted to a maximum number. A private company is legally obliged to have only one but the sole director cannot be the company secretary. As the initial directors will already have been appointed before

incorporation, the Articles can only provide the procedure for appointing subsequent directors.

Often the Articles of a small firm name directors as permanent directors. This is achieved either through private agreement within the company (which can be overturned by a resolution at a company meeting), or more securely by attaching enhanced voting rights to the directors' shares, thus enabling them to vote out any resolution tabled for their removal.

(f) Power of directors and remuneration   The power to run a company is normally vested in the directors who will exercise this function through resolutions passed at duly convened board meetings. In practice in small firms, however, decisions are taken on a daily basis by all directors.

The Articles usually contain a provision to vest in the directors the power to deal in company property, to mortgage company property, and to issue securities. It is possible, if required, to limit the total amount of debt the directors may incur on behalf of the company at any one time without the prior consent of the shareholders. Provision for directors' remuneration and expenses is made in the Articles; however, a contract of employment is usually drawn up separately to cover the directors' entitlements to salary, share of profits and expenses.

(g) Miscellaneous provisions   Further provisions in the Articles will deal variously with matters such as allocation of shares following the death of a shareholder; the procedures for calling and conducting general meetings; voting rights at company meetings; appointment and removal of directors and the company secretary; use of the company seal; payment of dividends on shares; and provisions governing the winding-up of the company.

Formal requirements for running a company

Every company must have a registered office, the location of which determines the tax office which will deal with the company's tax matters. Outside the registered office and every office or place of business of the company, the company's name must be permanently displayed. The registered office does not have to be the company's place of business; sometimes a company will nominate its solicitors or accountants to act in this capacity and give their address.

Company stationery
The company name must appear on all stationery including letters, cheques, invoices (which must also state the company VAT number), and receipts. Business letters must also show the address of the registered office, the place of registration and the registered number of the company.

Accounts
A company must decide a date on which all its accounts for the preceding year will be presented (the accounting reference period). The Registrar of Companies must be notified of this date, on form G224, within six months of incorporation.

The Companies Act 1985 imposes the requirement that accounts must be kept which are capable of showing with reasonable accuracy the financial position of the company at any given time. Accounts must show:

(1) All moneys paid and received by the company and the details of the transactions.
(2) The current assets and liabilities of the company.
(3) The level of stock held at the end of each financial year.
(4) Details of creditors and debtors.

Accounts must be laid before a general meeting of members within ten months of the accounting reference period.

The company auditor should be appointed before the first Annual General Meeting and must be a chartered or certified accountant, or a person authorized as an auditor by the Department of Trade and Industry. The auditor of a small company is often its accountant, but the liability to prepare accounts and make tax returns vests in the directors. The duty of the auditor is to inform the members of the accuracy of the company's accounts.

Company seal and statutory books

A formal register must be kept giving details of shares and shareholders; directors and the company secretary; directors' interests; and mortgages and charges. All share issues and issues and transfers must be documented in the register. A numbered share certificate will then be issued by the company secretary and pressed with the company seal. A minute book and a book of share certificates must also be maintained. A company must have a seal with its name engraved upon it. The seal must be used on formal company documents which would be made by deed if executed by an individual, e.g. mortgage documents, share certificates, debentures.

Meetings

The conduct of the business of the company is determined in meetings of directors and company members. The procedure for calling and conducting meetings is contained in the Articles of Association.

The meetings held by directors or 'board meetings' deal with the day to day conduct of the company's affairs. At the very first board meeting the directors should ensure that the formalities outlined above have been complied with or are under way.

At general meetings the members of the company exercise their power over company affairs by passing resolutions. An Annual General Meeting (AGM) must be held within 18 months of incorporation and every year thereafter. Members must have 21 days' notice of an AGM. The main functions carried out at AGMs are:

(1) The receipt of the company accounts and chairman's report.
(2) The proposal of a dividend on shares.
(3) The re-election of directors and other officers and the re-election of auditors.

Extraordinary general meetings (EGMs) may be called at 14 days' notice to deal with urgent business that cannot wait until the AGM to be dealt with. The procedure for proposing and voting on resolutions is similar to that used in AGMs.

Mortgages, debentures and charges

Every charge or mortgage created or debenture issued must be registered with the Registrar of Companies within 21 days of its commencement. Failure to register will result in the imposition of a fine.

The Registrar will issue a certificate of registration for every debenture issued, which must be endorsed on each debenture. When a charge has been satisfied a memorandum of satisfaction should be lodged with the Registrar.

Annual return

Within 14 days of each AGM an annual return must be lodged with the Registrar of Companies. This document states the address of the registered office; details of the company's shares and shareholders; details of the company's debts; a list of all members and changes in members since the last return and details of the directors and secretary. The return must be signed by a director and the company secretary and be submitted together with the correct registration fee.

Taxation

Corporation tax is charged on the profits of a company's accounting period and is payable nine months after the expiration of that period (1 April to 31 March). Therefore, if a company's accounting period straddles financial years for which different rates of corporation tax have been fixed, profits will be apportioned to the period falling either side of the end of the year. Tax returns are made quarterly and additionally on the annual accounting date if that does not coincide with a quarterly accounting date. By careful consideration of the first accounting reference period, the first payment of tax can be considerably lessened and cash flow improved for the first year. Professional advice should be taken in this respect.

VAT is dealt with separately and collected by HM Customs and Excise. VAT returns must be made quarterly on prescribed dates. Strict rules govern the keeping of VAT accounts and hefty fines are levied for late payment. VAT matters are invariably dealt with by the company accountant.

The imputation system

Where a company proposes to issue a dividend to shareholders, advance corporation tax is payable on the amount of the dividend. Payment of advance corporation tax must be made at the quarterly return date or on the annual accounting date. The amount of advance corporation tax paid will then be deducted from the overall tax liability for that period.

Notification of changes after incorporation

The Registrar of Companies must be notified of any of the following changes taking place after incorporation.

(1) Change of directors or secretary – notification within 14 days on form G288 by new director/s and company secretary.

(2) Change of registered office – notification on form G287 within 14 days signed by a director and the company secretary.

(3) Increase in company capital – notification within 15 days on form G123.

(4) Change in allotment of shares – notification within one month on form PUC2 where the change has taken place for cash consideration, or on form PUC3 where there has been no cash consideration. This form must be accompanied by the written contract together with the prescribed details on form G88(3).

(5) Change of company name together with a copy of the special resolution authorising the change.

(6) Changes in the Memorandum or Articles of Association together with the authorizing special resolution within 15 days.

Winding-up

A company can be wound up or dissolved by the members themselves or by the court. There are three routes to winding-up or liquidation.

- voluntary winding-up by the members
- voluntary winding-up by the creditors
- compulsory winding-up by the court.

The first two forms do not involve the intervention of the court. They are so named because it is either the members or the creditors who take the initiative in winding-up. This will either be done because the purposes for which the company was formed have been completed or exhausted, or because the company has run into financial trouble from which it cannot reasonably be expected to recover.

Upon liquidation the powers of the directors cease and the management of the company is taken over by a liquidator. The liquidator may be appointed by the members, creditors or court. The liquidator must use his best endeavours to satisfy as much of the company's indebtedness as possible, and must draw up accounts demonstrating what funds and/or assets are available for the satisfaction of the creditors.

The liquidator owes fiduciary duties to the company whose agent he is, i.e., he owes a duty to the company to do the best financially for it as he can. In a compulsory liquidation, he may be empowered to engage in litigation in the company's name, carry on such of the company's business as may be necessary and pay the company's debts or enter into such compromises or arrangements with creditors as are necessary. If there are sufficient funds within the company to satisfy all the creditors, the remainder will be divided among the shareholders according to their entitlements as laid out in the Articles of Association.

Striking-off the Register

A company may be struck off the Register where it appears to the Registrar that it has ceased trading. This inference will be raised where no annual return is filed. The directors of a company which has ceased trading and which has no assets or liabilities may initiate the striking-off of their own motion in order to avoid the possible expense of a voluntary liquidation.

Chapter 25

The Sale of Goods

The range of transactions which can be described as a sale of goods is enormous, and includes sales of goods worth from a few pence to millions of pounds. Yet the basic legal framework governing the diverse range of transactions is the same.

This area of law affects the pharmacist in his dual role as purchaser and seller of medicinal and other products. As a purchaser, the pharmacist will come into daily contact with this area of the law when he purchases medicines and other products from his wholesaler suppliers. The same law will regulate the pharmacist's onward sale of these products to the customer. The object of this section of the book is to provide a synopsis of the relevant law, much of which is to be found in the Sale of Goods Act 1979.

Unless otherwise stated, references to statutory sections in this chapter will refer to the Sale of Goods Act 1979.

The basic definition of a sale of goods is found in section 2(1), which defines it as a 'contract whereby the seller transfers or agrees to transfer the property in goods to the buyer for a money consideration, called the price'. 'Property in goods' is a way of describing what is commonly called ownership, but a sale of goods can include an agreement to sell whereby the ownership of the goods passes at a later date. 'Money consideration' generally means that the buyer must pay in money. A combination of money and goods in exchange, for example a trade-in on a new car, comes within this definition, but a pure exchange of goods does not.

Contracts for labour and materials supplied and contracts of hire-purchase do not fall within the law on sale of goods. In the former, the principal object of the contract is the provision of services. In the latter, the hirer (the buyer) does not acquire the ownership, but merely an option to purchase when all the instalments are paid. There is statutory protection for the customer in these circumstances outside the sale of goods law.

Formation of the contract

The precise moment when the contract is formed is critical, in that before the contract is formed either party is free to withdraw. The contract is made when an offer made by one party is accepted by the other. An offer is an offer to buy. The display of goods for sale in a shop, for example, is merely an invitation to make offers. The customer makes the offer when he produces the goods to the cashier, and it is accepted when the cashier accepts payment.

The Carbolic Smoke Ball

One of the principal cases in the law of contract concerned a proprietor of a medicinal product. In *Carlill* v. *Carbolic Smoke Ball Co.* (1893), the defendants, who were the owners of a medicinal product called 'The Carbolic Smoke Ball', issued an advertisement in which they offered to pay £100 to any person who succumbed to influenza after having used one of their smoke balls in a specified manner and for a specified period. They added that they had deposited a sum of £1000 with their bankers to show their sincerity. The plaintiff, on the faith of the advertisement, bought and used the ball as prescribed, but succeeded in catching influenza. She sued for the £100. The defendants argued that the advertisement was a mere 'puff', never intended to create a binding obligation, that there was no offer to any particular person, and that, even if there were, the plaintiff had failed to notify her acceptance. The Court of Appeal rejected these arguments. Although the offer was made to the world, the contract was made with that limited portion of the public who came forward and performed the condition on the faith of the advertisement. Accordingly, the plaintiff recovered the £100.

Using the post

When the buyer and seller transact a sale by post, special rules apply. Generally, when the means of communication is expected to be the post, the acceptance takes place when the letter of acceptance is posted; see *Household Fire & Carriage Insurance Co.* v. *Grant* (1879). When the chosen means of communication is instantaneous, such as telephone or fax, the acceptance takes effect when it is actually communicated to the offeror; see *Brinkibon Ltd* v. *Stahag Stahl* (1982).

Oral and written contracts

Section 4 provides that the contract of sale 'may be made in writing (either with or without seal), or by word of mouth, or it may be implied from the conduct of the parties'. Thus the form of the contract is something which is decided by the parties to it, and where the contract is not made in writing, a court may infer the existence of a contract from oral or any documentary evidence tending to show that a contract was made.

The price to be paid

The price to be paid is usually agreed between the parties, but where it is not, section 8(2) provides that 'where the price is not determined ... the buyer must pay a reasonable price'. Sometimes, however, the price to be paid for the goods is so fundamental an aspect of the contract that a court will refuse to enforce a contract where none has been agreed. If none has been agreed it may often be the case that the parties have done no more than agree to contract at some later date, and have not concluded an enforceable contract of sale. When deciding upon such issues, the court will look to all the surrounding circumstances to determine the intention of the parties at the time of the agreement in order to determine whether they intended to contract.

Cancelling the contract

As a general rule, once a contract has been concluded it cannot be cancelled. There are certain exceptions under the Consumer Protection (Cancellation of Contracts Conducted Away From Business Premises) Regulations, 1987, SI 1987 No. 2117, whereby customers who contract with unsolicited traders are entitled to a seven day cooling-off period in which the buyer may cancel the contract. However, the Regulations do not apply where:

(1) the price is less than £35
(2) the contract relates to the sale or provision of finance for the sale of land
(3) the contract relates to building construction or alteration
(4) the contract relates to the sale of food or drink.

There are also exceptions for certain mail order catalogues where separate rights are set out in the mail order contract. Where the purchase is made by the consumer with the assistance of credit, a separate statutory regime applies in the form of the Consumer Credit Act 1974 and the Consumer Protection Act 1987. This legislation falls outside the scope of this book.

The passing of property

The time at which ownership transfers from the seller to the buyer does not always coincide with the transfer of physical possession from one to another. Often, for example in shipping contracts, property passes before the buyer accepts delivery. It is important to determine when ownership vests in the buyer for a number of reasons:

(1) The 'risk' in the goods, i.e. the risk of them falling in value or perishing passes with ownership.
(2) The buyer cannot transfer ownership to a third party until such time as he has ownership himself.
(3) The seller cannot sue the buyer for the price of the goods until ownership has passed.
(4) If the buyer or seller become bankrupt, the rights of the other party will depend on who has ownership.

The rules governing the transfer of ownership are contained in sections 16 to 19, and their application depends upon whether the goods are specified or unspecified at the time of making the contract. Specified goods are those which are identified and agreed on at the time the contract of sale is made. A branded bottle of cough mixture taken from a display is therefore specific, but 100 grams of aqueous cream taken from a larger quantity is not specific as it cannot be said *which* 100 grams have been sold.

Section 17 provides that ownership of specific goods passes to the buyer at such time as the parties intended it to be transferred. If no specific provision has been agreed between the parties, then the court will look at all the surrounding circumstances to see what their intention was. If none can be found, the rules in sections 16–19 apply.

Section 16 provides that 'where there is a contract for the sale of unascertained goods no property is transferred to the buyer unless and until the goods are ascertained'. Thus until the goods can be specifically identified as those forming the subject matter of the contract, ownership cannot pass. For example, an English buyer contracts to buy 100 tonnes of senna leaves from the cargo of the ship *Empress* and the ship leaves India with 500 tonnes, 400 of which are firstly being delivered to Lisbon. If the 100 tonnes is mixed in with the bulk, it does not become ascertained until the 400 tonnes is unloaded. Once the goods are ascertained, ownership passes in accordance with the intention of the parties.

Rules set out in section 18 of the Act apply where the intention of the parties cannot be ascertained.

Rule 1   Where there is an unconditional contract for the sale of specific goods, in a deliverable state, the property in the goods passes to the buyer when the contract is made, and it is immaterial whether the time of payment, or the time of delivery, or both be postponed.

Thus, when the goods are specific and ready to be handed over, the buyer becomes the owner the moment the contract is made. However, if the goods are not in a deliverable state and require something doing to them before delivery, ownership cannot pass until they are in an appropriate condition (see below).

Rule 2   Where there is a contract for the sale of specific goods and the seller is bound to do something to the goods for the purpose of putting them in a deliverable state, the property does not pass until the thing is done, and the buyer has notice that it has been done.

'Notice' means actual knowledge that the goods are in a deliverable state.

Rule 3   Where there is a contract for sale of specific goods in a deliverable state, but the seller is bound to weigh, measure, test or do some other act or thing with reference to the goods for the purpose of ascertaining the price, the property does not pass until the act or thing is done and the buyer has notice that it has been done.

Rule 3 is self-explanatory, but it must be noted that it applies only where the seller is bound to do something to the goods.

Rule 4   When goods are delivered to the buyer on approval or on sale or return or similar terms, the property in the goods passes to the buyer:

(a)   When he signifies his approval or acceptance to the seller or does any other act adopting the transaction.
(b)   If he does not signify his approval or acceptance to the seller but retains the goods without giving notice of rejection, then if a time has been fixed for the return of the goods, on the expiration of that time and, if no time has been fixed, on the expiration of reasonable time.

In ascertaining whether the buyer has signified his approval or acceptance where he has not specifically stated to the seller that he has accepted the goods, he will be taken to have done so if he does something which substantially impedes his ability to return the goods by the end of the period. Pledging the goods to a pawnbroker for a period exceeding the time limit for refusal would satisfy this test. However, if he cannot return the goods because, for example, they have been stolen, this will operate as an excuse and property will not pass.

Rule 5 (1)   Where there is a contract for the sale of unascertained or future goods by description, and goods of that description and in a deliverable condition are unconditionally appropriated to the contract, either by the seller with the assent of the buyer, or by the buyer with the assent of the seller, the property in the goods then passes to the buyer; and the assent may be express or implied, and may be given before or after the appropriation is made.

Rule 5 (2)   Where, in pursuance of the contract, the seller delivers the goods to the buyer or to a carrier or other bailee or custodian for the purpose of transmission to the buyer, and does not reserve the right of disposal, he is taken to have unconditionally appropriated the goods to the contract.

Thus, for the operation of Rule 5 it is necessary that the goods complying with the contract be unconditionally appropriated to the contract, i.e. they become specified by one of the parties, and that the other party assents. Returning to the example of the cargo of senna leaves, if the contract was merely for the delivery of 100 tonnes of senna leaves, the goods would not become specified and accepted until the senna leaves were off-loaded and accepted by the buyer.

When goods have to be dispatched by a carrier, they will normally be unconditionally appropriated when they are handed over to the carrier. However, the same rules apply, and the goods must be specified in order for ownership to pass.

Section 19 provides that, if the seller reserves a right of disposal of the goods until certain conditions are fulfilled, ownership does not pass until those conditions are fulfilled. For example, if a seller dispatches goods to the buyer through a carrier with instructions that the goods cannot be handed over until the buyer has paid, the goods will remain the seller's property until the buyer has paid for them.

The Romalpa clause

In the case of *Aluminium Industrie Vaasen BV* v. *Romalpa Aluminium Ltd* (1976), the Court of Appeal had to consider the situation where the seller had sold a large quantity of materials to the buyer in the knowledge that the buyer would only be able to pay the seller when the materials had been used to manufacture goods, and the finished product sold. Before full payment was made the buyer became insolvent, some of the materials remained in their raw state, and some had been processed and mixed with other substances. The Court of Appeal upheld the validity of a clause in the contract of sale which reserved the ownership of the materials to the seller until they had been paid for or until they became processed with other materials, and which created a *fiduciary duty* (binding financial duty) in the buyer to repay the seller out of the proceeds of sale of the manufactured product the price of the raw materials. Thus a seller in such a situation can reserve ownership of the goods until they become transformed or sold onto a third party, and can create a right to be paid out of the proceeds of the buyer's subsequent sale to a third party. Such clauses have become commonly known as Romalpa clauses. They are sometimes found in the standard contracts used by perfume and cosmetic manufacturers.

Transfer of risk

As was stated above, the usual position is that the risk in the goods transfers with ownership unless the parties agree otherwise (section 20(1)). Therefore, if the goods are damaged or stolen, the loss falls on the seller if it occurs before ownership is transferred, otherwise it falls on the buyer.

There are two limitations on this rule. The first is created by section 20(2) which provides that '... where the delivery has been delayed though the fault of either the buyer or seller, the goods are at the risk of the party at fault as regards any loss which might not have occurred but for such fault'. The second is created by section 20(3) which provides that 'nothing in this section shall affect the duties or liabilities of either seller or buyer as a bailee or custodian of the goods of the other party'. The effect of this section is that the party in possession of the goods must take reasonable care of them, and if the goods are damaged or lost as a result of his negligence, he will have to bear that loss.

If the buyer has to bear some loss because the risk in the goods has passed to him, he must still carry out all his obligations under the contract. Thus if he withholds some of the purchase price he is in breach of the contract and can be sued for the remainder by the seller.

Perishing of goods

Section 6 provides that 'where there is a contract for the sale of specific goods, and the goods without the knowledge of the seller have perished at the time when the contract is made, the contract is void'. There can be no legally constituted contract for goods which have perished before the contract date. 'Perish' means more than slight deterioration not sufficient to change the commercial character of the goods. In *Asfar* v. *Blundell* (1896) it was held that dates which had been under water for two days and which had been contaminated with sewage had 'perished' and were no longer commercially valuable.

Section 7 provides that 'where there is an agreement to sell specific goods, and subsequently the goods, without any fault on the part of the seller or the buyer, perish before the risk passes to the buyer, the agreement is avoided'. This section applies the common law doctrine of frustration, whereby a contract is declared void if supervening events outside the control of either party render performance of the contract impossible. Section 7 applies only to specific goods, but the same considerations apply to unspecified goods as apply in the case of goods perishing before the making of the contract. The contract will not be frustrated if the origin of the unspecified goods is not specified.

It follows from this that once the risk in the goods has passed to the buyer, the contract cannot be avoided by section 7, or in the case of unspecified goods at common law by the doctrine of frustration. If the position were to be otherwise, the concept of the passing of risk would be meaningless.

When the contract is either avoided by the operation of section 6 or 7 or declared void at common law, the buyer need not pay for the goods and the seller need not deliver them. However, if the parties had provided for the eventuality which occurred, the terms of the contract would take precedence.

In the case where the buyer has paid some of the purchase price before the goods perished, if the contract is avoided by operation of section 6 or 7, then the buyer will recover the whole of the sums he has paid over. If the contract is frustrated at common law, i.e. the goods were unspecified, the Law Reform (Frustrated Contracts) Act 1943 empowers the court, before remitting the balance to the buyer, to deduct from the sums already paid to the seller a sum towards expenses incurred by the seller in performing the contract and to deduct any reasonable sum for any benefit the buyer has received under the contract.

Invalid title

The situation often arises where the seller of goods does not have proper title to the goods. This may occur where the goods are not his to sell, or where the contract by which he originally acquired the goods is voidable (discussed below). The general principle is contained in the maxim *nemo dat quod non habet*, in other words, you cannot give what you do not own. Section 2(1) provides that:

> '. . . where goods are sold by a person who is not their owner, and who does not sell them under the authority or with the consent of the owner, the buyer acquires no better title to the goods than the seller had, unless the owner of the goods is by his conduct precluded from denying the seller's authority to sell.'

Generally speaking, a seller cannot transfer to a buyer any better title than that which he already possesses. Where there has been a chain of sales, for example, where B, without authority, sells A's goods to C who in turn sells them to D, C and D have no better title to the goods than B had. In order to retrieve his goods A can take out an action (called an action for conversion) against D for the recovery of the goods. D may then sue C who may in turn sue B for breach of contract, for it will be an implied term of each contract that the seller had full title to the goods.

If, however, A represented by words or conduct that B had authority to sell his goods, then A will be prevented from asserting that the sale was unauthorized. For the representation to have this effect, it must have been made intentionally or negligently, it must have misled the innocent purchaser and the innocent purchaser must have bought the goods. For example, in *Eastern Distributors* v. *Goldring* (1957), a customer who wished to raise some money against his van conspired with a motor trader by pretending that he was buying the van from the motor trader. Both of them filled out their portions of the hire purchase forms. The customer subsequently sold the van to a third party and defaulted on the payments to the hire purchase company. The question then arose as to whether the hire purchase company had acquired title from the motor trader or the customer. It was held that as the customer had allowed the motor trader to represent the van as belonging to him, he was prevented from disputing that the title had passed to the hire purchase company.

Where the owner has signed a document purporting to transfer title, the document will usually be taken to have legal effect except in the rare circumstances where the owner can show both that he was radically mistaken about the nature and effect of the document, and where he can show that he was not careless in signing it.

Exceptions to the nemo dat principle

Mercantile agents

A mercantile agent is an independent agent to whom someone else entrusts his goods and to whom is usually transferred the authority to sell the goods, consign them, or to raise money on the security of the goods. Problems as to title may occur when the owner instructs the mercantile agent that his goods are not to be sold without his express authority. For example, a man may wish to place his sports car in the window of a car show room to see how many offers may be lodged, and to ascertain the level of offers made. The manager of the show room may be acting as a mercantile agent on a commission basis, but it may be agreed between the parties that the car is not to be sold without the owner's express permission.

Another exception to the *nemo dat* maxim is created by section 2(1) of the Factors Act 1889, by which a mercantile agent in possession of goods with the authority of the owner, but without the authority to sell, may pass a good title to a purchaser from him if the purchaser buys from him in good faith and without notice that he does not have authority to sell. In this situation the burden is on the purchaser to prove that he was acting bona fide and bought without knowledge of the absence of authority. Thus a purchaser can acquire good title to the sports car if he innocently believes the mercantile agent to be the true owner. The owner must then sue the agent for the market value of the car.

Sale where the owner's title is voidable

An exception to the *nemo dat* rule can occur where the owner's title is voidable. An example of what is meant by voidable title is where B has induced A to enter into a contract of sale by making some misrepresentation, for example that he is a respectable person whose cheque will be honoured, when in fact he is an impostor who has no funds to meet the cheque. Under these circumstances B has falsely induced A to enter into the contract and will acquire only a voidable title. A will retain the right to set the contract aside and claim his goods back. However, if B sells the goods to C before A realises that he has been misled, C will get a perfect title (provided he buys in good faith and without notice of B's dishonesty) by virtue of section 23.

Lawyers distinguish between a voidable contract and one which is void, i.e. not valid from the outset. Where the contract is void, C cannot acquire good title. This will occur when the following two conditions are met:

(1) The identity of the buyer was an essential fact to A when selling to B.

(2)   When making the contract A was intending to deal with someone other than B.

Thus in *Cundy* v. *Lindsay* (1878), a rogue purchaser ordered goods from the seller, Lindsay, in the name of Blenkarn of 37 Wood Street. The signature was written in such a way that it looked like the name of the reputable firm Blenkirn & Co. Assuming that he was dealing with a reputable firm, Lindsay dispatched the goods to Blenkirn & Co. at 37 Wood Street. Blenkarn received the goods but never paid for them, and sold them to Cundy who knew nothing of the fraud. The House of Lords held that the contract between Lindsay and Blenkarn was void and therefore the goods still belonged to Lindsay.

Seller retaining possession sells to third party

The situation may arise where the seller sells or agrees to sell goods to B and later sells or agrees to sell them to C. The question arises, to whom do the goods belong? Applying section 24 of the 1979 Act and section 8 of the Factors Act 1889, under certain circumstances C may acquire title to the goods following a previous sale to B. The conditions are as follows:

(1)   A must have been in possession of the goods or documents of title at the time of the sale to C. The point of this condition is that B could have safeguarded his position by taking immediate possession of the goods or documents of title.
(2)   There must be delivery to C of the goods or documents of title.
(3)   C must be acting in good faith and acting without notice of the previous contract with B.

The purpose of these provisions is to safeguard the position of C. B obviously retains the right to sue A for breach of contract when the goods are not delivered.

Buyer in possession without ownership sells to third party

The buyer usually has ownership of goods when he takes possession, but in some circumstances he may have possession without ownership. For example, a buyer may take delivery, but the agreement is that ownership does not pass until payment is made. What is the position of the third party purchaser who buys before the original buyer has paid the original seller and thereby acquired title?

The answer is that by operation of section 25 of the 1979 Act and section 9 of the Factors Act 1889, the subsequent purchaser will acquire good title where certain conditions are satisfied as follows.

(1)   The person selling must be someone who has bought or agreed to buy the goods. Purchasing an option or purchasing goods on hire purchase is not sufficient for this condition to be met.
(2)   The person selling the goods must have been a buyer in possession, in other words he must have obtained possession of, or documents of title to the goods with the consent of the seller.
(3)   There must be a delivery or transfer of the goods or documents of title to the innocent sub-purchaser.

(4)   The buyer in possession must have acted in the normal course of business of a mercantile agent. In other words the transaction with the sub-purchaser must be carried out in such a way as it would be carried out by a mercantile agent. This is a little absurd as the buyer in possession may not be a mercantile agent, but the requirement is implicit in the statutory section.
(5)   The sub-purchaser must be acting bona fide and unaware that the original seller has any rights in respect of the goods.

All the above requirements must be fulfilled in order for the sub-purchaser to acquire a good title.

Misrepresentation

A misrepresentation occurs when one party is induced into entering a contract as a result of something which has been represented by the other party which is in fact false. Statements amounting to a misrepresentation may be made orally or in writing; the essential factor is that it operates on the mind of the other party.

A distinction must be drawn between mere statement of opinion or trader's 'puff' and a genuine misrepresentation. A statement of opinion is something other than a statement of fact. Traders' puffs are, for example, claims that a particular product will 'cure smoking', or will 'protect against cardiac arrest', or some other serious illness.

The misrepresentation need not have been made fraudulently in order for it to be actionable; it may be made innocently or negligently. Accordingly, this area of the law may be particularly relevant to the community pharmacist who sells a product about which he has no personal knowledge. The misrepresentation must, however, be an influencing factor on the mind of the party induced.

The aggrieved party may succeed in rescinding the contract and/or in obtaining damages. The effect of rescission is to return the parties to the position they were in before the making of the contract. Thus goods and purchase price must be returned. Rescission is not available where to grant it would be unfair to one of the parties. For example:

(1)   Where the parties cannot be returned to their pre-contract position, e.g. where the goods have been consumed or used in a manufacturing process.
(2)   Where the goods of an innocent third party would be affected, e.g. where the goods have been sold on by the purchaser.
(3)   Where an unreasonable length of time has elapsed since the date of the contract.
(4)   Where the contract has been affirmed by the aggrieved party, e.g. where the purchaser of an unsound second-hand car restores the vehicle and drives it for six months before claiming rescission.

Damages may be available in addition to rescission to compensate any extra loss suffered by the aggrieved party, or they may be awarded as an alternative to rescission. However, damages are not normally allowable where the mis-representation was wholly innocent, e.g. where the misrepresentation is made upon the basis of information honestly believed to be true and by a person who cannot be expected to have known otherwise. The seller of a nicotine patch who states, in reliance upon the manufacturer's claim, that the patch will cure the purchaser from smoking, would make a wholly innocent representation if in fact the properties of the particular patch have no effect on the purchaser who wishes to stop smoking.

Some contracts seek to exclude liability for misrepresentation by means of exclusion clauses. These are invalid unless they satisfy the requirement of reasonableness in the Unfair Contract Terms Act 1977. The circumstances in which such clauses will be valid will be rare and probably confined to specialized markets where the buyer and seller are both expert in the goods being sold.

Terms of the contract

As a general rule, the parties to a contract will be bound by the terms they agree upon. However, in order for a term to be binding, it must be incorporated into the contract. This is often done by reducing the entire contract to writing, but contracts may be made orally. A written contract may also have terms incorporated into it by oral agreement. The requirement is either that the terms were expressly agreed by the parties, or that the party seeking to rely on the term took all reasonable steps to bring it to the attention of the other party. For example, one of the terms of a theatre-goer's contract with the theatre cloakroom may be that no liability is accepted for loss of or damage to coats. This term may be adequately incorporated by the position of a prominent notice which can be seen by potential customers.

Terms of the contract may be express or implied. Express terms are those specifically set out or agreed by the parties. Implied terms are those implied by operation of law. Terms may be implied by statute (see below), or they may be implied by the court to make sense of a contract, for example, where a contract makes no express stipulation as to the time in which goods must be delivered, a term will be implied whereby they must be delivered within a reasonable time.

Conditions and warranties

Contractual terms are classified as either conditions or warranties. Conditions are terms of the contract which are so fundamental to its performance that breach of the term would go to the root or essence of the contract. Warranties are other terms which, although they must be performed, are not so fundamental that a failure to perform goes to the substance of the contract. For example, if a second-hand car is sold purportedly running in good order, if it is delivered without an engine, the absence of an engine would be fundamental to the contract and would constitute a breach of condition. If, however, it was delivered requiring minor adjustments to the carburettor, this would amount to no more than a breach of warranty. The significance of this difference is that a breach of condition entitles the other party to treat the contract as repudiated, to return the goods and to sue for damages for any further losses incurred, whereas a breach of warranty merely entitles the aggrieved party to sue for compensation in damages, e.g. the cost of employing a mechanic to adjust the carburettor.

Terms implied by statute

In contracts for the sale of goods, sections 12 to 15 of the Sale of Goods Act 1979 imply some important terms into contracts for the benefit of the purchaser. The terms implied are expressly stated to be either conditions or warranties: different remedies apply according to the nature of the term breached.

Section 12(1) implies a condition on the part of the seller that he has a right to sell the goods. Section 12(2) implies warranties that

'... (a) the goods are free ... from any charge or encumbrance not disclosed or known to the buyer before the contract is made
(b) the buyer will enjoy quiet possession of the goods ...'

We have seen how issues are resolved when a bona fide purchaser buys goods from a seller with a questionable title. If the purchaser acquires ownership through the operation of those rules then there is no dispute with the seller. If, however, the original owner still has ownership, the buyer can sue the seller for breach of condition claiming damages and/or the purchase price.

Where a third party retains any rights over the goods, not amounting to ownership, which have not been disclosed to the buyer, the buyer may sue for damages for breach of warranty. This may occur, for example, where the goods are subject to a repairer's lien, i.e. a party who has carried out repairs to the goods may have acquired ownership of the goods in proportion to the sum outstanding for the cost of repairs carried out by him. In such a case the buyer can sue the seller for the sums still owed to the repairer and any additional sums incurred as a direct result.

Section 13 provides that:

'(1) Where there is a contract for the sale of goods by description, there is an implied condition that the goods will correspond to the description.'

This section is designed to cover the situation in which the buyer has not seen the goods for himself but has relied upon a description. Thus, where a car is described as a 'Herald, White Convertible 1961' when it emerges after the sale that in fact the vehicle is two cars welded together, one of which is older than 1961, a breach of condition occurs (*Beale* v. *Taylor* (1967)). Most packaged goods sold in pharmacies are sold by descriptions on the label; therefore, if the contents fail to match the label there is a breach of condition.

Section 14 implies two conditions. The first in section 14(2) provides that:

'Where the seller sells goods in the course of a business, there is an implied condition that the goods supplied under the contract are of merchantable quality, except that there is no such condition:

(a) as regards defects specifically drawn to the buyer's attention before the contract is made; or

(b) if the buyer examines the goods before the contract is made, as regards defects which the examination ought to reveal.

It is important to note that this section applies only to goods sold in the course of a business. In a private sale, unless such a term is expressly included, there is no such term implying merchantable quality. Further exceptions to the application of the section are included in the section itself, namely that if the buyer examines the goods himself or has the defects drawn to his attention, he cannot then complain that the goods are sub-standard.

'Merchantable quality' is defined in section 14(6) as meaning that the goods must be as fit for the purpose for which goods of that kind are commonly bought as it is reasonable to expect. Thus goods cannot be expected to be in immaculate condition, and the standard to be expected will vary according to the circumstances. For example, a second-hand car sold as 'in working mechanical condition' will not be of merchantable quality if the brakes fail immediately after purchase. If, however, the clutch needs replacing 500 miles after the purchase, the car will nonetheless be of merchantable quality as it can only be expected that parts will need to be replaced on second-hand cars.

Section 14(3) provides that:

'Where the buyer sells the goods in the course of a business and the buyer … makes known to the seller … any particular purpose for which the goods are being bought, there is an implied condition that the goods supplied under the contract are reasonably fit for the purpose, whether or not that is a purpose for which such goods are normally supplied.'

Section 14(3) could be particularly relevant to a pharmacist who counterprescribes a product in circumstances where the product is not licensed for the condition in question.

The section applies to transactions carried out in the course of a business. The expression 'reasonably fit' does not require the goods to be of the highest quality, merely that they are suitable for the job intended. This can cause difficulties for the purchaser where, for example, he has bought a washing machine which has cosmetic damage to it but which nonetheless functions perfectly in cleaning clothes. The retailer may in this situation be able to argue successfully that it is fit for its purpose. If the retailer is successful, the purchaser can then only sue for breach of an implied warranty that the machine would be in good cosmetic order. (The courts will only imply a term where it considers that term to have been intended to be included by the parties, or where the contract would not make sense without the inclusion of such a term.) It was established in *Slater and Slater (a firm)* v. *Finning Ltd* (1996) that where a purchaser fails to make known that goods are to be used for other than their normal purpose, the seller's obligation does not extend to anything beyond an assurance that the good are fit for the purpose for which they would ordinarily be used. There is no breach of the implied condition of fitness where the failure of the goods to meet the intended purpose arises from an abnormal feature or idiosyncrasy, not made known to the seller, on the part of the purchaser or the use to which the goods are to be put.

Section 15 provides that where the contract is a contract for sale by sample, e.g. where a quantity of senna leaves are bought having examined a sample from the bulk, there is an implied condition that:

(1) The bulk will correspond to the sample in quality.
(2) The buyer will have reasonable opportunity of comparing the bulk with the sample.
(3) The goods will be free from any defect, rendering them unmerchantable, which would not be apparent on reasonable examination of the sample.

The bulk must correspond to the sample and, where it does not, the buyer may treat the contract as repudiated and sue for the price and/or damages.

Implied terms in contracts other than those for sale of goods

The Supply of Goods and Services Act 1982 creates implied terms similar to those in the Sale of Goods Act 1979, which apply to contracts closely related to the sale of goods such as barter, contracts for repair and contracts for the provision of services.

Sections 2 to 5 of the 1982 Act give to customers in contracts of barter and contracts for repair (e.g. a contract where a roofer repairs a roof and supplies the materials used), rights in relation to title, description, quality and sample which are identical to those conferred by the Sale of Goods Act 1979. These rights relate specifically to the goods/materials supplied under such a contract. Sections 2 to 5 of the 1982 Act correspond only to sections 12 to 15 of the Sale of Goods Act 1979, and do not create any further rule concerning, for example, the passing of ownership and risk under a contract of barter.

Sections 6 to 10 of the 1982 Act imply similar conditions to those in sections 12 to 15 of the Sale of Goods Act 1979 into contracts of hire other than hire purchase agreements. Thus in contracts for the hire of cars or plant, for example, similar terms relating to title, merchantable quality, fitness for purpose and correspondence to sample apply.

Sections 13 to 15 deal specifically with contracts for the supply of services, and are fairly self explanatory.

Section 13 implies a term that '... where the supplier is acting in the course of a business, there is an implied term that the supplier will carry out the service with reasonable care and skill'. Where this term is breached, the customer can sue the supplier for damages, e.g. for the cost of having the defective work made good. A pharmacist would be caught by this section if, for example, he failed to take reasonable care in mixing solutions whilst dispensing a prescription for a patient.

Section 14 provides that where a time for performance of the contract for services is not specified in the contract, there is an implied term that the supplier will carry out the service within a reasonable time.

Section 15 provides that where the price is not specifically stated in the contract for services, there is an implied term that the customer will pay a reasonable price.

Exemption clauses

Clauses which purport to exclude or restrict the liability of one or other of the parties to a contract are termed exemption clauses. The validity of many such clauses is governed by the Unfair Contract Terms Act 1977, but common law rules also apply.

A clause is of no effect unless it is incorporated as a term of the contract, and incorporation must occur at the time of contracting. If the exemption clause is brought to the attention of the purchaser after the time of contracting, it is of no effect. Thus exemption clauses printed on receipts are usually of no effect.

As with all contractual terms, an exemption clause must be specifically incorporated into the contract to be of effect. Where the contract is written and signed by the buyer, he will be presumed to be bound. Where a clause is contained in an unsigned document, the party seeking to rely upon it must prove that it was brought to the attention of the other party, or that all reasonably necessary steps were taken to draw the other party's attention to it.

Where the exemption clause is displayed on a notice, as in a cloakroom or car park, the clause will only be incorporated if at the time of contracting the customer already knew of the existence of the term, or reasonable steps had been taken to draw it to his attention.

Where there has been a course of dealing between the parties on the same terms, the same terms will be presumed to be incorporated into later contracts, including exemption clauses.

A party other than a party to a contract cannot rely on an exclusion clause in that contract. Thus a manufacturer cannot rely on an exclusion clause incorporated into the contract of sale between a retailer and consumer.

Exemption clauses are always construed narrowly and against the party seeking to rely upon them. In this respect the law is plainly weighted in favour of the person prejudiced by the operation of the clause.

The Unfair Contract Terms Act 1977 curbs the operation of exemption clauses in many respects.

Section 6 of the Act prevents a seller from avoiding any liability imposed by sections 12–15 of the Sale of Goods Act 1979, i.e. the terms as to title, description, merchantable quality, fitness for purpose and sample, where the buyer deals as a consumer. A buyer deals as a consumer where he is not acting in the course of business, but where the seller is, and where the goods are of a type normally supplied for private use. Purchases at auctions or by competitive tenders are excluded.

Where the buyer is not dealing as a consumer, the seller cannot exclude himself from the liability imposed by section 12 of the Sale of Goods Act 1979 (implied terms as to title), but he can exclude liabilities imposed by sections 12 to 15 insofar as the exemption clause satisfies the requirement of reasonableness. This is in order that businessmen maintain freedom to contract on whatever terms they choose. Exemption clauses can be unreasonable in certain circumstances, however, especially where the parties are not in equal bargaining positions. Thus in determining the reasonableness or otherwise of such a clause, under Schedule 2 of the Unfair Contract Terms Act 1977, the court can take into account the strength of the bargaining positions of the parties; whether the customer was acting under an inducement to agree to the term; whether the customer knew or ought to have known of the existence of the term; whether, where the term excludes liability for the breach of some condition, it was reasonable at the time of the contract to expect that condition to be complied with; and whether the goods were made specifically to the order or specification of the customer.

Where the clause seeks to exclude liability from terms other than those imposed by the Sale of Goods Act 1979, it will be subject to the requirement of reasonableness where:

(1) The seller's liability is a business liability; *and*
(2) In buying the goods the buyer deals as a consumer or on the seller's written standard terms of business.

Where neither of the above applies, the exemption clause will be valid. Where either of them do apply, section 3 of the Unfair Contract Terms Act 1977 applies, by which the seller cannot:

> '... when in breach of contract, exclude or restrict any liability in respect of his breach; or ...
>   (b) claim to be entitled
>
>   (i) to render a contractual performance substantially different from that which was reasonably expected of him; or
>   (ii) in respect of the whole or any part of his contractual obligation, to render no performance at all,
>
> except in so far as the contract term satisfies the requirement of reasonableness.'

The courts have obviously a wide discretion in interpreting the reasonableness of exemption clauses in these circumstances, and each case will have to be considered on its facts bearing in mind the factors listed in Schedule 2 (see above).

Where the contract purports to exclude liability for negligence, section 2 of the Unfair Contract Terms Act 1977 provides that liability for death or personal injury caused by negligence cannot be excluded. However, liability for other loss or damage can be excluded, but only insofar as the clause satisfies the requirement of reasonableness.

The Unfair Contract Terms Act 1977 applies to contracts generally, and is not limited in its application to contracts for the sale of goods.

Remedies available to the seller – buyer in default

When the buyer is in default, the seller has personal remedies exercisable through the courts and remedies exercisable against the goods.

Personal remedies

The seller has two possible remedies under this head: damages for non-acceptance or an action for the price.

Section 49 of the Sale of Goods Act 1979 allows the seller to sue for the price of the goods where:

(1) The buyer has wrongfully refused or neglected to pay according to the terms of the contract; *and*

(2) Either the property has passed to the buyer or the price is payable on a certain day irrespective of delivery.

The most important thing to note about the above requirements is that the buyer's refusal to pay must be wrongful. If he has rightfully rejected the goods the seller's action fails. Furthermore, under section 28 the buyer is entitled to refuse payment until delivery (unless there has been a contrary agreement). If the specified date for payment has passed, however, the seller may bring an action. Under section 37, the seller may have a claim where the buyer does not take delivery of the goods within a reasonable time from when he has been informed that the seller is ready and able to deliver, and has been requested to take delivery.

If for some reason the seller cannot maintain an action under section 49, he may have a claim for damages under section 50 where 'the buyer wrongfully neglects or refuses to accept and pay for the goods'. Usually the damages under this head will be less than the price.

Remedies against the goods

The three possible remedies against the goods are lien, stoppage in transit and resale. These are available to the seller who is owed the whole of the price.

The seller's lien is a right to retain possession of the goods when ownership of the goods has passed to the buyer. Section 41(1) enables this right to be exercised:

(1) Where the goods have been sold without any stipulation as to credit.

(2) Where the goods have been sold on credit, but the term of the credit has expired.

(3) Where the buyer becomes insolvent.

The seller loses his lien where any of the following occurs:

(1) The seller is paid by the buyer.

(2) An innocent third party acquires title under one of the *nemo dat* exceptions (see above).

(3) The seller delivers the goods to any seller or carrier for the purpose of transmission to the buyer without reserving the right of disposal of the goods. However, even when this occurs, the seller may still exercise his right to stoppage in transit.

(4) The buyer or his agent lawfully obtains title to the goods.

(5) The seller waives his lien.

Under section 44, if the buyer has become insolvent and the goods are in transit, the seller can resume possession of the goods and retain them until payment is made. Transit ends when the buyer obtains delivery; the carrier acknowledges that he holds the goods on behalf of the buyer; or when the carrier wrongfully refuses to hand the goods to the buyer. The fact that part of the goods have been delivered does not stop the remainder being stopped in transit.

Under section 48, the seller is allowed to resell the goods where:

(1) they are of a perishable nature and the buyer does not tender the price within a reasonable time of being told that the unpaid seller intends to resell; *or*
(2) the seller expressly reserves the right of resale in case the buyer should default, and the buyer defaults.

When the right of resale is exercised, the contract is rescinded. When it is rescinded, if the title has passed to the buyer, it reverts to the seller. By section 48(2), if an unpaid seller resells the goods when he has exercised his seller's lien or stopped the goods in transit, the subsequent buyer acquires a good title to them as against the original buyer. The original buyer then has to bring an action against the seller for non-delivery, provided the seller did not have the right to resell.

Buyer's remedies

Specific performance

Section 52 allows the court to make an order that the goods be delivered to the buyer in the case of a contract to deliver specific or ascertained goods. Such an order can only be made where the specific goods are ascertained and where damages would not be an adequate remedy, e.g. when it is commercially essential that the buyer have the specific goods. When such an order is made, the seller does not have an option to deliver other goods or repay the price.

Rejection of the goods

Where the seller has breached a condition of the contract, as well as a right to damages, the buyer has a right to reject the goods (to treat the seller's breach as a repudiation of the contract). The buyer need not deliver the goods to the seller, but may inform him that he rejects the goods. Any storage expenses reasonably incurred will be recoverable from the seller.

Breach of a warranty will not entitle the buyer to reject the goods, but gives him an action for damages.

Where there has been a breach of condition, the buyer loses his right to reject the goods once he has accepted them. By section 35 acceptance is constituted when:

(1) The buyer informs the seller that he has accepted the goods.
(2) If after taking delivery, and following a reasonable time in which to examine the goods, the buyer carries out some act inconsistent with the seller being owner of them (e.g. he uses them in a manufacturing process).
(3) The buyer retains the goods for more than a reasonable length of time without telling the seller that he has rejected them.

The buyer may lose his right to reject the goods by waiving the right. This may occur where he knows that the seller is in breach of a condition before the date of delivery, but nevertheless accepts delivery in spite of the breach.

If the buyer rejects the goods, he can do so without treating the contract as repudiated, and therefore the seller remains at liberty to re-tender goods in accordance with the contract.

Damages

The buyer can claim damages for non-delivery or for breach of any other condition or warranty. This is in addition to any right to reject the goods and recover the purchase price.

The purchase price can be recovered where there has been a failure on the part of the seller to deliver. Where the buyer has rejected the goods or treated the contract as repudiated, he is entitled to the return of any payment made.

The measure of damages

In general, contract damages compensate any loss naturally arising from the breach, and any loss which, at the time of making the contract, the defendant could have predicted as likely to result from the breach of it. Some specific rules relate to contracts for the sale of goods.

Non-acceptance

Section 50 of the Sale of Goods Act 1979 provides that:

(1)   Where the buyer wrongfully neglects or refuses to accept and pay for the goods, the seller may maintain an action against him for damages for non-acceptance.
(2)   The measure of damages is the estimated loss directly and naturally resulting, in the ordinary course of events, from the breach of contract.
(3)   Where there is an available market for the goods in question, the measure of damages is prima facie to be ascertained by the difference between the contract price and the current market price at the time or times when the goods ought to have been accepted, or at the time of refusal to accept.

The principle behind this section is that if the seller is able to resell the goods he will receive only nominal damages if he could get a good price on resale. This section does not, however, exclude any further loss which was reasonably foreseeable. So, for example, the seller will be able to recover any extra storage expenses he had to incur.

Non-delivery

Section 51 provides that:

(1)   Where the seller wrongfully neglects or refuses to deliver the goods to the buyer, the buyer may maintain an action against the seller for damages for non-delivery.

(2)   The measure of the damages is the estimated loss directly and naturally resulting, in the ordinary course of events, from the seller's breach of contract.

(3)   Where there is an available market for the goods in question the measure of damages is prima facie to be ascertained by the difference between the contract and market price or current price of the goods at the time ... when they ought to have been delivered ... or at the time of refusal to deliver.

This is the converse of section 50, and provides that where the buyer may buy the goods elsewhere, his damages are limited to the difference between the contract price and the price elsewhere, plus any other reasonably foreseeable loss.

Anticipatory breach

Where one of the parties to a contract commits an anticipatory breach, e.g., before the date for performance of the contract the seller informs the buyer that he will not deliver, or the buyer informs the seller that he cannot pay, the other party has an option to treat the contract as repudiated immediately and to claim damages, or wait until there has been actual failure to perform and claim damages under the principles in either section 50 or section 51. If the former course is adopted, the innocent party is under a duty to minimize his loss by buying alternative goods at the best available price. If the price of the goods is currently rising, the damages will be assessed according to the best price the innocent party could have obtained as soon as reasonably practicable after the acceptance of the repudiation. However, if the innocent party refuses to accept the anticipatory breach as a repudiation, he is not under a duty to minimize his loss, and damages will be assessed according to the normal principles in section 50 or section 51.

Late delivery

Late delivery by the seller will normally be a breach of condition. If the buyer rejects the goods for breach of condition, his damages are assessed as in the case of non-delivery. If it is only a breach of warranty or if the buyer accepts the goods, the damages are prima facie assessed according to the difference between the value of the goods on the date they should have been delivered and their value (if lower) when actually delivered.

Breach of warranty

Section 53(2) and (3) provides:

'(2) The measure of damages for breach of warranty is the estimated loss directly and naturally resulting, in the ordinary course of events, from the breach of warranty.

(3) In the case of breach of warranty of quality such loss is prima facie the difference between the value of the goods at the time of delivery to the buyer and the value they would have had if they had fulfilled the warranty.'

Under this section the buyer has a choice as to claiming his capital loss or his loss of profit. He cannot claim both. In *Cullinane* v. *British Rema* (1953) the sellers had warranted that a clay pulverising machine would process clay at six tons per hour. In fact it could not do so. The buyer claimed first for capital loss and secondly for loss of profits, being the difference between those profits actually made and those that would have been made had the machine performed as promised. The Court of Appeal held that both claims could not succeed, and disallowed the smaller of the claims. The Appeal Court also stated that loss of profits could have been claimed for the whole of the useful life of the machine.

Subsection 3 provides that only the prima facie amount can be claimed. In addition to the losses discussed above, the buyer may also claim any loss which could reasonably have been predicted by both parties as likely to occur in the event of the breach. The question is, 'had the seller been aware of the defect at the time of the contract, what type of damage could the seller at the time of contract have reasonably predicted?'

In *Parsons* v. *Uttley Ingham* (1978) the sellers sold a hopper to a farmer for the storage of pig nuts. When it was installed, the ventilator was not opened by the installers. As a result, the pig nuts became mouldy and the pigs died as a result of eating them. The sellers were held liable for the loss of the pigs, the Court of Appeal taking the view that the loss of the pigs was a reasonably foreseeable consequence of the failure to ensure that the ventilator was working correctly.

Under section 55(1), the buyer may set off damages due to him for breach of warranty against the price he owes the seller, but retains the right to sue for any excess.

Mitigation of loss

In all cases of breach of contract, whether or not in a contract for the sale of goods, the innocent party is under a duty to take reasonable steps to minimize his loss. Failure to do so will result in the loss which could have been avoided being deducted from the damages. The requirement is one to act reasonably in the particular circumstances. For example, if the seller delivers defective goods but offers to buy them back at a reasonable price, the buyer will normally be under a duty to accept the offer. This does not prejudice his claim for the excess. The seller cannot force the buyer to accept defective goods. If the buyer rejects the goods and the market price is climbing, the buyer will usually be under an obligation to minimize his loss by purchasing alternative goods as soon as reasonably practicable. However, if alternative goods are not available, e.g. the goods were being made especially for the buyer, the buyer cannot reasonably be expected to buy alternative goods which will not suit his purpose.

Penalty clauses

Some contracts contain a clause which stipulates how much is to be paid by the party in breach; e.g. £50 for every day payment fails to be made after the due date. The general rule is that such a clause is binding on the party in breach if it is a genuine attempt by the parties to estimate the actual loss which will be caused to the innocent party during the period of breach. Thus, if the sum claimed is extravagant and unconscionable in comparison with the amount of the actual loss, the clause will be of no effect. However, if the penalty clause is void, the innocent party may nevertheless sue for his loss in the normal way.

Product liability

Fundamental to the English law of contract is the doctrine of *privity of contract*. This means that no one other than a party to a contract can sue on it. This has particular implications where damage has been caused by a product to a consumer or a third party. If damage is caused to a consumer, he can sue the retailer under one of the implied terms in the Sale of Goods Act 1979. He cannot, however, sue the manufacturer under normal contractual principles as he has no contract with him. In any event, the measure of damages under the contract is limited to putting the parties back into the positions they would have enjoyed had the contract never been made. If the product is, for example, a defective medicine, contractual damages will not cover damages for personal injury and loss of earnings incurred by the consumer. Furthermore, if the person harmed is someone other than the buyer, he has no right to sue on the contract of sale at all.

The traditional remedy for such an occurrence was to sue for negligence in the law of tort. Damages in negligence compensate the aggrieved party for all the reasonably foreseeable losses incurred as a result of the negligence. The main problem for the consumer, however, is that he bears the burden of proving that the manufacturer was negligent, a task which is often by no means easy.

Consumer Protection Act 1987

The law in this area was considerably advanced by the Consumer Protection Act 1987, which implemented an EC (now EU) Directive on product liability. Under the Act, any person who is injured by a defective product can sue the manufacturer for compensation whether or not the manufacturer was negligent.

To succeed the consumer must establish four things:

- that the product contained a defect
- that the plaintiff suffered damage
- that the damage was caused by the defect
- that the defendant was producer, own-brander or importer into the EU of the product.

A product is defective if its safety is not such as persons generally are entitled to expect. Safety includes not only safety in the context of death or personal injury, but also the risk of damage to property. In determining the defectiveness of the product, section 39(2) of the Act requires that the nature of the product, any instructions, what use might reasonably be expected for the product and the time when the product was supplied by the producer, must all be considered.

The term 'product' is very wide and covers everything which can be considered a product, including gas and electricity. There are exceptions relating to land, some agricultural produce and game.

Under the 1987 Act damages may be claimed for death, personal injury or damage to property (including land) which is ordinarily intended for private use, occupation or consumption; and intended by the person suffering the loss or damage mainly for his private use, occupation or consumption.

Thus damage to business property cannot be claimed under the Act (and must therefore be claimed for in negligence). Furthermore, only claims worth over £275 can be entertained. The final qualification is that under the Act a claim cannot be made for the cost of the defective product itself – this must be made under the contract of sale.

Claims can be brought against the manufacturer or, in the case of products which are abstracted from the earth such as coal, the abstracter. An 'own-brander' is someone who holds themselves out as a producer. Pharmacies which carry their own brand name on goods fall into this category. The only importers who are liable are those who import the goods from outside the EU into the EU.

Defences

Section 4 of the Act provides the following defences which, if relied upon, must be proved by the defendant:

(1) The defect is due to compliance with a statutory regulation or EU rule.
(2) The defendant did not supply the product.
(3) The defendant supplied the product otherwise than in the course of business and did not produce it with a view to profit, e.g. the defendant gave to friends a bottle of his home-made wine which had become contaminated.
(4) The defect did not exist in the product at the time of supply.
(5) The defect is in the design of the overall product and the defendant is merely the manufacturer of a component.
(6) The defect was such 'that the state of scientific and technical knowledge at the relevant time was not such that a producer of products of the same description as the product in question might be expected to have discovered the defect if it had existed in his products while they were under his control'. This 'state of the art' defence protects the producer who can show that the defect was not such that it could have been discovered at the time the product was made, abstracted or imported.

Furthermore, it is open to the producer to argue that part of the damage was due to the contributory negligence of the consumer, e.g. when the purchaser of a lawn mower fails to read the safety instructions and suffers an injury which he would not have suffered if he had read the instructions. If this is proved, then the damages will be reduced in proportion to the culpability of the consumer.

Under the Act the producer is prohibited from excluding liability imposed by the Act. However, any claim must be made within three years of the date of the injury or damage occurring, and in any event within ten years of the producer supplying the product.

Chapter 26

Employment Law

The contract of employment

A pharmacist needs to be aware of the basic principles of employment law. He may employ members of staff, perhaps a locum pharmacist, dispenser or shop assistant; or alternatively he may himself be an employee of a limited company, sole trader or partnership.

A contract of employment is approached legally in the same way as any other commercial contract. Over the years, however, there have developed particular regulations relating to the formation of such a contract, the conditions of service and termination of the contract. Much of the law in this area is contained in the Employment Rights Act 1996 (ERA), though some common law rules remain. Thus contracts of employment are subject to rigorous controls from the beginning to the end of the employment. The rules are complex, and they need to be examined in considerable detail in order for their application to be fully grasped.

Contract of service or contract for services?

There is a fundamental difference between a contract *of* service (employment) and a contract *for* services, i.e. between the existence of an employer/employee relationship, and the relationship between a party and a self-employed contractor. This distinction is important as most of the relevant legislation applies only to the employer/employee relationship. The system of taxation is also different. The duties of the employer towards his employee are far more onerous. There are certain terms which are only implied into a contract *of employment* and which are not implied into a contract *for services*. Further, in some situations where the employee has committed an unlawful act, his employer will be vicariously liable for his wrongdoing; no such principle applies where the contract is merely one for services.

The distinction is not always an easy one to draw, and in the past the courts have experienced difficulty in devising a satisfactory test to discern the difference. Having tried tests which look to the level of control exercised by the employer, or the extent to which the employee is integrated into the employer's business, a three stage 'economic reality' test has been developed.

In *Ready Mix Concrete Ltd* v. *Minister of Pensions and National Insurance* (1968), the court held that a contract of employment can only exist where:

(1) the employee agrees to provide his own work and skill
(2) there is some element of control exercisable by the employer; *and*
(3) the other terms of the contract are not inconsistent with a contract of employment.

This case involved the question of whether the driver of a lorry who had obtained it on hire-purchase from the plaintiff company was an employee. He was required to paint the lorry in the company livery, but could use substitute drivers if he was unwell or away. The court found that the provision for the use of substitute drivers rendered the driver an independent contractor.

Form of the contract of employment

There is no formal requirement that the entire contract of employment be evidenced in writing: therefore valid contracts can be made orally. However, section 1 of the ERA 1996 requires the employer to produce a written statement within two months of the commencement of employment containing the following information:

(1) the names of the parties and the date upon which the period of employment began
(2) the rate of remuneration and the method for calculating it
(3) the intervals at which remuneration is to be paid
(4) the terms relating to hours of work
(5) the terms concerning entitlement to holiday
(6) terms relating to provision for inability to work through sickness and details of sick pay arrangements
(7) the periods of notice required for either party to terminate the contract
(8) the terms concerning pension arrangements
(9) the job title/description.

The employee must also be provided with details of:

(1) any applicable disciplinary rules
(2) the person to whom he can apply should he be unhappy with the operation of any disciplinary procedure
(3) the person to whom he can apply if he has any grievance with his employment generally
(4) whether a contracting-out certificate (under the provisions of the Social Security Pensions Act 1975) is in force in relation to that employment.

All the above information may be included in one document to which the employer may then draw the employee's attention. The written statement is not itself the contract of employment, but is strong prima facie evidence of the terms agreed upon by the parties. There is nothing to prevent the parties from altering the terms set out in the statement at a later date, in which case the subsequent agreement will take precedence.

Terms of the contract of employment

Apart from the conditions implied by statute, the contract of employment will usually consist of a written or an oral agreement between the parties setting out the basic conditions of employment. Express statements made prior to the contract may also be incorporated, and deviation from such statements will constitute breach of contract unless there has been specific agreement to be contrary. Attempts to vary the terms or conditions of employment after the contract has been made will only be effectual if they are specifically agreed to by the parties.

Collective agreements

Many contracts of employment consist partly or wholly of terms which have been arrived at collectively by means of negotiations with a trade union. Such collective agreements may be incorporated into the contract of employment by express incorporation, or may be implied by statute. For example, under the ERA 1996 there is provision for collective agreements to replace the statutory provisions for the right to claim unfair dismissal or the right to claim statutory redundancy payment. Should the S of S approve the collective agreement, the terms negotiated between the trade union and the employers will replace those created and implied by statute.

Company rules

Where there is a company rule book, those rules may be incorporated into the individual contract of employment subject to the following principles.

(1) If the employee agrees before the making of the contract that the rules are to form part of the contract, then they are expressly incorporated into the contract.
(2) The rules may be incorporated if he is given other notice, i.e. the posting of a large notice, that they are to be included in the contract. However, the matter is usually decided as a matter of custom and practice.
(3) Not all rules automatically become terms of the contract. This may be so where, for example, rules have become out of date. It is a matter of construction of the specific rules as to whether they are terms of the contract or merely guidelines as to how the work should be performed.

The nebulous nature of this area of law is further emphasized by the part which custom plays in determining terms of the contract of employment. In *Marshall* v. *English Electric Co. Ltd* (1945) it was stated as a matter of general principle that 'established practice at a particular factory may be incorporated into a workman's contract of service, and whether he knew it or not, it must be presumed that he accepted employment on the same terms as applied to other workers in the same factory'. The range of customs is potentially wide and may even relate to such matters as dismissals procedure. Examples of the incorporation of custom can be seen in case law. In *Sagar* v. *Ridehalgh and Son Ltd* (1931), it was held that the customs of the Lancashire weaving trade were incorporated into the contract of employment of an individual weaver. Therefore customary deductions for faulty workmanship were held to be lawfully deductible. *Davson* v. *France* (1959) shows the operation of the principle in the converse manner. A musician who had received one week's notice to quit was held to have been wrongfully dismissed as the customary period in the trade was 14 days.

Continuity of employment

Once an employee has commenced employment, he acquires various rights if continuity of employment is maintained. For example, although an employee is always entitled to sue for breach of his contract of employment in an action for wrongful dismissal (i.e. dismissal that is in breach of the terms of the contract of employment), the right to complain to an industrial tribunal for unfair dismissal (a much wider concept the conditions for which are contained in the Industrial Tribunals Act 1996 (ITA) and discussed below) is only acquired after two years' continuous employment.

Part XIV of the ERA 1996 deals with the continuity of employment, and section 218(2) prescribes that:

'If a trade or business, or an undertaking (whether or not established by or under an Act) is transferred from one person to another –

(a) the period of employment of an employee in the trade or business or undertaking at the time of the transfer counts as a period of employment with the transferee, and

(b) the transfer does not break the continuity of the period of employment.'

Special categories of employee

There are several categories of employee to whom special considerations apply.

Company directors

Company directors are usually considered as employees if they have a written service contract with the company, but non-executive directors are usually not. The question as to whether such a person is or is not an employee is always a matter of law to be decided upon the test for the incidents of employment (see above). Where, for example, a non-executive director did not have anything in writing referring to him as an employee, and where he had not been paid remuneration for a period due to the financial condition of the company, the Employment Appeal Tribunal would be unable to find that he was an employee.

Partners

Partners in a firm are not employees. However, those employed by partnerships may be employees.

Civil servants

Civil servants were long thought not to be employees, but the position now seems to be that they enjoy a relationship similar to that created under a contract of employment, subject to the right of the Crown to dismiss its servants at its pleasure. This is not as harsh as it sounds, as many of the legal protections accorded to other employees, including the ERA 1996 provisions for unfair dismissal, apply equally to Crown servants. Police officers and prison officers are exceptions to this, however, and cannot claim unfair dismissal. Similarly, members of the armed forces are specifically excluded from statutory protection.

Minors

Minors (i.e. persons under the age of 18) are bound by the contract of employment subject to the same proviso affecting any other contract, that it must be substantially for their benefit when taken as a whole. This is a matter to be decided by the court, and is a measure designed to stop an unfair advantage being taken of young persons.

   Children under the age of 13 cannot be employed. Between the ages of 13 and 16 a minor may work part-time subject to a strict limit on hours. 'Young persons' between the ages of 16 and 18 may work subject to various restrictions, e.g. those contained in the Factories Act 1961, which limit the hours of work and the nature of work which may be undertaken.

Temporary staff

Temporary workers who are drafted in to replace regular employees who are absent through illness or maternity leave, are not normally regarded as unfairly dismissed if the regular employee returns to work.

Probationary staff

Probationary employees can be dismissed in accordance with the conditions of their probation, but if the probationary period extends to two years of continuous employment, the statutory rights will be acquired and the employer will be subject to the statutory requirement of showing that the dismissal was fair.

Staff over 65

Section 109 of the ERA 1996 provides that persons over the age of 65 are unable to claim unfair dismissal. By section 156 of the ERA 1996, men over 65 and women over 60 are excluded from the right to claim a statutory redundancy payment. Implementation of recent EU case law may equalize the position between the sexes.

Employee's duties under the contract of employment

The duties upon the employee which are commonly implied into the contract of employment by historical operation of the common law are the duties:

- to be ready and willing to work
- to use reasonable care and skill

- to obey lawful orders
- to take care of the employer's property *and*
- to act in good faith.

Ready and willing to work

The duty to be ready and willing to work needs little explanation. It is the duty of the employee to present himself for work and to abide by the terms of his employment. If the employee fails to attend for work, it constitutes a breach of the contract of employment and the employer may act accordingly. The employer may withhold pay with just cause if the employee is failing in his contractual duties, but withholding pay for no just cause is a breach of contract which gives the employee the option to repudiate the contract and sue for damages.

Reasonable care

The duty to use reasonable care and skill can be described as a twofold duty, i.e. not to be unduly negligent *and* to be reasonably competent.

Where a third party takes an action against an employer for the negligent act of an employee, the employer will be vicariously liable (liable on the employee's behalf), but if the employer can prove that the employee was in breach of the implied term in his contract not to be unduly negligent, the employee may be held liable to the employer for all or a portion of the damages. The duty to be reasonably competent requires that the employee is able and competent at the job. Therefore if someone holds himself out as skilled in a trade in which he has no experience, the employer will be entitled to claim that the employee has breached his duty of competence.

Lawful orders

Disobedience to orders which are in the scope of the contract of employment can amount to a breach of contract and may in certain circumstances justify summary dismissal. However, in order for such action to be justified, the order must have been within the scope of the contract. Although employees are not obliged to obey orders falling outside their contract, they will be obliged to adapt to new machinery and working techniques if the appropriate training is given. Whether the extent of the change is unreasonable is a matter which can only be decided in specific circumstances. An employee may lawfully disobey an order which is prima facie within the scope of his contract if either the execution of the order involves exceptional danger for which there is no extra payment, or the execution of the order constitutes a criminal offence. (Most cases involving dismissal for disobedience to an order come before the industrial tribunal. Under the ERA 1996 the employer must show that the dismissal was reasonable, therefore the nature of the order will be subject to the test of reasonableness – see below.)

Care of the employer's property

The duty to take care of the employer's property is self-explanatory. Where the employee's breach of the implied term to take care of the employer's property results in the employer sustaining loss, the employee is liable to indemnify him.

Act in good faith

The duty to act in good faith towards an employer has several aspects.

There is a duty not to make a secret profit which entails an obligation on the employee not to make a personal profit in the course of his employment. If such profits are discovered, the employee will be liable to repay them.

There is a duty to disclose certain information. For example, in an action by the widow of an epileptic building worker, the court found that the employee had breached his duty to inform his employer of his condition. As the employee's death resulted from his suffering a fit at height, the claim for compensation failed.

There is a general duty on the employee not to disclose confidential information gained from his employer. Information is confidential if the owner believes that the release of the information could be injurious to him and if the information is not publicly known. Whether particular information satisfies these requirements will depend on the particular circumstances, including the availability of the information within the profession and generally. Contracts of employment relating to work in areas where confidential information is handled will usually contain a specific term dealing with the duty not to disclose. Problems often arise when employees leave their employment and seek to use information gained whilst employed. The duty not to disclose confidential information does extend to ex-employees, but it is not so wide as to extend to 'know-how'. In *Faccenda Chicken* v. *Fowler* (1986), the Court of Appeal stated that the distinction between confidential information and know-how is based on:

(1) The nature of the employment, i.e. whether information known to be secret is dealt with by the employee.
(2) The nature of the information, i.e. whether it is such as to constitute a trade secret.
(3) Whether the employee was informed by the employer that the information was confidential.
(4) Whether the confidential information was easily distinguishable from other information which the employee was free to disclose.

These are common sense principles which will be applied to each specific situation.

Restraint of trade covenants

Employers are often keen that the employee does not use the expertise gained whilst in employment to aid competing concerns when he leaves his employment. Thus covenants in restraint of trade may be included in the contract of employment, whereby the employee promises:

- not to establish a competing business within a certain distance from his former employer, or within a specified period of time from terminating his employment; *or*
- not to use his expertise to the benefit of a competing concern within a certain period of the termination of his employment.

Such covenants (which are merely terms of the contract which have continuing effect after the termination of the period of employment) are subject to the requirement of reasonableness. If an employer sues a former employee for breach of his covenant, the issue of reasonableness will be decided by reference to the following factors:

(1) *Time* – the covenant will be held invalid if it purports to run for an excessive period of time.
(2) *Area* – the covenant must normally be limited to the area within which the former employee worked. (An action for breach of an express or implied term forbidding the former employee from using confidential information is distinct from an action for breach of restraint of trade covenant. In the former case the duty will attach notwithstanding the whereabouts of the former employee.)
(3) *Nature of the competing business* – the covenant must be limited to similar business in competition with the former employer.
(4) *The public interest in not fettering the activities and marketability of a skilled man* – thus a balance always has to be struck between the gaining of an unfair advantage by an employee, and the public interest in free trade and availability of services.

If an employee is thought by the former employer to be in breach of his covenant, an application may be made to the courts for an injunction restraining the employee from acting in continuing breach of the covenant.

If during the period of employment the employer breaches the contract of employment by unfairly dismissing the employee, the employee may thereafter disregard the effect of the restraint of trade clause.

Employer's duties under the contract of employment

Both common law and statute have created a variety of obligations which must be fulfilled by the employer. The main obligations are as follows:

(1) The duty to pay remuneration.
(2) The duty to pay sick pay.
(3) The duty to treat the employee with trust and confidence.
(4) The duty not to require the employee to work beyond agreed hours or hours prescribed by statute.
(5) The duty to allow time off work for the purpose of carrying out certain public functions.
(6) The duty to indemnify legitimate expenses.
(7) The duty to provide a safe working environment.

Remuneration

This is normally determined by reference to the contract. Failure to pay the agreed rate is a breach of contract which may entitle the employee in certain circumstances to claim constructive dismissal (see below under 'unfair dismissal').

Minimum pay

The National Minimum Wage Act 1998 provides for a statutory minimum wage of £3.60 an hour before deductions for most workers. Those aged between 18 and 21 are only entitled to £3 an hour and trainees in their first six months to £3.20. Although there are some exceptions (such as apprentices and 16 and 17 year olds) the Act's application to 'workers' goes beyond the unfair dismissal legislation in applying to home workers and agency temps. In the context of community pharmacy, this means that the legislation will apply to collection and delivery drivers who may not be employed by a pharmacy under a formal contract of employment.

Workers paid less than the minimum wage will be able to complain of an unauthorized deduction in the industrial tribunal or bring a civil action for breach of contract. Workers are entitled to access to records and the right not to be victimized for asserting their rights under this legislation in good faith. The Act also provides for enforcement by government agency and for criminal penalties. The detailed provisions are complex and may be found in the National Minimum Wage Regulations 1999. They address situations where workers are paid by reference to output rather than time, are on standby, etc.

Sick pay

The contract of employment will normally specify the terms relating to the payment of sick pay. If it does not do so, terms may be implied. There is no general presumption that sick pay is to be paid, but the court or industrial tribunal will attempt to construe the intentions of the parties at the time of contracting. However, under the Social Security and Housing Benefits Act 1982, as amended by Schedule 2 para 13 of the ERA 1996, all employers are obliged to pay their employees up to eight weeks sick pay in any one tax year. To qualify for statutory sick pay the employee must be:

(1) At least 16 years of age and gainfully employed.
(2) He must have been incapable of work for a period of at least four days.
(3) The claim must be made for a period when the employee would have been working but for the incapacity.

The current rates of Statutory Sick Pay (SSP) are:

Weekly Earnings	Sick Pay per week
£195 or more	£52.50
Under £195	£46.95

Should the employer fail to pay statutory sick pay, a complaint may be made to the employer. Should the employer fail to give adequate reasons for failing to pay, the matter may be referred to an insurance officer, whose decision can be in turn appealed to the DSS.

Trust and confidence

This duty has grown up as a result of case law involving constructive dismissal, i.e. a claim by the employee that the behaviour of the employer was such that it left no reasonable alternative but to leave the employment. In *Courtalds Northern Textiles Ltd* v. *Andrew* (1978), the Employment Appeal Tribunal held that in a contract of employment there was an implied term that an employer 'would not without reasonable cause, conduct (himself) in a manner calculated to be likely to destroy or seriously damage the relationship of trust and confidence between the parties'. Breach of such a term is likely only to be argued in a dismissal claim; in other words, when the relationship between the employer and the employee has broken down.

Hours of duty

The hours to be worked will be included in the contract of employment. However, there are statutory maxima which apply to limit the total hours allowable.

Minimum hours

The Working Time Regulations 1998 provide for:

(a) a minimum daily rest period of 11 consecutive hours
(b) an additional minimum weekly rest period of 24 hours
(c) a rest break in any working day over six hours
(d) maximum average working week of 48 hours (over a four-month reference period)
(e) minimum four weeks' annual paid holiday
(f) night workers' normal working hours should not exceed eight in 24.

The Working Time Regulations 1998 provide for enforcement by the Health and Safety Executive and local authorities. However, in *Barber* v. *RJB Mining (UK) Ltd* (1999) the High Court held that employees may also seek a declaration and injunction restraining their employer from requiring them to work an average of 48 hours per week.

Time off for public functions

These include being a magistrate; a member of a local authority; a member of a statutory tribunal; a member of an HA; a member of the governing body of a local authority maintained establishment; or being a member of a water authority. Time off must also be allowed for jury service. Under section 55 of the ERA 1996 a pregnant employee must also be allowed a reasonable amount of time off for the purposes of receiving ante-natal care.

Incurred expenses

There is a duty on employers to indemnify employees for expenses incurred in executing their duties.

Safe working environment

Control of Substances Hazardous to Health Regulations 1988
The Control of Substances Hazardous to Health (COSHH) Regulations 1988 came into force on 1 October 1989. They affect the use of hazardous substances in a work situation, by laying down measures which an employer must take to control hazardous substances and to protect people who are exposed to such substances.
  Regulation 6 requires that an employer may not carry on any work that is liable to expose any person to any substance hazardous to health, unless a suitable and sufficient assessment of the risks has been made.

Hazardous substances   A substance hazardous to health is defined as:

  'any natural or artificial substance: solid, liquid, gas, vapour or hazardous micro-organism, and certain dust levels'.

Substances hazardous to health can include:

(1) Any substance classed under the Chemicals (Hazard Information and Packaging) Regulations 1994, SI 1994 No. 3247 as 'toxic, very toxic, harmful, corrosive, irritant, carcinogenic, mutagenic, toxic for reproduction, sensitizing'.
(2) Any micro-organism.
(3) Any dust.
(4) Any substance which has a prescribed maximum exposure limit, e.g. formaldehyde.
(5) Any other substance which can adversely affect the health.

In other words, *any* substance used or present at work.

  Helpfully, the COSHH Regulations state that a substance is *not* hazardous when it is at a level that nearly all the population can be exposed to it, repeatedly, without ill effect.

Exclusions   Certain situations are specifically excluded from COSHH:

(1) Those covered by the Control of Lead at Work Regulations 1980.
(2) Those covered by the Control of Asbestos at Work Regulations 1987.
(3) When the hazard is radioactivity.
(4) When the hazard is the explosive or flammable properties of the substance.
(5) Underground mines.
(6) Medicines administered to patients.

Employer's duties   The employer must first of all decide whether or not any substance is potentially hazardous. This must be done by a competent person. The employer must then:

(1)   Assess the risk to health from the use of the substance in the workplace.
(2)   Decide what precautions are needed.
(3)   Introduce appropriate measures to control the risk.
(4)   Inform and train employees about the risks and about the precautions to be taken.
(5)   Ensure the measures are actually taken.
(6)   In some cases, monitor any exposure of workers to hazardous substances.

Detailed guidance on such assessment is given in the Management of Health and Safety at Work Regulations 1992, SI 1992 No. 2051 which require all employers to assess the risk to employees while at work, and are made under the Health and Safety at Work, etc. Act 1974.

Records   All records should be available for inspection by the Health and Safety Executive.

The Manual Handling Operations Regulations 1992, SI 1992 No. 2793

These require the employer to take steps to avoid hazardous manual handling operations; to assess the safety of any operations which are necessary; to reduce the risk of injury from those operations so far as is reasonably practicable. Employees are required to follow specified systems of work.

The Electricity at Work Regulations 1989

These require employers to take all reasonably practicable steps to avoid danger from electrical installations. The Regulations do not specifically require annual tests of equipment, although this is one way of minimizing risk.

The Health and Safety (Display Screen Equipment) Regulations 1992, SI No. 2792

These implement a European Directive 90/270/EEC on health and safety. They require an employer to assess the risks in the use of computers, and to minimize those risks. This is to be done by ensuring that equipment, including desks, hardware and software is suitable and appropriate. Eyesight tests are to be provided for employees on request.

The Safety Representative and Safety Committee Regulations 1977

An employer must consult with all staff, either directly or where appropriate through a recognized trade union, on health and safety matters. This includes telling staff about new measures, and taking account of their views. A 'competent person' must be appointed to liaise with staff.

Wages issues

Deductions

The Wages Act of 1986 regulated the payment of wages, and created a system based upon the contract of employment. The Act abolished the old requirement that wages be paid in cash, thus permitting cashless payment. Now subsumed by Part II of the ERA 1996, deductions from wages can only be made in order to comply with a statutory provision (e.g. tax or national insurance), or by prior agreement.

Itemized pay statement

An employee has a right to an itemized pay statement giving particulars of the amount of gross pay and deductions made.

Lay-off periods

During periods when an employee is laid off because there is no work, Part III of the ERA 1996 provides for a system of guaranteed payments during the period of the lay-off. In order to be eligible for such a payment the employee must have been continuously employed for at least one month when the lay-off occurs; he must have been laid off for the whole of his normal working hours on a day he is normally required to work; he must not have refused a reasonable offer of alternative employment; he must comply with any requirements imposed by the employer with a view to ensuring that his services are available; he must not have been laid off as a result of industrial action; and he must have been available for employment on the day. If the above conditions are fulfilled, then the employee is entitled to be paid for the number of hours per day for which he was laid off, or £14.50 per day, whichever is the lesser sum. Failure to pay the guaranteed payment may be made the subject of a complaint to the industrial tribunal.

If an employee is suspended from work as a result of the operation of certain statutory provisions (listed in section 64(3) of the ERA 1996), for example, if his workshop is temporarily closed as a result of a notice served under the Health and Safety at Work Act 1974, he is entitled to remuneration. To qualify, the employee must have been continuously employed by the employer for one month, he must not be incapable of work through sickness; he must not have unreasonably refused suitable alternative work; and he must not have refused to comply with reasonable requirements imposed by the employer with a view to ensuring that his services are available. The maximum period for such pay is 26 weeks.

Maternity issues

Maternity pay

Part VIII of the ERA 1996 provides the framework for maternity pay and leave.
In order to qualify for maternity pay an employee:

(1) Must continue to be employed by her employer until the beginning of the eleventh week before the expected week of confinement
(2) Must have been employed for at least two years by the employer at the beginning of the eleventh week before the expected week of confinement *and*
(3) Have produced a medical certificate confirming the expected week of confinement if required to do so by her employer.

The entitlement is to 18 weeks' maternity pay. The rate of pay is 90% of full wages minus the maternity allowance payable by the Department of Social Security. A complaint about non-payment may be made to the industrial tribunal. (An employer who has paid maternity leave in accordance with these provisions is entitled to recover the full amount from the Maternity Pay Fund which is maintained by class 1 social security contributions.)

Return to work

The employee has the right to return to work after the birth if at least 21 days prior to her absence (or as soon as reasonably practicable thereafter), she informs the employer in writing of her expected absence; of her intention to return to work; and of the expected week of confinement. Not later than 49 days after the start of the week of confinement, the employer may write to the employee asking for written confirmation of the intention to return to work. Confirmation must be made within 14 days of the request.

The right to return to work may be exercised before the expiration of 29 weeks from the actual week of confinement, and includes the right to return to the same job on terms no less favourable than those previously enjoyed. If the employer can prove that by the time the employee intended lawfully to return there was no suitable position, she will be entitled to a redundancy payment. There will be no such entitlement if she refuses a suitable vacancy.

Unlawful dismissal

If, in breach of her right to return, the employee is not allowed to return to work, or if she has been made redundant and not been offered a suitable available alternative position, the employee may claim to have been unlawfully dismissed, subject to the employer's defence that he acted reasonably because of something which happened in the employee's absence.

Postponed return

The employer has the right to postpone the return of the employee for up to four weeks. The employee may postpone her return if either she is ill (in which case the postponement can be for up to four weeks), or if there is an interruption in work (such as a strike), which renders it unreasonable to expect the employee to return to work on that day.

Maternity leave

Irrespective of any entitlement to maternity pay, section 71 of ERA 1996 establishes a general right to 14 weeks' maternity leave for all employees, regardless of length of service, hours of work or size of firm, during which an employee is entitled to the benefit of all her normal contractual rights, except for remuneration, which is specifically excluded. This right to maternity leave was introduced in 1993, implementing the requirements of a European Directive on the introduction of measures to encourage improvements in the safety and health at work of pregnant workers and workers who have recently given birth or are breast-feeding. It is additional to the right of employees with at least two years' continuous employment to return to work after up to 29 weeks' maternity absence, and like the right to return it is subject to detailed notice requirements. An employee with a separate contractual right to maternity leave is entitled to exercise a 'composite' right by taking advantage of whichever right is, in any particular respect, the more favourable.

Insolvent employer

If an employer becomes insolvent, Part XII of the ERA 1996 provides that the employee becomes a preferential creditor in respect of up to four months' wages, or such limit as may be set by the S of S. Other payments such as guarantee payments and payments for time off during ante-natal care are also classed as preferential debts. The employee may claim from the S of S certain sums due from his employer, comprising arrears of up to eight weeks' wages, six weeks' holiday pay and wages during the statutory minimum period of notice. The employee also has the right to ask the S of S to pay pensions contributions which have not been paid due to the employer's insolvency. If the employee does not receive the sums to which he believes he is entitled from the S of S, he has the right to make a complaint to an industrial tribunal.

Equal pay and discrimination

Equal pay

Article 119 of the Treaty of Rome, the Treaty which was signed by the UK on joining the then EEC, provides that:

'Each member state shall … maintain the application of the principle that men and women should receive equal pay for equal work.

For the purpose of this Article, "pay" means the ordinary basic or minimum wage or salary and any other consideration, whether in cash or in kind, which the worker receives, directly or indirectly, in respect of his employment from his employer.'

The spirit of Article 119 is now embodied in the Equal Pay Act 1970 (as amended by the Equal Pay (Amendment) Regulations 1983, SI 1983 No. 1794).

The Act is broadly designed to ensure that men and women employed in similar work receive equal remuneration.

By section 1(1) of the Act an 'equality clause' is implied into a woman's contract of employment if one has not already been included. A woman thus has the right to equal pay with men in three situations:

(1) Where the woman is carrying out 'like work' with a man in the same employment (section 1(2)(a)).
(2) Where her work is 'rated as equivalent' to that done by a man following a job evaluation study (section 1(2)(b)).
(3) Where her work is of 'equal value' in terms of the demands made upon her, to that of a man in the same employment.

Each of these situations must be examined in turn.

Like work

Where a woman claims to be entitled to equal pay on the grounds that her work is 'like work' with a man in the same employment, she must show that the work done by them both is of a broadly similar nature, and that any differences are not of practical importance in relation to terms and conditions of employment. The nature and extent of any differences will have to be closely examined in each individual case. However, the Act is so worded as to prevent irrelevant or insignificant differences in jobs from precluding equal pay. For example, in *Coombs Holdings* v. *Shields* (1978) a female teller in a betting shop claimed equal pay with a male employee doing the same job. On behalf of the employer it was urged that the male employee deserved greater remuneration because he was expected to deal with any trouble that arose. The tribunal found that the difference did not justify a finding that they were not doing like work.

Rated as equivalent

A claim for equal pay based on a finding that the work carried out by the woman is rated as equivalent to that carried out by a male employee invariably follows a job evaluation study. An employer is not obliged to authorize or commission such a study, but once he does he will be bound by the findings.

Section 1(5) of the Act provides that:

'A woman is to be regarded as employed on work rated as equivalent with that of any men if, but only if, her job and their job have been given an equal value, in terms of the demands made on the worker ... or would have been given an equal value but for the evaluation being made on a system setting different values for men and women on the same demand under any heading.'

Equal value

By an amendment made in 1983, section 1(2)(c) of the 1970 Act states that an equality clause is to be implied into a contract of employment:

'Where a woman is employed on work which ... is, in terms of the demand made on her (for instance under such headings as effort, skill and decision), of equal value to that of a man in the same employment.'

This clause is operative only where the provisions relating to like work and work rated as equivalent have no application, for example, where a cook in a shipyard canteen claims to be entitled to equal pay with male shipyard workers (*Hayward* v. *Cammell Laird Shipbuilders Ltd* (1984)). In order to adjudicate on this matter the industrial tribunal must first be satisfied that there are reasonable grounds for determining that the work is of equal value. If there are not, the claim will automatically be dismissed. Secondly, the tribunal must require a panel of experts (to be appointed by the Advisory, Conciliation and Arbitration Service (ACAS)) to compile a report on whether the work is of equal value. The tribunal will then consider the findings in the report in deciding whether the work is of equal value.

The general approach is for the work of the complainant to be compared with that of the 'comparator' male, with whom the complainant alleges she is entitled to equal pay. Percentage points are awarded, taking the output of the comparator as 100%. For example, in *Wells* v. *F. Smales and Son (Fish Merchants) Ltd* (1985), there were 14 female applicants. The ACAS assessor said that nine of them scored higher than the comparator, but five scored lower (between 79% and 95% of the comparator's score). The tribunal found that they all scored so closely that they should all be entitled to equal pay.

The House of Lords in *British Coal Corporation* v. *Smith* (1996) ruled that common terms and conditions meant terms and conditions which were substantially comparable on a broad basis. It is sufficient for the applicant to show that her comparators at another establishment and at her establishment were or would be employed on broadly similar terms.

Employer's defences

Section 1(3) of the 1970 Act provides a defence to an employer against a claim for equal pay where he can prove that the variation in pay is genuinely due to a material factor which is not the difference of sex. That factor must be a material difference between the woman's case and the man's, except where work is alleged to be of equal value, in which case the difference *may* be such a material difference. In other words, where there is a claim based on an allegation of equal value the employer may be able to base his defence arguments on economics. For example, where there are existing females doing a skilled job and, in order to attract other skilled workers into the job, the employer offers more money to new employees who happen to be male, the employer may successfully defend the disparity in wages on the grounds of economic necessity. In the case of *Bilka-Kaufhaus GmbH* v. *Weber von Hartz* (1986), the European Court of Justice held that the disparity in pay must be objectively justified, and must be reasonably necessary in order to cope with a particular set of circumstances (like those previously described). Therefore matters of mere convenience are prevented from justifying a departure from equal terms in a woman's contract.

An employee wishing to make a complaint must do so by making an application to the industrial tribunal. If the tribunal finds in the employee's favour, it may make a declaration to the effect that equal pay must be paid, and up to two years of back pay may be awarded.

Sex discrimination

The Sex Discrimination Act 1975 outlaws discrimination on the grounds of sex and/or the fact that a person is married. There are certain exceptions to the prohibition on discrimination contained in the Act as follows:

(1) 'Special treatment' of women on the grounds of pregnancy and childbirth (section 2).
(2) Discrimination in favour of members of a sex of which in the previous year there were few or no members in the particular job (section 48).
(3) Discrimination in selection, promoting or training where being a man or a woman is a 'genuine occupational qualification'.
(4) Discrimination in certain specified professions such as the police and prison service (section 17–20).
(5) Discrimination in respect of provisions relating to death or retirement.

In relation to (5) above there is still a certain amount of uncertainty. Until recently the position was that if there was a fixed retirement age for men with a particular employer, a woman could not be compelled to retire at a lower age.

The Act covers the following areas of employment:

(1) The selection, interviewing and offering of a job (section 6(1)(a)).
(2) The terms upon which employment is offered (as opposed to the terms of employment once it has commenced) (section 6(1)(a)).
(3) Access to promotion, training, transfer or any other benefit, facility or service (section 6(2)(a)).
(4) Dismissal or the subjecting of any person to any detriment (section 6(2)(b)).

Under section 38(1) it is unlawful to publish any advertisement which might reasonably be taken as displaying an intention to commit an act which is contrary to the Act. Job descriptions which specify the sex of candidates are therefore unlawful.

The categories of discrimination

There are two categories of discrimination in the Act.

Direct discrimination   Less favourable treatment on the grounds of sex or being married. For this to be shown, a direct comparison between the treatment of men and women in the same employment must be possible.

Indirect discrimination   A person discriminates against a woman if:

'he applies to her a requirement which he applies or would apply to a man but

   (i)   which is such that the proportion of women who can comply with it is considerably smaller than the proportion of men who can comply with it, *and*
  (ii)   which he cannot show to be justifiable irrespective of the sex of the person to whom it is applied, *and*
 (iii)   which is to her detriment because she cannot comply with it.'

An example of indirect discrimination would be where candidates are required to be at least 65 kg in weight where that requirement cannot be shown to be justifiable in order to fulfil (ii) above. For example, in *Price* v. *Civil Service Commission* (1978) a condition that all job applicants be under 28 years of age, was held to be discriminatory as many women have time off to have children in their late twenties.

Direct discrimination is unlawful *per se*, but indirect discrimination is not unlawful if it can be shown to be justifiable. 'Justifiable' was defined in *Panesar* v. *Nestlé Co. Ltd* (1980) as 'reasonable commercial necessity' and not 'absolutely necessary'.

In *Ojutiku* v. *Manpower Services Commission* (1982) Lord Keith said: 'I decline to put any gloss on the word "justifiable" ... except that I would say that it clearly applies a lower standard than the word "necessary". There should be sound and tolerable reasons.' Thus commercial considerations will often be capable of defeating a claim based on an allegation of indirect discrimination.

Financial compensation

When the sex and race discrimination legislation was enacted, Parliament provided that financial compensation may not be awarded in cases of indirect discrimination unless it is established that the discrimination was intentional. The law has been developed further in respect of sex discrimination by virtue of the Sex Discrimination and Equal Pay (Miscellaneous Amendments) Regulations 1996. These Regulations provide that industrial tribunals in indirect sex discrimination cases may now award compensation regardless of whether or not the indirect sex discrimination is intentional or not. The Regulations respond to recent criticism that the law was out of line with the requirements of the EC Equal Treatment Directive 76/207. As a consequence the provisions of the Sex Discrimination Act 1975 which preclude the award of damages in cases of unintentional indirect sex discrimination must now be read as amended by the Regulations.

Discrimination on the grounds of race

The Race Relations Act 1976 renders unlawful discrimination on grounds of 'colour, race, nationality or ethnic or national origin'. As with the Sex Discrimination Act 1975 there are defences available to an employer, for example, where it can be proved that being a member of a certain racial group is a 'genuine occupational qualification'. Thus it would not be unlawful for the owner of an Indian restaurant to discriminate against applicants for the job of a waiter where the aim of the restaurant is to create a particular ambience (see section 5(2) of the 1976 Act).

A person who wishes to make a complaint may complain to the industrial tribunal. If the tribunal finds in the applicant's favour, it may make a declaration of rights of the respective parties, and may order compensation. The employer may also be ordered to take certain steps to reduce the effect of the discrimination on the complainant.

The Commission for Racial Equality

The Commission for Racial Equality has extensive investigatory powers, and may conduct formal investigations of employers. Where appropriate the Commission may issue a non-discrimination notice against the employer it has investigated, requiring him to take steps to remedy the situation. Where the notice is not acted upon, the Commission may seek a High Court injunction to enforce compliance. The Commission may issue codes of practice for employers to encourage compliance with the terms of the Act. It also encourages employers to adopt an equal opportunities policy. The position is slightly different under various Acts with respect to Northern Ireland, where in some types of employment employers are obliged to discriminate positively in favour of persons belonging to certain religious groups.

Disability discrimination

The Disability Discrimination Act 1995 introduced new rights for disabled people where discrimination occurs during the course of employment. Where an employer employs at least 15 people, he is placed under a statutory duty to accommodate the needs of a disabled person at work, by considering what adjustments are needed for a particular individual. The duty applies to the situation where a person becomes disabled during the course of his employment, as well as to the situation where an employer interviews a disabled person at the recruitment stage.

A disabled person is one who has 'a physical or mental impairment which has substantial and long-term adverse affects on his or her ability to carry out day-to-day activities'. An 'impairment' will be regarded as affecting normal daily activities if it affects mobility, dexterity, coordination, continence, ability to carry, speech, hearing, eyesight, memory, ability to concentrate, and perception of the risk of personal danger. This will include depression since it is a recognized clinical illness causing impairment.

Self-induced illnesses are specifically excluded from the Act. These include abuse of an addictive substance (alcohol, drugs, nicotine) and complications resulting from deliberate disfigurement (tattoos, body piercing).

In addition to accommodating the needs of a disabled person, the Act provides that reasons for dismissing an employee must not be discriminatory on the grounds of disability. However, this does not mean that employment can never be terminated on grounds of ill-health. If, for example, an employee developed multiple sclerosis or Parkinson's disease, it would be acceptable for an employer to terminate the employment, but only where the illness made it impossible for an employee to perform the main functions of his job and it was not reasonable and practical for an employer to make an adjustment.

In this context the kind of adjustments that an employer should consider include adjustments to premises, re-allocating some of the disabled employee's duties to another employee, altering the employee's working hours, assigning the employee to a different place of work or a different activity at work, allowing the employee reasonable time away from work for rehabilitation and treatment, acquiring or modifying equipment, and where necessary providing supervision.

Discrimination against part-time workers

A part-time worker may complain to an industrial tribunal where an employer discriminates against him because he is part-time. Regulation 5 of the Part-time Workers (Prevention of Less Favourable Treatment) Regulations 2000 gives a part-time worker a right not to be treated less favourably than the employer treats a comparable full-time worker as regards the terms of his contract, or by being subjected to any other detriment by any act or deliberate failure to act.

The starting point for assessing whether a part-time worker is being treated less favourably is to determine who the correct comparable full-time worker should be. The regulations state that a full-time worker is comparable to a part-time worker if, at the time when the treatment alleged to be less favourable to the part-time worker takes place, both workers have been employed by the same employer doing the same work with similar levels of qualification, skills and experience.

The definition of a worker for the purposes of the regulations is sufficiently wide to include a self-employed worker who does not genuinely run his own business. Moreover, there is no prescribed maximum number of hours to be worked by a part-time worker before he can be said to become a full-time worker for the purposes of the regulations. A worker is full-time if he is paid wholly or in part by reference to the time he works, and, having regard to custom and practice of the employer in relation to workers employed by him under the same type of contract, is identified as a full-time worker. There is no minimum number of hours to be worked before a worker qualifies as a part-time worker.

Examples of where an employer in a pharmacy might treat a part-time worker less favourably are:

- where a part-time worker's workload is re-organised and he is given more or less work on a pro rata basis
- where a part-time worker is not considered as a candidate for promotion because he is part-time
- where a part-time worker's pay is less pro rata
- where a part-time worker is not afforded equivalent contractual sick pay and maternity pay
- where a part-time worker does not have equal access to an occupational pension scheme, or other benefits such as health insurance, staff discounts, etc.
- where a part-time worker is not given equal access to training
- where a part-time worker is selected for redundancy because he is part-time
- where a part-time worker is not afforded his statutory entitlement to annual leave and parental leave.

Bringing the employment to an end

Dismissal

The position at common law is that an employer could lawfully dismiss an employee by giving notice in accordance with the period prescribed by the contract of employment. To a certain extent this still remains the case, but as will be seen below, in a few circumstances an employee will be entitled to compensation for loss of his job even though notice was given.

The requisite period of notice required to effect a dismissal may be expressly stated in the contract of employment, or may be implied into the contract by custom in the trade or profession. Where no such period can be implied, a court may arrive at a reasonable period which will be determined by taking all the surrounding circumstances into account, including the age of the employee and the length of service. As a fall-back, section 86 of the ERA 1996 provides a minimum period of notice of one week for an employee who has been continuously employed for between one week and two years, and for an employee who has been employed for over two years, the period is one week for every full year of employment.

Summary dismissal

Where an employer dismisses an employee without notice, it is termed 'summary dismissal'. If there is no justification for the dismissal it is wrongful, and an action for damages may be brought in the county court for breach of the contract of employment. Alternatively, the dismissal may be sufficiently unjustified to merit a complaint of unfair dismissal to an industrial tribunal (although both actions cannot be taken in respect of the same incident).

As a general rule, summary dismissal is only justifiable where the conduct of the employee is such that it prevents 'further satisfactory continuance of the relationship'. For example, in the case of *Sinclair* v. *Neighbour* (1967), the manager of a betting shop borrowed some money from the till, without attempting to hide the fact and with every intention of paying it back. His summary dismissal was nevertheless justified as he was also fully aware that the practice was forbidden.

Resignation

If the employee wishes to leave his employment, he must also comply with the notice procedures. Where none is expressly contained in the contract of employment or can be implied, the same statutory notice periods apply as apply to an employer, except that where the employee has been continuously employed for at least one month, he must give at least one week's notice. However, in a situation where an employee feels forced to leave immediately through the behaviour of his employer, he may make a claim for 'constructive dismissal' (see below).

The employment may be terminated by agreement, in which case the termination will not qualify as a dismissal for the purposes of an unfair dismissal or redundancy claim, although to achieve this result the employment must not be terminated as a result of pressure being applied to the employee to encourage him to leave. Further, the employment may come to an end where it is 'frustrated', i.e. where sickness or imprisonment prevent the employee from returning to work. However, the negative effect of finding a contract of employment frustrated through sickness is that frustration brings a contract to an end: therefore, the employee will not be entitled to statutory sick pay from his employer, and will have to rely on state benefits.

Action for wrongful dismissal

Where an employee alleges that he has been wrongfully dismissed, i.e., where he has been unjustifiably dismissed without, or without the requisite period of, notice by his employer, he may bring an action in the civil courts for wages lost through insufficient notice being given. For this purpose the wages are calculated in accordance with the amount the employee could reasonably be expected to have earned in the notice period (including income such as commission which does not come directly from the employer). Deductions will be made for:

(1) Other sums earned in alternative employment during the dismissal period.
(2) Any state benefits received during the same period.
(3) Sums representing the tax and national insurance contributions that would have been paid out of the wages in the notice period.

Unfair dismissal

The most common form of action taken against an employer is an action for unfair dismissal in the industrial tribunal. Section 94 of the ERA 1996 gives every employee the right not to be unfairly dismissed. This applies whether the dismissal was in accordance with the contract of employment or not. (This procedure is open to all employees except for a few categories, the most important of which are persons over retiring age, policemen, employees on certain 'fixed term' contracts, share fishermen and employees who mainly work outside the UK.)

Proving unfair dismissal

In order to prove unfair dismissal, the employee must first show that there was a dismissal. In most cases this will be obvious. In some cases, however, the employee will have to allege 'constructive dismissal', i.e. the behaviour of the employer was such that the employee could not reasonably be expected to have continued in the employment.

For some time an industrial tribunal would only find constructive dismissal where the employer could be shown to have breached the terms of the contract of employment. However, this was not adequate to cover situations where employers 'squeezed out' employees without committing any specific breach. The modern approach is therefore to imply a term that the employer will not breach the 'relationship of trust and confidence' between himself and the employee and to find constructive dismissal where that term is breached. In the case of *Woods* v. *W.M. Car Service* (1981) it was said that '... an employer who persistently attempts to vary an employee's conditions of services with a view to getting rid of the employee or varying the employee's conditions of service, does an act in a manner calculated to destroy the relationship of confidence and trust between [them]'. Such an employer has therefore breached an implied term.

Unfairness

Having established dismissal, the tribunal must then decide the issue of unfairness. In order to determine the unfairness or otherwise of the dismissal, the reasonableness of the employer's actions are examined. It is for the employer to establish the reasons for the dismissal. Section 98(4) of the ERA 1996 provides that the tribunal must then decide whether:

'in the circumstances (including the size and administrative resources of the employer's undertaking) the employer acted reasonably or unreasonably in treating it as a sufficient reason for dismissing the employee; and that question shall be determined in accordance with the equity and substantial merits of the case.'

Thus the employer is under a duty to act reasonably both substantively and procedurally.

In determining the reasonableness of the dismissal, the tribunal must consider the surrounding circumstances and the provisions of the ACAS code of conduct *Disciplinary Practice and Procedures in Employment*. This provides for various steps to be taken before dismissal such as warnings for offences which are not of the utmost gravity, and a fair hearing before dismissal.

Reasonableness of the dismissal
The employer may rely on one of five categories of reasons to justify the dismissal as reasonable.

Capability or qualifications   The employer may show that the employee was incompetent or not suitably qualified for the employment, but even where this is proved, the employer remains under a duty to comply with the procedural requirements for dismissal in order to render the dismissal reasonable.

Conduct   Where there has been misconduct on the part of the employee, the employer may act reasonably in dismissing him. The ACAS code of practice deals with the procedures which should be adopted by employers, and provides, for example, that only 'serious misconduct' justifies dismissal for a first breach of discipline. The categories of misconduct are wide, but would include for example, drunkenness, dishonesty, sexual harassment and criminal convictions outside the employment.

Redundancy   This is discussed in further detail below, but where an employer can show that the reason for the dismissal was that the employee had genuinely been rendered redundant, the dismissal will not be unfair. Dismissal for redundancy may be rendered unfair in certain situations where the procedure for choosing specific employees for redundancy in similar occupations may have been carried out unfairly. Thus employers are obliged to operate redundancy criteria, and to apply the criteria fairly. Such criteria are often decided in conjunction with trade unions, and where this is the case they may be considered by the tribunal.

Illegality of continued employment   Where it would be illegal for an employee to carry on his employment, e.g. where a solicitor has lost his practising certificate and so can no longer act for clients, dismissal may be justified on the ground of reasonableness.

Other substantial reasons   This is an open category to accommodate particular circumstances. Thus dismissal has been held as justified in cases where employees have unreasonably refused to agree to alterations in working arrangements and hours; where there has been an insurmountable conflict of personalities between employer and employee; and where the work was only of a temporary nature and came to an end.

Pregnancy
A dismissal on the grounds of pregnancy alone will be unfair. The employer can only justify a dismissal in such circumstances where he can show that the employee is, or will have become incapable of doing the work required, or that the employee will not be able to do the work without contravening a legal requirement.

Trade union membership
Except in certain limited circumstances, it is unfair to dismiss an employee for belonging to a trade union. However, membership of trade unions in specific employment is illegal, e.g. the security services.

Procedure
An employee who wishes to allege that a dismissal has been carried out unfairly must make a complaint to the industrial tribunal on form IT1 within three months of the termination of employment (although this period is extendible at the discretion of the tribunal). A copy of the complaint is then sent to the employer who may contest the allegation by replying within 14 days. ACAS is also informed of the complaint, and an attempt to organize a reconciliation between the parties without the need for a formal hearing is made. The procedure governing applications to the industrial tribunal is set out in the Industrial Tribunals Act 1996.

Powers of the tribunal
When a finding of unfair dismissal has been made, the tribunal has a number of remedies available. When the finding has been made, the employee has the option (where practical) to be reinstated (in the same job), or re-engaged (in similar employment). Where it is practicable to make such an order for reinstatement or re-engagement, and the employer only partially complies or fails to comply with the order, the tribunal may make an award of compensation of between 13 and 26 weeks' pay (or 52 weeks' pay in the case of sexual or racial discrimination). The existence of such compensatory awards is designed to encourage the employer to comply with the terms of the order.

Where re-instatement or re-engagement are not appropriate, an award of compensation will be made. The compensation will consist of a basic award and a compensatory award. The maximum basic award is £6600 and is calculated on the basis of the table below.

Age of Employee	Amount of Award (calculated in weeks' pay for each year of continuous employment)
18–21	0.5
22–40	1
41–65	1.5

The compensatory award will invariably be larger, and is subject to a current maximum of £50 000. The heads of loss compensated are as follows:

(1) Expenses directly incurred as a result of the dismissal including loss of perks and fringe benefits.
(2) Lost earnings up to the hearing date.
(3) Estimated future loss of earnings.
(4) The manner of the dismissal, i.e. if the manner of the dismissal will have made the employee less attractive to subsequent employers, compensation may be awarded.
(5) Loss of the protection afforded against unfair dismissal by two years of continuous employment, i.e. the risk of being unfairly dismissed during the first two years of subsequent employment without the protection of the ERA 1996 may be compensated for in small amount.
(6) Loss of pension rights.

There is no upper limit for the compensatory award in unfair dismissal proceedings where the dismissal is attributable to discrimination under the EEC Directive for equal pay and equal treatment for men and women, as regards access to employment, vocational training and working conditions; see *Marshall* v. *Southampton and SW Hampshire AHA* (1993).

The employee is under a duty to minimize his loss by taking all reasonable steps to find and accept offers of reasonable alternative employment. Further, if the tribunal finds that the employee contributed to the loss of his employment, it may make a deduction from the overall sum of the compensatory award.

Redundancy

Under the ERA 1996, all persons who work under a contract of employment are entitled to an award on being made redundant with exceptions as follows:

(1) Employees of less than two years' standing.
(2) Persons over retirement age.
(3) Persons under 18 years.
(4) Share fishermen.
(5) Persons on 'fixed term' contracts of longer than two years who have agreed in writing to forgo their right to a redundancy payment.
(6) Persons normally working outside the UK.
(7) Those covered by an approved redundancy agreement.

An employee can only claim to have been made redundant where he can be shown to have been dismissed. Once dismissal has been proved, there is a presumption by virtue of section 163(2) of the ERA 1996 that the reason for the dismissal was redundancy. It is then for the employer to show that the dismissal was for some reason other than redundancy (e.g. misconduct). By section 139(1) of the ERA 1996, there is a redundancy where the dismissal is attributable to:

'(a) the fact that the employer has ceased, or intends to cease, to carry on the business for the purposes of which the employee was employed by him; ... (or)
(b) the fact that the requirements of that business for employees to carry out work of a particular kind ... have ceased or diminished or are expected to cease or diminish.'

Where the employer has asked for volunteers for redundancy, and the employee accepts a redundancy package voluntarily, the right to claim a redundancy payment under the ERA 1996 is lost.

Where an employee is laid off or put on short time, and there is no provision for such an eventuality in the contract of employment, the employee is entitled to claim to have been made redundant. If the contract of employment does make provision for such eventualities, but the employee is laid off or on short time for four consecutive weeks or for six of the preceding 13 weeks, the employee may claim redundancy.

This is done by sending written notice of intention to claim redundancy to the employer. The employer then issues a counter notice within seven days stating that there is a reasonable chance within the following four weeks that the employee will commence a period of 13 weeks consecutive employment. If the promise is not fulfilled, the employee is entitled to a redundancy payment.

If an employee is offered suitable alternative employment by his employer, he will lose his right to a redundancy payment if he unreasonably refuses it.

Redundancy awards

An employee who considers that he has been made redundant must make a written claim for a payment to his employer. If the employer refuses to make the payment, the employee can refer the matter to the industrial tribunal within six months of the termination of the employment. The amount of the award is calculated in accordance with the table set out above which is also used for calculating the basic award in unfair dismissal proceedings. However, for each month a claimant is over the age of 64, the overall amount is reduced by one twelfth for each complete month worked and the maximum weekly figure for earnings used in calculating the payment is £220, and the maximum number of years for which payment can be claimed is 20.

Some large employers agree their own schemes for redundancy with employees and trade unions. With the consent of the S of S, they can thereby contract out of the legislation.

Where the employee is a member of an independent trade union, the employer is usually under a duty to discuss proposed redundancy with a union representative. Particular rules requiring consultation apply when the number of employees facing redundancy is greater than ten. If the employer fails to carry out the necessary consultation process, the trade union may make a complaint to the industrial tribunal and seek a declaration of the parties' respective rights. The tribunal may also make a 'protective award' whereby the employees concerned must be paid during a specific period not exceeding 90 days. This is designed to protect the employees' interests during the consultation period. If the employer fails to comply with an order for a protective award, the employee may make a complaint to the tribunal as an individual.

There is therefore fairly comprehensive provision for compensatory payments to employees who are made redundant, but unless the employee has been working for many years, the size of the statutory award is likely to be relatively small. An employee who has been notified of forthcoming redundancy is entitled to reasonable time off work in order to look for alternative employment, but only if he has been in continuous employment for two years.

Human rights at work

One of the areas forecast to be most affected by the Human Rights Act 1998 is employment law. Although the Act does not create direct obligations by an employer to an employee, industrial tribunals will be required to interpret existing UK employment law in line with the principles of the European Convention on Human Rights and its associated case law.

Employee privacy is a key area, since Article 8 of the Convention provides for the right to respect for private and family life, home and correspondence. Interference with this right is only permitted if it is 'in accordance with the law' and 'necessary in a democratic society' and is effected for a legitimate purpose, such as the prevention of crime or the protection of health.

The case law under the Convention makes it clear that employees cannot complain if they are made aware that their employer reserves the right to conduct monitoring of telephone, e-mail and other communication facilities. Since working in a pharmacy exposes a dishonest employee to a vista of temptations (*viz.* unlawful sales of medicines, fraudulent prescription claims, etc.) pharmacists would be well advised to insert a clause to this effect in an employee's contract of employment.

The use of CCTV and other monitoring equipment may be permitted; however, a crucial point is that measures conflicting with the right to privacy can only be taken where 'proportionate', in the sense that the interference must be reasonable and justifiable in the circumstances. Indiscriminate monitoring may not be permitted.

Dress codes are frequently discussed in the light of Article 10 of the Convention, which guarantees freedom of expression. One of the leading cases on this point concerned an employee who was dismissed for insisting upon wearing a number of badges to work proclaiming that she was a lesbian. Her unfair dismissal claim failed on the basis that the employer could decide, after sensible consideration, what was likely to offend fellow customers and employees. The result of this case is unlikely to be different now that the Human Rights Act 1998 is in force. Community pharmacists have reasonable grounds to impose a sensible dress code to operate their pharmacy, provided that the code is reasonable and justifiable, or proportionate, in all the circumstances.

Only time will tell how much the principles of the Act will affect the approach of industrial tribunals to their application of UK employment law. Although many of the issues covered by the Act are already addressed by domestic law, inevitably there will be some cases where the Human Rights Act 1998 will give rise to some expanded arguments on the part of an aggrieved employee.

Definitions

Analysis: includes microbiological assay but no other form of biological assay, and analyse has a corresponding meaning.

Animal: includes any bird, fish or reptile. [It therefore excludes other classes of animal, e.g. insect.]

Animal test certificate: Section 32 of the MA 1968 is a certificate which is issued by the MCA and which certifies that, subject to the provisions on the face of the certificate, the licensing authority has consented to the test in question. It authorizes the sale or supply of a medicinal product, its procurement, manufacture or assembly for the purposes of a medicinal test on animals. Such a sale would otherwise be unlawful by virtue of section 32(1).

Appliance: means an appliance included in a list for the time being approved by the S of S for the purposes of section 41 of the NHS Act 1977 (as amended). [NHS (PS) Regulations 1992.]

Appropriate committee: means whichever one of the committees established under section 4 of the MA 1968 (known as Section 4 Committees) is appropriate in the circumstances being considered.

Appropriate Ministers: means the M(H), the Secretary of State concerned with health in Scotland, and the Minister of Health and Social Services for Northern Ireland where the function considered is one concerned with matters of human health alone.

Where the matter is concerned with veterinary drugs and the treatment of diseases of animals 'the appropriate Ministers' means the Health Ministers listed above, plus the Agriculture Ministers, i.e. the Minister of Agriculture, Fisheries and Food, the Secretary of State concerned with agriculture in Scotland, and the Minister of Agriculture for Northern Ireland.

Approved non-proprietary name: means a non-proprietary name which is not mentioned in Sch. 10 to the GMS Regulations or, except where the conditions in paragraph 44(2) of the doctors' terms of service are satisfied, in Sch. 11 to those Regulations. [NHS (PS) Regulations 1992.]

Assemble: in relation to a medicinal product means: enclosing the product in a container which is labelled before the product is sold or supplied, *or* labelling the container which already contains the product.

Business: includes a professional practice and includes any activity carried on by a body of persons, whether corporate or incorporate.

Chemist: (1) means in the NHS (PS) Regulations:

(a) A registered pharmacist.
(b) A person lawfully conducting a RPB in accordance with section 69 of the MA 1968.
(c) A supplier of appliances. [NHS (PS) Regulations 1992.]

(2) means in the NHS (Charges) Regulations 1989:

Any person, other than a doctor, providing pharmaceutical services.

Clinical trial, clinical trial certificate: section 31 of the MA 1968.

The Commission: the Medicines Commission.

Composition: means the ingredients of which a medicinal product consists and the proportions, and the degrees of strength, quality and purity, in which those ingredients are contained in the medicinal product.

Container: the bottle, jar, box, packet, or other receptacle which contains the medicinal product. It excludes a capsule, cachet or other article in which the product is or is to be administered. Where the bottle, jar, etc., is or is to be contained in another receptacle – an outer packaging – the term 'container' does not include the outer packaging.

Contravention: includes failure to comply.

Controlled locality: means an area which an HA or, on appeal, the S of S has determined is rural in character in accordance with Reg. 9 or, as the case may be, Reg. 10. [NHS (PS) Regulations 1992.]

Dentist: means a person registered in the Dentists' Register under the Dentists Act 1957.

Disease: includes any injury, ailment or adverse condition, whether of body or mind.

Doctor:

(1)   Means a fully registered person within the meaning of the Medical Act 1956. [MA1968.]
(2)   Means a medical practitioner. [NHS (PS) Regulations 1992.]
(3)   Means a registered medical practitioner. [NHS (GMS) Regulations 1992.]
(4)   Means a registered medical practitioner, other than one acting in the capacity of an opththalmic medical practitioner [NHS (Service Committees and Tribunal) Regulations 1992.]

Drugs:

(1)   Includes medicines. [NHS (PS) Regulations 1992.]
(2)   Includes medicines, but does not include contraceptive substances. [NHS (Charges) Regulations 1989.]

Enforcement authority: means any Minister or body on whom a duty or power to enforce any provisions of the MA 1968 or of any regulations or order made thereunder is imposed or conferred by or under sections 108 to 110 of the Act.

Export: means export from the UK by land, sea or air.

Food and drugs authority: Section 83, Food and Drugs Act 1955.

The Gazette: the London, Edinburgh and Belfast Gazettes.

Group practice: means an association of not less than two doctors both or all of whom:

(1)   Have their names included in an HAs medical list.
(2)   Coordinate, in the course of regular contact between them, their respective obligations under the terms of service for doctors to provide personal medical services to their patients.
(3)   Conduct and manage their practices from at least one common set of practice premises [NHS (GMS) Regulations 1992.]

Health prescription: means a prescription issued under or by virtue of:

(1)   In England and Wales, the NHS Act 1977.
(2)   In Scotland, the NHS (Scotland) Act 1978.

(3) In Northern Ireland, the Health and Personal Social Services (Northern Ireland) Order 1972. [POM 1983.]

Herbal remedy: a medicinal product consisting of a substance produced by drying or crushing a plant or plants, or subjecting them to any other process; *or* a mixture of one or more such substances together with water or some other inert substance.
Herd: includes a flock.
Hospital:

(1) Includes a clinic, nursing home or similar institution. [but is otherwise not defined] (MA 1968).
(2) Means

(a) Any institution for the reception and treatment of persons suffering from illness.
(b) Any maternity home.
(c) Any institution for the reception and treatment of persons during convalescence or persons requiring medical rehabilitation,

and includes clinics, dispensaries and out-patient departments maintained in connection with any such home or institution, and hospital accommodation shall be construed accordingly. [NHS Act 1977.]

Hover vehicle: means a vehicle designed to be supported on a cushion of air. [Appears in the MA 1968, section 111, dealing with rights of entry of medicines inspectors.)
Illness: includes mental disorder within the meaning of the Mental Health Act 1983 and any injury or disability requiring medical or dental treatment or nursing. [NHS Act 1977.]
Ingredient: in relation to the manufacture or preparation of a substance, includes anything which is the sole active ingredient of that substance as manufactured or prepared. [Ingredient includes the sole active. Presumably the term extends beyond actives to non-actives – in other words, ingredients are the substances from which the product is created.]
Label: is the notice describing or relating to the contents, which is affixed to or otherwise displayed on a container or package of medicinal products.
Leaflet: includes any written information.
Licensing authority: the body of Ministers concerned with health and agriculture. The MCA acts on behalf of Ministers as the UK licensing authority.
Listed drugs and medicines: means the drugs and medicines included in a list for the time being approved by the S of S for the purposes of section 41(c) of the NHS Act 1977. [NHS (PS) Regulations 1992.]
Locality: except in the expression 'controlled locality' means the locality for which an HA is established. [NHS (PS) Regulations 1992.]
Manufacture: includes any process carried out in the course of *making* the product. It does not include dissolving, dispersing, diluting or mixing with a vehicle for the purpose of administering the product. Thus the reconstitution of an injection from powder and water is not manufacture. Neither is the dissolving of a tablet in water to form a solution to drink. However the production of a medicine from its ingredients will be manufacture, regardless of the scale of the production.
Manufacturer's licence: subject to a number of exceptions, no person shall, in the course of a business carried on by him, manufacture or assemble any medicinal product except in accordance with a manufacturer's licence.
Medical: includes surgical. [NHS Act 1977.]
Medical records: means the records maintained in respect of any patient pursuant to paragraph 36 of the doctors' terms of service [NHS (GMS) Regulations 1992.]

Medicine: includes such chemical reagents as are included in a list for the time being approved by the S of S for the purposes of section 41 of the NHS Act 1977.

Non-proprietary name: in relation to a drug means:

(1) Where the drug is described in a monograph in the current edition (as specified in section 103(5) of the MA 1968), as in force at the time of the supply of the drug, of the EP, BP, BPC, BNF, International Pharmacopoeia (IP), the Cumulative List of Recommended International Non-proprietary names or the DPF, any name, or abbreviation of such name, at the head of that monograph or, where such name consists of two or more words, any name derived from a suitable inversion of such words which is permitted by that publication; *or*

(2) Where the drug is not so described but has an approved name, being the name which appears in the current edition (as defined in section 103(5) of the MA 1968) of the list of names prepared and published under section 100 of that Act, as in force at the time of the supply of the drug, such approved name. [NHS (PS) Regulations 1992.]

Package: the box or wrapping in which the 'container' is placed.

Parenteral adminstration: means administration by breach of the skin or mucous membrane. [POM 1983.]

Patient:

(1) Paragraph 4 of Sch. 2 to GMS Regulations 1992, SI 1992 No.635, gives a long list of the persons who are 'a doctor's patients', e.g. temporary residents.

(2) means:

    (a) Any person for whose treatment a doctor is responsible under his terms of service.

    (b) Any person who applies to a chemist for the provision of pharmaceutical services including a person who applies on behalf of another person.

    (c) A person who pays or undertakes to pay on behalf of another person a charge for which these Regulations provide. [NHS (Charges) Regulations 1989.]

(3) Includes an expectant or nursing mother and a lying-in woman [NHS Act 1977.]

Pharmaceutical Society: RPSGB or PSNI.

Pharmacist:

(1) In Great Britain: a person registered in the register of pharmaceutical chemists, established under the Pharmacy Act 1852 and maintained under section 2(1) of the Pharmacy Act 1954.

(2) In Northern Ireland: a person registered in the register of pharmaceutical chemists for Northern Ireland, made out and maintained under section 9 of the Pharmacy and Poisons Act (Northern Ireland) 1925. [MA 1968.]

(3) A registered pharmacist, other than a supplier of appliances only, whose name is included in the list of an HA under section 42 of the NHS Act 1977 or who is employed by any person (including a body corporate) who is so included. [NHS (PS) Regulations 1992.]

(4) Means a registered pharmacist. [NHS Service Committees and Tribunal) Regulations 1992.]

Pharmacy: means any premises where drugs are provided by a pharmacist pursuant to arrangements made under section 41 of the NHS Act 1977. [NHS (PS) Regulations 1992.]

Plant: includes any part of a plant.

Poultry: means domestic fowls, turkeys, geese, ducks, guinea-fowls, pigeons, pheasants and partridges.

Practice area: means the area in which a doctor is under an obligation to visit patients, by virtue either of his application for inclusion in the medical list or of any variation to it pursuant to these Regulations or the terms of service. [NHS (GMS) Regulations 1992.]

Practitioner:

(1) Doctor, dentist or vet. [MA 1968.]
(2) Means a doctor, dentist, opththalmic medical practitioner, optician or chemist against whom a complaint has been made or in respect of whom a matter has been referred under Regs. 7 or 8. [NHS (Service Committees and Tribunal) Regulations 1992.]

Prescribed: prescribed by Regulations made under the MA 1968.

Prescription form:

(1) A form provided by an HA or by an FHSA and issued to enable a person to obtain pharmaceutical services. [NHS (PS) Regulations 1992.]
(2) A form on which the provision of pharmaceutical services may be ordered by:

    (a) A doctor in pursuance of a health authority's functions; *or*
    (b) A doctor or dental practitioner under the provisions of their terms of service,

and which contains on its reverse side a form of declaration of entitlement to exemption. [NHS (Charges) Regulations 1989.]

Product licence: is a licence granted for the purposes of section 7 of the MA 1968. Subject to a number of exceptions, commercial activities related to a medicinal product are unlawful unless a product licence is in existence.

Registered pharmacist: means a pharmacist registered in the register of pharmaceutical chemists. [NHS Act 1977.]

Registered pharmacy: means premises for the time being entered in the Register of Premises kept by the Registrar of the RSPGB. [It is the premises which constitute a 'registered pharmacy', not the business or practice.]

Relevant service:

(1) Wholetime service in the armed forces of the Crown in a national emergency, whether as a volunteer or otherwise.
(2) Compulsory wholetime service in those forces, including service resulting from any reserve liability.
(3) Any equivalent service by a person liable for compulsory wholetime service in those forces.

Retail pharmacy business: means a business which: consists of the retail sale of P or POM, or includes the retail sale of P or POM. It does not include the professional practice of a practitioner, i.e. doctor, dentist or vet.

It does not matter whether GSL medicines are sold by retail as well; it is the inclusion of the retail sale of P or POM which makes a business an RPB.

Scheduled drug: means a drug or other substance specified in Sch. 10 to the GMS Regulations 1992 or except where the conditions in paragraph 44(2) of the doctors' terms of service are satisfied, Sch. 11 to those Regulations. [NHS (PS) Regulations 1992.]

Substance: means any natural or artificial substance, whether in solid or liquid form or in the form of a gas or vapour.

Supply: means supply in circumstances corresponding to retail sale as defined in the MA 1968. [POM 1983.]

Treatment:

(1) In relation to disease, includes anything done or provided for alleviating the effects of the disease, whether it is done or provided by way of cure or not. [MA 1968.]
(2) Means medical attendance and treatment, but does not include child health surveillance services, contraceptive services, maternity medical services or minor surgery services, unless the doctor has undertaken to provide such services to the person concerned in accordance with these Regulations. [NHS (GMS) Regulations 1992.]

Venereal disease: syphilis, gonorrhea or soft chancre (Venereal Disease Act 1917).

Veterinary drug: means a medicinal product which is manufactured, sold, supplied, imported or exported for the purpose of being administered to animals, but not for the purpose of being administered to human beings.

Veterinary practitioner: means a person registered in the supplementary veterinary register kept under section 8 of the Veterinary Surgeons Act 1966.

Veterinary surgeon: means a person registered in the register of veterinary surgeons kept under section 2 of the Veterinary Surgeons Act 1966.

Wholesale dealer's licence: no person shall, in the course of a business carried on by him, sell, or offer for sale, any medicinal product except in accordance with a licence granted for the purpose. There are a number of exceptions.

Writing: includes any form of notation, whether by hand or by printing, typewriting or any similar process, and 'written' has a corresponding meaning. [This definition includes the use of rubber stamps and the like. The legislation must use a phrase such as 'in his own handwriting' if it is to be restrictive. By extension, the use of a word processor comes within the definition of writing. The question of distant printers, faxes, etc., is still unclear.]

Appendix 2

National Health Service Act 1977 Sections 1, 8, 15, 42 & 43

Functions of the Secretary of State

1 Secretary of State's duty as to health service

(1) It is the Secretary of State's duty to continue the promotion in England and Wales of a comprehensive health service designed to secure improvement —

   (a)   in the physical and mental health of the people of those countries, and

   (b)   in the prevention, diagnosis and treatment of illness,

and for that purpose to provide or secure the effective provision of services in accordance with this Act.

(2) The services so provided shall be free of charge except in so far as the making and recovery of charges is expressly provided for by or under any enactment, whenever passed.

Local administration

8 Health Authorities

(1) It is the duty of the Secretary of State by order to establish, in accordance with Part I of Schedule 5 to this Act, authorities to be called Health Authorities.

(2) Subject to subsection (4) below, a Health Authority shall act for such area of England or of Wales as is specified in the order establishing the authority.

(3) A Health Authority shall be known by such name, in addition to the title 'Health Authority', as —

   (a)   appears to the Secretary of State appropriately to signify the connection of the Health Authority with the area for which the authority are to act; and

   (b)   is specified in the order establishing the authority.

(4) The Secretary of State may by order —

   (a)   vary a Health Authority's area;

   (b)   abolish a Health Authority; or

   (c)   establish a new Health Authority.

(5) The Secretary of State shall act under this section so as to secure —

   (a)   that the areas for which Health Authorities are at any time acting together comprise the whole of England and Wales; but

   (b)   that no area for which a Health Authority act extends both into England and Wales.

(6) The power to make incidental or supplemental provision conferred by section 126(4) below includes in particular, in its application to orders made under this section, power to make provision for the transfer of staff, property, rights and liabilities.''

(2) Subject fo section 8, subsection (1) shall not come into force until 1st April 1996.

15 Duty of Health Authority

(1) It is the duty of each Health Authority, in accordance with regulations

[(*a*) to administer the arrangements made in pursuance of this Act for the provision of general medical services, general dental services, general ophthalmic services and pharmaceutical services for their area;]

(*b*) to perform such [management and] other functions relating to those services as may be prescribed.

(1B) In relation to a medical practitioner, any reference in this Act or the National Health Service and Community Care Act 1990 to the relevant Health Authority shall be construed as follows, —

(*a*) if he practises in partnership with other medical practitioners, the relevant Health Authority is that Health Authority on whose medical list the members of the practice are included and, if some are included on one Health Authority's medical list and some on another's or if any of the members is included in the medical lists of two or more Health Authorities, the relevant Health Authority is that Health Authority in whose area resides the largest number of individuals who are on the lists of patients of the members of the practice; and

(*b*) in any other case, the relevant Health Authority is that Health Authority on whose medical list he is included and, if there is more than one, that one of them in whose area resides the largest number of individuals who are on his list of patients.]

(2) . . .

s. 41 Arrangements for pharmaceutical services

It is the duty of every Health Authority, in accordance with regulations which shall be made for the purpose, to arrange as respects their area for the provision to persons who are in that locality of —

(*a*) proper and sufficient drugs and medicines and listed appliances which are ordered for those persons by a medical practitioner in pursuance of his functions in the health service, the Scottish health service, the Northern Ireland health service or the armed forces of the Crown;

(*b*) proper and sufficient drugs and medicines which are ordered for those persons by a dental practitioner in pursuance of –

   (i)   his functions in the health service, the Scottish health service or the Northern Ireland health service (other than functions exercised in pursuance of the provision of services mentioned in paragraph (*c*)); or

   (ii) his functions in the armed forces of the Crown;

(*c*) listed drugs and medicines which are ordered for those persons by a dental practitioner in pursuance of the provision of general dental services or equivalent services in the Scottish health services or the Northern Ireland health service;

(*d*) such drugs and medicines and such listed appliances as may be determined by the Secretary of State for the purposes of this paragraph which are ordered for those persons by a prescribed description of person in accordance with such conditions, if any as may be prescribed, in pursuance of functions in the health service, the Scottish health service, the Northern Ireland health service or the armed forces of the Crown; and

(*e*) such other services as may be prescribed.

[42 Regulations as to pharmaceutical services

(1) Regulations shall provide for securing that arrangements made by a Health Authority under section 41 above will enable persons in the Health Authority's area for whom drugs, medicines or appliances mentioned in that section are ordered as there mentioned to receive them from persons with whom such arrangements have been made.

(2) The regulations shall include provision—

(a) for the preparation and publication by a Health Authority of one or more lists of persons, other than medical practitioners and dental practitioners, who undertake to provide pharmaceutical services from premises in the Health Authority's area;

(b) that an application to a Health Authority for inclusion in such a list shall be made in the prescribed manner and shall state—

  (i) the services which the applicant will undertake to provide and, if they consist of or include the supply of appliances, which appliances he will undertake to supply; and

  (ii) the premises from which he will undertake to provide those services;

(c) that, except in prescribed cases—

  (i) an application for inclusion in such a list by a person not already included; and

  (ii) an application by a person already included in such a list for inclusion also in respect of services or premises other than those already listed in relation to him,

  shall be granted only if the Health Authority is satisfied, in accordance with the regulations, that it is necessary or desirable to grant it in order to secure in the neighbourhood in which the premises are located the adequate provision by persons included in the list of the services, or some of the services, specified in the application; and

(d) for the removal of an entry in respect of premises from a list if it has been determined in the prescribed manner that the person to whom the entry relates—

  (i) has never provided from those premises; or

  (ii) has ceased to provide from them.

  the services, or any of the services, which he is listed as undertaking to provide from them.

(3) The regulations may include provision—

(a) that an application to a Health Authority may be granted in respect of some only of the services specified in it;

(b) that an application to a Health Authority relating to services of a prescribed description shall be granted only if it appears to the Health Authority that the applicant has satisfied such conditions with regard to the provision of those services as may be prescribed;

[(ba) that an application to a Health Authority by a person who qualified to have his name registered under the Pharmacy Act 1954 by virtue of section 4A of that Act (qualification by European diploma) shall not be granted unless the applicant satisfies the Health Authority that he has the knowledge of English which, in the interests of himself and persons making use of the services to which the application relates, is necessary for the provision of pharmaceutical services in the Health Authority's area

(c) that the inclusion of a person in a list in pursuance of such an application may be for a fixed period;

(d) that, where the premises from which an application states that the applicant will undertake to provide services are in an area of a prescribed description, the applicant shall not be included in the list unless his inclusion is approved by reference to prescribed criteria by the Health Authority in whose area the premises are situated; and]

(e) that that Health Authority may give its approval subject to conditions.

(4) The regulations shall include provision conferring on such persons as may be prescribed rights of appeal from decisions made by virtue of this section.

(5) The regulations shall be so framed as to preclude—

(*a*)   a person included in a list published under subsection (2)(*a*) above; and

(*b*)   an employee of such a person;

from taking part in the decision whether an application such is as mentioned in subsection (2)(*c*) above should be granted or an appeal against such a decision brought by virtue of subsection (4) above should be allowed.

43 Persons authorised to provide pharmaceutical services

(1) No arrangements shall be made by a Health Authority (except as may be provided by or under regulations) with a medical practitioner or dental practitioner under which he is required or agrees to provide pharmaceutical services to any person to whom he is rendering general medical services or general dental services.

(2) No arrangements for the dispensing of medicines shall be made (except as may be provided by or under regulations) with persons other than persons who are registered pharmacists, or are persons lawfully conducting a retail pharmacy business in accordance with section 69 of the Medicines Act 1968 and who undertake that all medicines supplied by them under the arrangements made under this Part of this Act shall be dispensed either by or under the direct supervision of a registered pharmacist.

(3) No arrangements for the provision of pharmaceutical services falling within section 41(*d*) above shall be made with persons other than those who are registered pharmacists or are of a prescribed description.

Appendix 3

Medicines Act 1968
Sections 7, 8, 9, 10 & 52–60

7 General provisions as to dealing with medicinal products

(1) The following provisions of this section shall have effect subject to—

(a) any exemption conferred by or under this Part of this Act;

(b) the provisions of this Part of this Act relating to clinical trials and medicinal tests on animals; and

(c) the provisions of section 48 of this Act.

(2) Except in accordance with a licence granted for the purposes of this section (in this Act referred to as a 'product licence') no person shall, in the course of a business carried on by him, and in circumstances to which this subsection applies,—

(a) sell, supply or export any medicinal product, or

(b) procure the sale, supply or exportation of any medicinal product, or

(c) procure the manufacture or assembly of any medicinal product for sale, supply or exportation.

(3) No person shall import any medicinal product except in accordance with a product licence.

(4) In relation to an imported medicinal product, subsection (2) of this section applies to circumstances in which the person selling, supplying or exporting the medicinal product in question, or procuring the sale, supply or exportation or the manufacture or assembly for sale, supply or exportation of that product, has himself imported the product or procured its importation.

(5) In relation to any medicinal product which has not been imported, subsection (2) of this section applies to any circumstances in which the person selling, supplying or exporting the medicinal product in question, or procuring the sale, supply or exportation or the manufacture or assembly for sale, supply or exportation of that product, is responsible for the composition of the product.

(6) For the purposes of subsection (5) of this section a person shall be taken to be responsible for the composition of a medicinal product if (but only if) in the course of a business carried on by him—

(a) he procures the manufacture of the product to his order by another person, where the order specifies, or incorporates by reference to some other document, particulars of the composition of the product ordered, whether those particulars amount to a complete specification or not, or

(b) he manufactures the product otherwise than in pursuance of an order which fulfils the conditions specified in the preceding paragraph.

8 Provisions as to manufacture and wholesale dealing

(1) The following provisions of this section shall have effect without prejudice to the operation of section 7 of this Act, but subject to the exemptions and provisions referred to in paragraphs (a) to (c) of subsection (1) of that section.

(2) No person shall, in the course of a business carried on by him, manufacture or assemble any medicinal product except in accordance with a licence granted for the purposes of this subsection (in this Act referred to as a 'manufacturer's licence').

(3) No person shall, in the course of a business carried on by him, sell, or offer for sale, any medicinal product by way of wholesale dealing except in accordance with a licence granted for the purposes of this subsection (in this Act referred to as a 'wholesale dealer's licence').

9 Exemptions for doctors, dentists, veterinary surgeons and veterinary practitioners

(1) The restrictions imposed by sections 7 and 8 of this Act do not apply to anything done by a doctor or dentist which—

(a) relates to a medicinal product specially prepared, or specially imported by him or to his order, for administration to a particular patient of his, and consists of manufacturing or assembling, or procuring the manufacture or assembly of, the product, or of selling or supplying, or procuring the sale or supply of, the product to that patient or to a person under whose care that patient is, or

(b) relates to a medicinal product specially prepared at the request of another doctor or dentist, or specially imported by him or to his order at the request of another doctor or dentist, for administration to a particular patient of that other doctor or dentist, and consists of manufacturing or assembling, or procuring the manufacture or assembly of, the product, or of selling or supplying, or procuring the sale or supply of, the product to that other doctor or dentist or to that patient or to a person under whose care that patient is.

(2) Subject to subsection (3) of this section, the restrictions imposed by sections 7 and 8 of this Act do not apply to anything done by a veterinary surgeon or veterinary practitioner which—

(a) relates to a medicinal product specially prepared for administration to a particular animal or herd which is under his care, and consists of manufacturing or assembling, or procuring the manufacture or assembly of, the product, or of selling or supplying, or procuring the sale or supply of, the product to a person having the possession or control of that animal or herd, or

(b) relates to a medicinal product specially prepared at the request of another veterinary surgeon or veterinary practitioner for administration to a particular animal or herd which is under the care of that other veterinary surgeon or veterinary practitioner, and consists of manufacturing or assembling, or procuring the manufacture or assembly of, the product, or of selling or supplying, or procuring the sale or supply of, the product to that other veterinary surgeon or veterinary practitioner or to a person having the possession or control of that animal or herd.

(3) The last preceding subsection shall not have effect so as to exempt from the restrictions imposed by sections 7 and 8 of this Act anything done by a veterinary surgeon or veterinary practitioner—

(a) in relation to a vaccine specially prepared for administration to poultry, or

(b) in relation to any other vaccine, unless the vaccine is specially prepared for administration to the animal from which it is derived, or

(c) in relation to plasma or a serum, unless the plasma or serum is specially prepared for administration to one or more animals in the herd from which it is derived.

10 Exemptions for pharmacists

(1) Subject to the next following subsection, the restrictions imposed by sections 7 and 8 of this Act do not apply to anything which is done in a registered pharmacy, a hospital or a health centre and is done there by or under the supervision of a pharmacist and consists of—

(*a*) preparing or dispensing a medicinal product in accordance with a prescription given by a practitioner, or

(*b*) assembling a medicinal product;

and those restrictions do not apply to anything done by or under the supervision of a pharmacist which consists of procuring the preparation or dispensing of a medicinal product in accordance with a prescription given by a practitioner, or of procuring the assembly of a medicinal product.

(2) The exemption conferred by the preceding subsection does not apply to a vaccine specially prepared for administration to poultry, and does not apply to any other vaccine or any plasma or serum prepared or dispensed for administration to an animal or herd unless —

(*a*) in the case of a vaccine, it is specially prepared for administration to the animal from which it is derived, or

(*b*) in the case of plasma or a serum, it is specially prepared for administration to one or more animals in the herd from which it is derived,

and (in either case) it is so prepared in accordance with a prescription given by a veterinary surgeon or veterinary practitioner.

(3) Those restrictions do not apply to the preparation or dispensing in a registered pharmacy of a medicinal product by or under the supervision of a pharmacist in accordance with a specification furnished by the person to whom the product is or is to be sold or supplied, where —

(*a*) the product is prepared or dispensed for administration to that person or to a person under his care, or

(*b*) the product, not being a vaccine, plasma or serum, is prepared or dispensed for administration to an animal or herd which is in the possession or under the control of that person.

(4) Without prejudice to the preceding subsections, the restrictions imposed by sections 7 and 8 of this Act do not apply to anything which is done in a registered pharmacy by or under the supervision of a pharmacist and consists of —

(*a*) preparing or dispensing a medicinal product for administration to a person where the pharmacist is requested by or on behalf of that person to do so in accordance with the pharmacist's own judgment as to the treatment required, and that person is present in the pharmacy at the time of the request in pursuance of which that product is prepared or dispensed, or

(*b*) preparing a stock of medicinal products with a view to dispensing them as mentioned in subsection (1)(*a*) or subsection (3) of this section or in paragraph (*a*) of this subsection;

and those restrictions do not apply to anything which is done in a hospital or a health centre by or under the supervision of a pharmacist and consists of preparing a stock of medicinal products with a view to dispensing them as mentioned in subsection (1)(*a*) of this section.

52 Sale or supply of medicinal products not on general sale list

Subject to any exemption conferred by or under this Part of this Act, on and after such day as the Ministers may by order appoint for the purposes of this section (in this Part of this Act referred to as 'the appointed day') no person shall, in the course of a business carried on by him, sell by retail, offer or expose for sale by retail, or supply in circumstances corresponding to retail sale, any medicinal product which is not a medicinal product on a general sale list, unless —

(*a*) that person is, in respect of that business, a person lawfully conducting a retail pharmacy business;

(*b*) the product is sold, offered or exposed for sale, or supplied, on premises which are a registered pharmacy; and

(c)   that person, or, if the transaction is carried out on his behalf by another person, then that other person, is, or acts under the supervision of, a pharmacist.

53 Sale or supply of medicinal products on general sale list

(1) Subject to any exemption conferred by or under this Part of this Act, on and after the appointed day no person shall, in the course of a business carried on by him, sell by retail, or offer or expose for sale by retail, or supply in circumstances corresponding to retail sale, any medicinal product on a general sale list elsewhere than at a registered pharmacy, unless the conditions specified in the following provisions of this section are fulfilled.

(2) The place at which the medicinal product is sold, offered, exposed or supplied as mentioned in the preceding subsection must be premises of which the person carrying on the business in question is the occupier and which he is able to close so as to exclude the public, unless either —

(a)   the product is sold, offered, exposed for sale or supplied by means of an automatic machine and the product is a medicinal product in the automatic machines section of a general sale list, or

(b)   the product is a veterinary drug.

(3) The medicinal product must have been made up for sale in a container elsewhere than at the place at which it is sold, offered, exposed for sale or supplied as mentioned in subsection (1) of this section and the container must not have been opened since the product was made up for sale in it.

(4) The business, so far as concerns the sale or supply of medicinal products, must be carried on in accordance with such conditions (if any) as may be prescribed for the purposes of this section.

54 Sale of medicinal products from automatic machines

(1) On and after the appointed day no person shall sell, or offer or expose for sale, any medicinal product by means of an automatic machine unless it is a medicinal product in the automatic machines section of a general sale list.

(2) The appropriate Ministers may by order provide that no person shall by means of an automatic machine sell, or offer or expose for sale, any medicinal product to which the order applies unless the container in which it is sold, or offered or exposed for sale, complies with such restrictions as to the quantity of the medicinal product, or the number of medicinal products, which it contains as may be specified in the order.

(3) An order under subsection (2) of this section may be made either in respect of medicinal products generally or in respect of medicinal products of a particular description or falling within a particular class specified in the order.

Exemptions from sections 52 and 53

55 Exemptions for doctors, dentists, veterinary surgeons and veterinary practitioners

(1) The restrictions imposed by sections 52 and 53 of this Act do not apply to the sale, offer for sale, or supply of a medicinal product —

(a)   by a doctor or dentist to a patient of his or to a person under whose care such a patient is, or

(b)   in the course of the business of a hospital or health centre, where the product is sold, offered for sale or supplied for the purpose of being administered (whether in the hospital or health centre or elsewhere) in accordance with the directions of a doctor or dentist.

(2) Those restrictions also do not apply —

(a)   to the sale or supply of a medicinal product of a description, or falling within a class, specified in an order made by the Health Ministers for the purposes of this paragraph, where the product is sold or supplied by a registered nurse in the course of her professional practice, or

(b) to the sale or supply of a medicinal product of a description, or falling within a class, specified in an order made by the Health Ministers for the purposes of this paragraph, where the product either is sold or supplied by a certified midwife (or, in relation to England and Wales, by a certified midwife or exempted midwife) in the course of her professional practice or is delivered or administered by such a midwife on being supplied in pursuance of arrangements made by a local health authority in Great Britain or by a health authority in Northern Ireland.

(3) The restrictions imposed by those sections do not apply to the sale, offer for sale, or supply of a medicinal product by a veterinary surgeon or veterinary practitioner for administration by him or under his direction to an animal or herd which is under his care.

(4) Expressions to which a meaning is assigned by sub-section (2) of section 11 of this Act have the same meanings in this section as in that section.

56 Exemptions in respect of herbal remedies

(1) Subject to the following provisions of this section, the restrictions imposed by sections 52 and 53 of this Act do not apply to anything done at premises of which the person carrying on the business in question is the occupier and which he is able to close so as to exclude the public, and which consists of the sale, or offer or exposure for sale, or the supply in circumstances corresponding to retail sale, of a herbal remedy where the processes to which the plant or plants are subjected consist of drying, crushing or comminuting, with or without any subsequent process of tabletting, pill-making, compressing or diluting with water, but not any other process.

(2) Without prejudice to the preceding subsection, but subject to subsection (3) of this section, those restrictions do not apply to the sale or supply of a herbal remedy where the person selling or supplying the remedy sells or supplies it for administration to a particular person after being requested by or on behalf of that person and in that person's presence to use his own judgment as to the treatment required.

(3) The appropriate Ministers may by order provide that subsections (1) and (2) of this section shall not have effect in relation to herbal remedies of a description, or falling within a class, specified in the order.

57 Power to extend or modify exemptions

(1) The appropriate Ministers may by order provide that section 52 or section 53 of this Act, or both of those sections, shall have effect subject to such exemptions (other than those for the time being having effect by virtue of sections 55 and 56 of this Act) as may be specified in the order.

(2) Any exemption conferred by an order under the preceding subsection may be conferred subject to such conditions or limitations as may be specified in the order.

(3) The appropriate Ministers may by order provide that subsection (1)(b) or subsection (2) of section 55 of this Act shall cease to have effect, or shall have effect subject to such exceptions or modifications as may be specified in the order.

(4) No order shall be made under subsection (3) of this section unless a draft of the order has been laid before Parliament and approved by a resolution of each House of Parliament.

Additional provisions

58 Medicinal products on prescription only

(1) The appropriate Ministers may by order specify descriptions or classes of medicinal

products for the purposes of this section; and, in relation to any description or class so specified, the order shall state which of the following, that is to say –

(a) doctors,

(b) dentists, and

(c) veterinary surgeons and veterinary practitioners,

(d) registered nurses, midwives and health visitors who are of such description and comply with such conditions as may be specified in the order, and

(e) other persons who are of such a description and comply with such conditions as may be specified in the order.

(1A) The descriptions of persons which may be specified in an order by virtue of subsection (1)(e) are the following, or any sub-category of such a description –

(a) Persons who are registered by any board established under the Professions Supplementary to Medicine Act 1960;

(b) persons who are pharmacists;

(c) persons whose names are entered in a roll or record established by the General dental council by virtue of section 45 of the Dentists Act 1984 (dental auxiliaries);

(d) persons who are registered in either of the registers of ophthalmic opticians kept under section 7(a) of the Opticians Act 1989;

(e) persons who are registered osteopaths within the meaning of the Osteopaths Act 1993;

(f) persons who are registered chiropractors within the meaning of the Chiropractors Act 1994;

(g) persons who are registered in any register established, continued or maintained under an Order in Council under section 60(1) of the Health Act 1999;

(h) any other description of persons which appears to the appropriate ministers to be a description of persons whose profession is regulated by or under a provision of, or made under, and Act of the Scottish Parliament or Northern Ireland legislation and which the appropriate Ministers consider it appropriate to specify.

(1B) Where an order under this section includes provision by virtue of subsection (1)(e) the order shall specify such conditions as are necessary to secure that any person who is an appropriate practitioner by virtue of the provision may prescribe, give directions or administer only in respect of human use.

(2) Subject to the following provisions of this section –

(a) no person shall sell by retail, or supply in circumstances corresponding to retail sale, a medicinal product of a description, or falling within a class, specified in an order under this section except in accordance with a prescription given by an appropriate practitioner; and

(b) no person shall administer (otherwise than to himself) any such medicinal product unless he is an appropriate practitioner or a person acting in accordance with the directions of an appropriate practitioner.

(3) Subsection (2)(a) of this section shall not apply –

(a) to the sale or supply of a medicinal product to a patient of his by a doctor or dentist who is an appropriate practitioner, or

(b) to the sale or supply of a medicinal product, for administration to an animal or herd under his care, by a veterinary surgeon or veterinary practitioner who is an appropriate practitioner.

(4) Without prejudice to the last preceding subsection, any order made by the appropriate Ministers for the purposes of this section may provide –

(a) that paragraph (a) or paragraph (b) of subsection (2) of this section, or both those paragraphs, shall have effect subject to such exemptions as may be specified in the order, or, where the appropriate practitioner is a registered nurse, midwife or health visitor, or is an appropriate practitioner by virtue of provision made under subsection (1)(e) of this section, such modifications as may be so specified;

(b) that, for the purpose of paragraph (*a*) of that sub-section, a medicinal product shall not be taken to be sold or supplied in accordance with a prescription given by an appropriate practitioner unless such conditions as are prescribed by the order are fulfilled.

(4A) An order under this section may provide, in relation to a person who is an appropriate practitioner by virtue of subsection (1)(*d*) or (*e*), that such a person may —

(*a*) give a prescription for a medicinal product falling within a description or class specified in the order;

(*b*) administer any such medicinal product; or

(*c*) give directions for the administration of any such medicinal product, only where he complies with such conditions as may be specified in the order in respect of the cases or circumstances in which he may do so.

(4B) An order under this section may provide, in relation to a condition specified by virtue of subsection (4A), for the condition to have effect subject to such exemptions as may be specified in the order.

(4C) where a condition is specified by virtue of subsection (4A), any prescription or direction given by a person in contravention of the condition is not (subject to such exemptions or modifications as may be specified in the order by virtue of subsection (4)(*e*) of this section) given by an appropriate practitioner for the purposes of subsection (2)(*a*) or (*b*) of this section.

(5) Any exemption conferred or modification made by an order in accordance with subsection (4)(*a*) or (4B) of this section may be conferred or made subject to such conditions or limitations as may be specified in the order.

(6) Before making an order under this section the appropriate Ministers shall consult the appropriate committee, or, if for the time being there is no such committee, shall consult the Commission.

59 Special provisions in relation to new medicinal products

(1) The following provisions of this section shall have effect where an order under section 58 of this Act is made so as to apply to all medicinal products which fall within a class specified in the order and are of a description in respect of which the following conditions are fulfilled, that is to say, that —

(*a*) medicinal products of that description were not effectively on the market in the United Kingdom immediately before the first appointed day;

(*b*) a product licence granted under Part II of this Act (whether before, on or after the date on which the order comes into operation) applies to medicinal products of that description (whether it also applies to medicinal products of any other description or not); and

(*c*) before the grant of that licence, no product licence had been granted which was applicable to medicinal products of that description.

(2) Where such an order is made in accordance with the preceding subsection —

(*a*) the restrictions imposed by section 58(2) of this Act shall not apply by virtue of the order to medicinal products of any description except during a period beginning with the date which, in relation to medicinal products of that description, is the relevant date and of such duration from that date as may be specified in the order;

(*b*) in section 58(4)(*a*) of this Act the reference to exemptions specified in the order shall, in relation to that order, be construed as including a reference to any exemption specified in a direction given by the appropriate Ministers and relating to medicinal products of a particular description specified in that direction.

(3) In subsection (2)(*a*) of this section 'the relevant date', in relation to medicinal products of any description to which an order made in accordance with subsection (1) of this section applies, means the date on which the order comes into operation, or the date

on which the product licence applicable to medicinal products of that description (as mentioned in subsection (1)(*b*) of this section) comes into operation, whichever is the later.

60 Restricted sale, supply and administration of certain medicinal products

(1) Subject to the following provisions of this section, regulations made by the appropriate Ministers may provide that no person shall sell by retail, or supply in circumstances corresponding to retail sale, a medicinal product of a description specified in the regulations, or falling within a class so specified, unless—

(*a*) he is a practitioner holding a certificate issued for the purposes of this section by the appropriate Ministers in respect of medicinal products of that description or falling within that class, or a person acting in accordance with the directions of such a practitioner, and the product is so sold or supplied for the purpose of being administered in accordance with the directions of that practitioner, or

(*b*) he is a person lawfully conducting a retail pharmacy business and the product is so sold or supplied in accordance with a prescription given by such a practitioner.

(2) Any regulations made under this section may provide that no person shall administer (otherwise than to himself) a medicinal product of a description specified in the regulations, or falling within a class so specified, unless he is such a practitioner as is mentioned in subsection (1)(*a*) of this section or a person acting in accordance with the directions of such a practitioner.

(3) The powers conferred by the preceding subsections shall not be exercisable in respect of medicinal products of a particular description, or falling within a particular class, except where it appears to the appropriate Ministers that the sale by retail, or supply in circumstances corresponding to retail sale, or the administration, of such products requires specialised knowledge on the part of the practitioner by whom or under whose directions they are sold, supplied or administered.

(4) Any regulations made under this section in respect of a particular description or class of medicinal products may specify the qualifications and experience which an applicant for a certificate in respect of that description or class of medicinal products must have, and may provide for the appointment of a committee to advise the appropriate Ministers, in such cases as may be prescribed by or determined in accordance with the regulations, with respect to the grant, renewal, suspension and revocation of such certificates.

(5) Any such regulations shall include provision as to the grant, duration, renewal, suspension and revocation of certificates for the purposes of this section, including provision for affording—

(*a*) to an applicant for the grant or renewal of such a certificate, where the appropriate Ministers propose to refuse to grant or renew it, and

(*b*) to the holder of such a certificate, where the appropriate Ministers propose to suspend or revoke it,

an opportunity of appearing before, and being heard by, a person appointed for the purpose by the appropriate Ministers or of making representations in writing to those Ministers with respect to that proposal.

(6) Regulations made under this section may provide that, for the purposes of paragraph (*b*) of subsection (1) of this section, a medicinal product shall not be taken to be sold or supplied in accordance with a prescription as mentioned in that paragraph unless such conditions as are prescribed by the regulations are fulfilled.

(7) Before making any regulations under this section the appropriate Ministers shall consult the appropriate committee, or, if for the time being there is no such committee, shall consult the Commission.

The Medicines (Products Other Than Veterinary Drugs) (Prescription Only) Order 1983, ST 1983 No. 1212

1 Citation, commencement and interpretation

(1) This order may be cited as the Medicines (Products Other Than Veterinary Drugs) (Prescription Only) Order 1983 and shall come into operation on 14th September 1983.

(2) In this order, unless the context otherwise requires —

(*a*) 'the Act' means the Medicines Act 1968;

'aerosol' means a product which is dispersed from its container by a propellent gas or liquid;

'controlled drug' has the meaning assigned to it by section 2 of the Misuse of Drugs Act 1971(**a**);

'dosage unit' means —

(i) where a medicinal product is in the form of a tablet or capsule or is an article in some other similar pharmaceutical form, that tablet, capsule or other article, or

(ii) where a medicinal product is not in any such form, that quantity of the product which is used as the unit by reference to which the dose is measured;

'external use' means application to the skin, hair, teeth, mucosa of the mouth, throat, nose, ear, eye, vagina or anal canal when a local action only is intended and extensive systemic absorption is unlikely to occur; and references to medicinal products for external use shall be read accordingly except that such references shall not include throat sprays, throat pastilles, throat lozenges, throat tablets, nasal drops, nasal sprays, nasal inhalations or teething preparations;

'health prescription' means a prescription issued by a doctor or dentist under or by virtue of —

(i) in England and Wales, the National Health Service Act 1977(**b**),

(ii) in Scotland, the National Health Service (Scotland) Act 1978(**c**), and

(iii) in Northern Ireland, the Health and Personal Social Services (Northern Ireland) Order 1972(**d**):

'inhaler' does not include an aerosol;

'master' has the same meaning as in the Merchant Shipping Act 1894(**e**);

(**a**) 1971 c. 38
(**b**) 1977 c. 49.
(**c**) 1978 c. 29
(**d**) SI 1972/1265 (NI 14).
(**e**) 1894 c. 60.

'maximum daily dose' or 'MDD' means the maximum quantity of a substance contained in the amount of a medicinal product for internal use which it is recommended should be taken or administered in a period of 24 hours;

'maximum dose' or 'MD' means the maximum quantity of a substance contained in the amount of a medicinal product for internal use which it is recommended should be taken or administered at any one time;

'maximum strength' means such of the following as may be specified —

(i) the maximum quantity of a substance by weight or volume contained in a dosage unit of a medicinal product, and

(ii) the maximum percentage of a substance contained in a medicinal product calculated in terms of weight in weight, weight in volume, volume in weight or volume in volume, as appropriate;

'medicinal product' has the same meaning as in the Act except that it does not include a medicinal product which is a veterinary drug as defined in section 132(1) of the Act;

'the Misuse of Drugs Regulations' means, in relation to England, Wales and Scotland, the Misuse of Drugs Regulations 1973(**a**) and, in relation to Northern Ireland, the Misuse of Drugs (Northern Ireland) Regulations 1974(**b**);

'occupational health scheme' means a scheme in which a person, in the course of a business carried on by him, provides facilities for his employees for the treatment or prevention of disease;

'operator', in relation to an aircraft, means the person for the time being having the management of the aircraft;

'parenteral administration' means administration by breach of the skin or mucous membrane;

'prescription only medicine' means a medicinal product of a description or falling within a class specified in Article 3 of this order;

'registered ophthalmic optician' means a person who is registered in either of the registers of ophthalmic opticians established and maintained under section 2(*a*) of the Opticians Act 1958(**c**);

'repeatable prescription' means a prescription which contains a direction that it may be dispensed more than once;

'sell' means sell by retail as defined in section 131 of the Act and 'sale' has a corresponding meaning;

'soap' means any compound of a fatty acid with an alkali or amine;

'state registered chiropodist' means a person who is registered in the register established and maintained under section 2(1) of the Professions Supplementary to Medicine Act 1960(**d**) by the Chiropodists Board;

'supply' means supply in circumstances corresponding to retail sale as defined in section 131 of the Act;

'unit preparation' means a preparation, including a mother tincture, prepared by a process of solution, extraction or trituration with a view to being diluted tenfold or one hundredfold, either once or repeatedly, in an inert diluent, and then used either in this diluted form or, where applicable, by impregnating tablets, granules, powders or other inert substances; and

(*b*) a reference —

(i) to a numbered section is to the section of the Act which bears that number,

---

(**a**) SI 1973/797; relevant amending instruments are SI 1975/499, 1623, 1977/1380 and 1979/326.
(**b**) SR (NI) 1974 No. 272, amended by SR (NI) 1975 No. 140, 326 and 1977 No. 290.
(**c**) 1958 c. 32.
(**d**) 1960 c. 66.

(ii) to a numbered Article or Schedule is to the Article of, or Schedule to, this order which bears that number,

(iii) in an Article or in a Part of a Schedule to a numbered paragraph is to the paragraph of that Article or that Part of that Schedule which bears that number, and

(iv) in a paragraph to a lettered sub-paragraph is to the sub-paragraph of that paragraph which bears that letter.

(3) In Schedule 1 —

(a) entries specified in columns 2, 3 and 4 of Parts I and II relate to the substances listed in column 1 against which they appear and where, in relation to a particular substance listed in column 1, an entry in column 2, 3 or 4 bears a number or letter it relates only to such entries in the other of those columns as bear the same number or letter;

(b) the entries in column 4 of Part I shall be read subject to the note at the end of that Part; and

(c) the following abbreviations are used:
  'g' for gram.
  'mcg' for microgram,
  'mg' for milligram,
  'ml' for millilitre.

2 Appropriate Practitioners

For the purposes of section 58 (medicinal products on prescription only), doctors, dentists, veterinary surgeons and veterinary practitioners shall be appropriate practitioners in relation to all the descriptions and classes of medicinal products specified for the purposes of that section in Article 3.

3 Medicinal products on prescription only

(1) There are hereby specified descriptions and classes of medicinal products for the purposes of section 58, namely —

(a) subject to Article 4(1), medicinal products consisting of or containing a substance listed in column 1 of Part I of Schedule 1;

(b) subject to Article 4(2) and Part II of Schedule 1, medicinal products that are controlled drugs;

(c) medicinal products specified in Part III of Schedule 1;

(d) subject to Article 4(3), medicinal products that are for parenteral administration whether or not they fall within sub-paragaph (a) or (b);

(e) medicinal products —

  (i) which are not of a description and do not fall within a class specified in any of sub-paragraphs (a), (b), (c) or (d),

  (ii) which are of a description in respect of which the conditions specified in section 59(1) are fulfilled, and

  (iii) in respect of which a product licence is granted after the date of coming into operation of this order containing a provision to the effect that the method of sale or supply of the medicinal product is to be only in accordance with a prescription given by an appropriate practitioner.

(2) For the purposes of section 59(2)(a) (duration of restrictions for certain new products) the duration shall be a period of five years.

4 Medicinal products that are not prescription only

(1) Notwithstanding Article 3(1)(a), a medicinal product shall not be a prescription only

medicine by reason that it consists of or contains a particular substance listed in column 1 of Part 1 of Schedule 1 where—

(*a*)   in relation to that substance there is an entry in one or more of columns 2, 3 and 4;

(*b*)   the maximum strength in the product of that substance does not exceed the maximum strength, if any, specified in column 2; and

(*c*)   the medicinal product is sold or supplied—

   (i)   if a pharmaceutical form or a route of administration is specified in column 3, in such pharmaceutical form, and for administration only by such route, as may be so specified,

  (ii)   if a use is specified in column 3, in a container or package labelled to show a use so specified to which the medicinal product is to be put but no use not so specified,

 (iii)   if a maximum dose is specified in column 4, in a container or package labelled to show a maximum dose not exceeding that specified, and

 (iv)   if a maximum daily dose is specified in column 4, in a container or package labelled to show a maximum daily dose not exceeding that specified.

(2) Notwithstanding Article 3(1)(*b*), a medicinal product shall not be a prescription only medicine by reason that it is a controlled drug where it—

(*a*)   contains not more than one of the substances listed in column 1 of Part II of Schedule 1 (which substances are amongst the controlled drugs listed in Schedule 2 to the Misuse of Drugs Act 1971) and no other controlled drug;

(*b*)   contains that substance at a strength that does not exceed the maximum strength specified in column 2; and

(*c*)   is sold or supplied—

   (i)   in such pharmaceutical form as may be specified in column 3, and

  (ii)   in or from a container or package labelled to show a maximum dose not exceeding that specified in column 4.

(3) Notwithstanding Article 3(1)(*d*), the following medicinal products for parenteral administration shall not be prescription only medicines—

Biphasic Insulin Injection
Globlin Zinc Insulin Injection
Insulin Injection
Insulin Zinc Suspension
Insulin Zinc Suspension (Amorphous)
Insulin Zinc Suspension (Crystalline)
Isophane Insulin Injection
Neutral Insulin Injection
Protamine Zinc Insulin Injection.

5 Exemption for parenteral administration to human beings of certain prescription only medicines

The restriction imposed by section 58(2)(*b*) (restriction on administration) shall not apply to the administration to human beings of any of the following medicinal products for parenteral administration—

Adrenaline Injection BP
Atropine Sulphate Injection
Chlorpheniramine Injection
Cobalt Edetate Injection
Dextrose Injection Strong B.P.C.
Diphenhydramine Injection
Hydrocortisone Injection
Mepyramine Injection

Promethazine Hydrochloride Injection
Snake Venom Antiserum
Sodium Nitrite Injection
Sodium Thiosulphate Injection
Sterile Pralidoxime
if and so long as the administration is for the purpose of saving life in an emergency.

6 Exemptions for emergency sale or supply

(1) The restrictions imposed by section 58(2)(*a*) (restrictions on sale and supply) shall not apply to the sale or supply of a prescription only medicine by a person lawfully conducting a retail pharmacy business if and so long as the conditions specified in paragraph (2) are fulfilled.

(2) The conditions referred to in paragraph (1) are—

(*a*) that the pharmacist by or under whose supervision the prescription only medicine is to be sold or supplied is satisfied that the sale or supply has been requested by a doctor who by reason of any emergency is unable to furnish a prescription immediately;

(*b*) that that doctor has undertaken to furnish the person lawfully conducting a retail pharmacy business with a prescription within 72 hours;

(*c*) that the prescription only medicine is sold or supplied in accordance with the directions of the doctor requesting it;

(*d*) subject to paragraph (5), that the prescription only medicine is not a controlled drug specified in Schedule 2, 3 or 4 to the Misuse of Drugs Regulations;

(*e*) that an entry is made in the register kept under regulation 6 of the Medicines (Sale or Supply) (Miscellaneous Provisions) Regulations 1980(**a**) within the time specified in that regulation stating the particulars set out in paragraph 1 of Schedule 2 to those regulations.

(3) The restrictions imposed by section 58(2)(*a*) also shall not apply to the sale or supply of a prescription only medicine by a person lawfully conducting a retail pharmacy business if and so long as the conditions specified in paragraph (4) are fulfilled.

(4) The conditions referred to in paragraph (3) are—

(*a*) that the pharmacist by or under whose supervision the prescription only medicine is to be sold or supplied has interviewed the person requesting a prescription only medicine and has satisfied himself—

  (i) that there is an immediate need for the prescription only medicine requested to be sold or supplied and that it is impracticable in the circumstances to obtain a prescription without undue delay,

  (ii) that treatment with the prescription only medicine requested has on a previous occasion been prescribed by a doctor for the person requesting it, and

  (iii) as to the dose which in the circumstances it would be appropriate for that person to take;

(*b*) that no greater quantity of the prescription only medicine than will provide 5 days' treatment is sold or supplied except that there may be sold or supplied where the prescription only medicine—

  (i) is an aerosol for the relief of asthma, an ointment or a cream, and has been made up for sale in a container elsewhere than at the place of sale or supply, the smallest pack that the pharmacist has available for sale or supply,

  (ii) is an oral contraceptive, sufficient for a full cycle,

  (iii) is an antibiotic for oral administration in liquid form, the smallest quantity that will provide a full course of treatment;

(**a**) SI 1980/1923, to which there are amendments not relevant to this Order.

(c) subject to paragraph (5), that the prescription only medicine does not consist of or contain a substance specified in Schedule 2 to this order and is not a controlled drug specified in Schedule 2, 3 or 4 to the Misuse of Drugs Regulations;

(d) that an entry is made in the register kept under regulation 6 of the Medicines (Sale or Supply) (Miscellaneous Provisions) Regulations 1980 within the time specified in that regulation stating the particulars set out in paragraph 3 of Schedule 2 to those regulations;

(e) that the container or package of the prescription only medicine is labelled so as to show —
   (i) the date on which the prescription only medicine is sold or supplied,
   (ii) the name, quantity and, except where it is apparent from the name, the pharmaceutical form and strength of the prescription only medicine,
   (iii) the name of the person requesting the prescription only medicine,
   (iv) the name and address of the registered pharmacy from which the prescription only medicine was sold or supplied, and
   (v) the words 'Emergency Supply'.

(5) The conditions specified in paragraphs (2)(d) and (4)(c) shall not apply where the prescription only medicine consists of or contains Phenobarbitone or Phenobarbitone Sodium (but no other substance specified in Schedule 2 to this order or Schedule 2, 3 or 4 to the Misuse of Drugs Regulations) and is sold or supplied for use in the treatment of epilepsy.

7 Exemption for non-parenteral administration to human beings

The restriction imposed by section 58(2)(b) (restriction on administration) shall not apply to the administration to human beings of a prescription only medicine which is not for parenteral administration.

8 Exemption for medicinal products at high dilutions

The restrictions imposed by section 58(2) (restrictions on sale, supply and administration) shall not apply to the sale, supply or administration of a medicinal product which is not for parenteral administration and which consists of or contains, of the substances listed in column 1 of Part I or Part II of Schedule 1, only one or more unit preparations of such substances, if —

(a) each such unit preparation has been diluted to at least one part in a million (6x), and the person selling, supplying or administering the medicinal product has been requested by or on behalf of a particular person and in that person's presence to use his own judgment as to the treatment required, or

(b) each such unit preparation has been diluted to at least one part in a million million (6c).

9 Exemptions for certain persons

(1) The restrictions imposed by section 58(2)(a) (restrictions on sale and supply) shall not apply —

(a) to the sale or supply by a person listed in column 1 of Part I of Schedule 3, or

(b) to the supply by a person listed in column 1 of Part II of Schedule 3

of the prescription only medicines listed in column 2 of Part I or Part II, as the case may be, of Schedule 3 in relation to that person if and so long as the conditions specified in the corresponding paragraphs in column 3 of Part I or Part II, as the case may be, of Schedule 3 are fulfilled.

(2) The restriction imposed by section 58(2)(b) (restriction on administration) shall not apply to the administration by a person listed in column 1 of Part III of Schedule 3 of the prescription only medicines for parenteral administration listed in column 2 of that Part in

relation to that person if and so long as the conditions specified in the corresponding paragraphs in column 3 of that Part are fulfilled.

10 Exemption for sale or supply in hospitals
The restrictions imposed by section 58(2)(*a*) (restrictions on sale and supply) shall not apply to the sale or supply of any prescription only medicine in the course of the business of a hospital where the prescription only medicine is sold or supplied in accordance with the written directions of a doctor or dentist notwithstanding that those directions do not fulfil the conditions specified in Article 12(2).

11 Exemption in cases involving another's default
The restrictions imposed by section 58(2)(*a*) (restrictions on sale and supply) shall not apply to the sale or supply of a prescription only medicine by a person who, having exercised all due diligence, believes on reasonable grounds that the product sold or supplied is not a prescription only medicine, where it is due to the act or default of another person that the product is a product to which section 58(2)(*a*) applies.

12 Prescriptions
(1) For the purposes of section 58(2)(*a*) a prescription only medicine shall not be taken to be sold or supplied in accordance with a prescription given by a practitioner unless the conditions specified in paragraph (2) are fulfilled.

(2) The conditions referred to in paragraph (1) are that the presciption —

(*a*) shall be signed in ink with his own name by the practitioner giving it;

(*b*) shall, without prejudice to sub-paragraph (*a*), be written in ink or otherwise so as to be indelible, unless it is a health prescription which is not for a controlled drug specified in Schedule 2, 3 or 4 to the Misuse of Drugs Regulations, in which case it may be written by means of carbon paper or similar material;

(*c*) shall contain the following particulars —

    (i) the address of the practitioner giving it,

    (ii) the appropriate date,

    (iii) such particulars as indicate whether the practitioner giving it is a doctor, a dentist, a veterinary surgeon or a veterinary practitioner,

    (iv) where the practitioner giving it is a doctor or dentist, the name, address and the age, if under 12, of the person for whose treatment it is given, and

    (v) where the practitioner giving it is a veterinary surgeon or a veterinary practitioner, the name and address of the person to whom the prescription only medicine is to be delivered and a declaration by the veterinary surgeon or veterinary practitioner giving it that the prescription only medicine is prescribed for an animal or herd under his care;

(*d*) shall not be dispensed after the end of the period of six months from the appropriate date, unless it is a repeatable prescription in which case it shall not be dispensed for the first time after the end of that period nor otherwise than in accordance with the direction contained in the repeatable prescription;

(*e*) in the case of a repeatable prescription that does not specify the number of times it may be dispensed, shall not be dispensed on more than two occasions unless it is a prescription for oral contraceptives in which case it may be dispensed six times before the end of the period of six months from the appropriate date.

(3) The restrictions imposed by section 58(2)(*a*) (restrictions on sale and supply) shall not apply to a sale or supply of a prescription only medicine which is not in accordance with a prescription given by an appropriate practitioner by reason only that a condition specified in paragraph (2) is not fulfilled, where the person selling or supplying the

prescription only medicine, having exercised all due diligence, believes on reasonable grounds that that condition is fulfilled in relation to that sale or supply.

(4) In paragraph (2) 'the appropriate date' means—

(a) in the case of a health prescription, the date on which it was signed by the practitioner giving it or a date indicated by him as being the date before which it shall not be dispensed, and

(b) in every other case, the date on which the prescription was signed by the practitioner giving it;

and, for the purposes of sub-paragraphs (a) and (e) of that paragraph, where a health prescription bears both the date on which it was signed and a date indicated as being that before which it shall not be dispensed, the appropriate date is the later of those dates.

13 Revocations and transitional provision

(1) The orders specified in Schedule 4 are hereby revoked.

(2) Where immediately before the coming into operation of this order, the restrictions imposed by section 58 applied to the sale, supply or administration of a medicinal product of a particular description either by reason that the product fell within a class specified in Article 3(1)(e) (certain new products), or by virtue of Article 14(2) (transitional provision), of the Medicines (Prescription Only) Order 1980(**a**), those restrictions shall continue to apply to products of that description as though Article 3(1)(e) and (2), or, as the case may be, Article 14(2) of that order had remained in force.

(**a**) SI 1980/1921, relevant amending instrument is SI 1982/29.

Appendix 5

NHS (PS) Regulation 1992
Schedule 2

SCHEDULE 2

PART I

GENERAL

1 Interpretation

In this Schedule, unless the context otherwise requires, any reference in a paragraph to a numbered sub-paragraph is a reference to the sub-paragraph bearing that number in that paragraph.

2 Incorporation of provisions

Any provisions of the following affecting the rights and obligations of chemists or doctors who provide pharmaceutical services shall be deemed to form part of the terms of service for chemists or, as the case may be, of the terms of service for doctors who provide pharmaceutical services—

(a) the Regulations;

(b) the Drug Tariff in so far as it lists drugs and appliances for the purposes of section 41 of the Act;

(c) so much of Part II of the National Health Service (Service Committees and Tribunal) Regulations 1992(a) as relates to—

   (i) the investigation of questions arising between chemists and persons receiving pharmaceutical services and other investigations to be made by the pharmaceutical discipline committee and the joint discipline committee and the action which may be taken by the HA as a result of such investigations, and,

   (ii) appeals to the Secretary of State from decisions of the HA.

Directed services

2A A chemist with whom a Health Authority makes an arrangement for the provision of any directed service shall comply with the terms and conditions of the arrangement.

PART II
TERMS OF SERVICE FOR CHEMISTS

3 Provision of pharmaceutical services

(1) Where any person presents on a prescription form—

(a) an order for drugs, not being Scheduled drugs, or appliances, signed by a doctor; or

(b) an order for a drug specified in Schedule 11 to the Medical Regulations, signed by, and endorsed on its face with the reference "SLS" by, a doctor, or

---

(a) SI 1992/664.

(c) an order for listed drugs or medicines, signed by a dentist or his deputy or assistant; or

(d) an order for listed drugs or medicines, or listed appliances, signed by a nurse prescriber

a chemist shall, with reasonable promptness, provide the drugs or medicines so ordered, and such of the appliances so ordered as he supplies in the normal course of his business.

(1A) If a person presenting the prescription form asks the chemist to do so —

(a) he shall give an estimate of the time when the drugs, medicines or appliances will be ready; and

(b) if they are not ready by then, he shall give a revised estimate of the time when they will be ready (and so on).

(1B) Where a chemist reasonably believes that a form presented to him as a prescription form in accordance with paragraph 3(1) is not a genuine order for the person named on the form (for example because he reasonably believes the form has been stolen or forged), he may refuse to provide the drugs or medicines or listed appliances specified on the form presented.

(1C) Before providing the drugs or medicines or listed appliances ordered on a prescription form as specified in paragraph 3(1) —

(a) the chemist shall ask any person who makes a declaration on the prescription form that the person named on the prescription form does not have to pay the charges specified in regulation 3(1) of the Charges Regulations by virtue of either —

(i) entitlement to exemption under any of the sub-paragraphs (d) to (g) of regulation 6(1) of the Charges Regulations; or

(ii) entitlement to remission of such charges under regulation 3 of the Remission of Charges Regulations,

to produce satisfactory evidence of such entitlement unless the declaration is in respect of entitlement to exemption by virtue of sub-paragraph (d), (e) or (f) of regulation 6(1) of the Charges Regulations, and at the time of the declaration the chemist already has such evidence available to him; and

(b) if no satisfactory evidence is produced to the chemist (and, where it is relevant, none is already available to him as mentioned in sub-paragraph (a)) the chemist shall endorse the prescription form to that effect.

(2) Any drug which is provided as part of pharmaceutical services and included in the Drug Tariff, the British National Formulary, the Dental Practitioner's Formulary, the European Pharmaceopoeia or the British Pharmaceutical Codex, shall comply with the standard or formula specified therein.

(3) Subject to any regulations in force under the Weights and Measures Act 1985(a) and subject to sub-paragraphs (4) to (12) a chemist shall provide pharmaceutical services only in response to and in accordance with an order on a prescription form, signed as specified in sub-paragraph (1).

(4) Where an order, not being an order to which the Poisons Rules 1982(b) or the Misuse of Drugs Regulations 1985(c) applies, which is issued by a doctor or a dentist on a prescription form for drugs does not prescribe their quantity, strength or dosage, a chemist may provide the drugs in such strength and dosage as in the exercise of his professional skill, knowledge and care he considers to be appropriate and, subject to sub-pargraph (3), in such quantity as he considers to be appropriate for a course of treatment, for the patient to whom the order relates, for a period not exceeding five days.

(5) Where an order to which sub-paragraph (3) applies is for —

(a) an oral contraceptive substance;

(a) 1985 c. 72.
(b) SI 1982/218, amended by SI 1985/1077, 1986/10 and 1986/1704.
(c) SI 1985/2066, amended by SI 1986/2330, 1988/916 and 1989/1460.

(b)   a drug, which is available for supply as part of pharmaceutical services only together with one or more drugs; or

(c)   an antibiotic in a liquid form for oral administration in respect of which pharmaceutical considerations require its provision in an unopened package,

which is not available for provision as part of pharmaceutical services except in such packages that the minimum available package contains a quantity appropriate to a course of treatment for a patient for a period of more than 5 days, the chemist may provide that minimum available package.

(6) Where any drug, not being one to which the Misuse of Drugs Regulations 1985 apply, ordered by a doctor or dentist on a prescription form, is available for provision by a chemist in a pack in a quantity which is different to the quantity which has been so ordered, and that drug is —

(a)   sterile;

(b)   effervescent or hygroscopic;

(c)   a liquid preparation for addition to bath water;

(d)   a coal tar preparation;

(e)   a viscous preparation; or

(f)   packed at the time of its manufacture in a calendar pack or special container,

the chemist shall, subject to sub-paragraph (7), provide the drug in the pack whose quantity is nearest to the quantity which has been so ordered.

(7) A chemist shall not provide, pursuant to sub-paragraph (6), a drug in a calendar pack where, in his opinion, it was the intention of the doctor or dentist who ordered the drug that it should be provided only in the exact quantity ordered.

(8) In this paragraph —

(a)   'calendar pack' means a blister or strip pack showing the days of the week or month against each of the several units in the pack; and

(b)   'special container' means any container with an integral means of application or from which it is not practicable to dispense an exact quantity.

(9) Where, in a case of urgency, a doctor personally known to a chemist requests him to provide a drug, the chemist may provide that drug before receiving a prescription form, provided that —

(a)   that drug is not a Scheduled drug;

(b)   that drug is not a controlled drug within the meaning of the Misuse of Drugs Act 1971(**a**), other than a drug which is for the time being specified in Schedule 4 or 5 to the Misuse of Drugs Regulations 1985(**b**); and

(c)   the doctor undertakes to give the chemist such a prescription form within 72 hours.

(10) Except as provided in sub-paragraph (11), a chemist shall not provide a Scheduled drug, by way of pharmaceutical services or otherwise, in response to an order by name, formula or other description on a prescription form.

(11) Where a drug has an appropriate non-proprietary name and it is ordered on a prescription form either by that name or by its formula, a chemist may provide which has the same specification notwithstanding that it is a Scheduled drug, provided that where a Scheduled drug is a pack which consists of a drug in more than one strength, such provision does not involve the supply of part only of the pack.

(12) Where a drug which is ordered as specified in sub-paragraph (11) combines more than one drug, that sub-paragraph shall apply only if the combination has an appropriate non-proprietary name, whether the individual drugs which it combines do so or not.

(13) A chemist shall provide any drug which he is required to provide under this paragraph in a suitable container.

(14) A chemist shall not give, promise or offer to any person any gift or reward

---

(a)   1971 c. 38.
(b)   SI 1985/2066.

(whether by way of a share of or dividend on the profits of the business or by way of discount or rebate or otherwise) as an inducement to or in consideration of his presenting an order for drugs or appliances on a prescription form.

4 Premises and hours

(1) Pharmaceutical services shall be provided at each of the premises from which the chemist has undertaken to provide pharmaceutical services at such times as, following an application in writing by the chemist, shall have been approved in his case by an HA or, on appeal, the Secretary of State, in accordance with the following provisions of this paragraph.

(2) An HA shall not approve any application submitted by a chemist in relation to the times at which he is to provide pharmaceutical services unless it is satisfied that —
- (a) the times proposed are such that a pharmacist will normally be available —
  - (i) subject to sub-paragraph (4), for no less than 30 hours in any week, and
  - (ii) on 5 days in any such week; and
- (b) the hours when a pharmacist will normally be available in any week are to be allocated between the days on which he will normally be available in that week in such a manner as is likely to meet the needs of persons in the neighbourhood for pharmaceutical services on working days between the hours of 09.00 and 17.30 (or 13.00 on an early closing day).

(3) In this paragraph 'available' means, in relation to a pharmacist, available to provide pharmaceutical services of the kind he has undertaken to provide and 'availability' shall be construed accordingly; 'working day' means Monday to Saturday excluding Good Friday, Christmas Day or a bank holiday which falls on any such day; and 'an early closing day' means any working day when most shops in the neighbourhood are habitually closed after the hour of 13.00.

(4) The HA may approve an application to provide pharmaceutical services for less than 30 hours in any week provided that it is satisfied that the provision of pharmaceutical services in the neighbourhood is likely to be adequate to meet the need for such services on working days between the hours of 09.00 and 17.30 (or 13.00 on an early closing day) at times when the pharmacist is not available.

(5) An application for approval pursuant to sub-paragraph (2) shall be made in writing to a Health Authority.

(6) The HA shall determine an application within 30 days of receiving it.

(7) Subject to sub-paragraph (8), in determining any application, the HA shall either —
- (a) grant approval;
- (b) grant approval subject to any requirements that it considers appropriate for the purpose of ensuring that a pharmacist is available for the provision of pharmaceutical services at such times as are necessary to meet the need for such services on working days between the hours of 09.00 and 17.30 (or 13.00 on an early closing day); or
- (c) refuse approval.

(8) Where the HA is considering whether to grant approval subject to any requirements, as mentioned in sub-paragraph (7)(b), it shall consult the Local Pharmaceutical Committee before determining the application.

(9) An HA shall notify the chemist in writing of its determination, and, where it refuses an application or grants an application subject to any requirements under sub-paragraph 7(b), it shall send the chemist a statement in writing of the reasons for its determination or, as the case may be, for the imposition of the requirements and of the chemist's right of appeal under sub-paragraph (10).

(10) A chemist may, within 30 days of receiving a notification pursuant to sub-

paragraph (9), appeal in writing to the Secretary of State against any refusal of approval or against any condition imposed pursuant to sub-paragraph (7)(b).

(11) The Secretary of State may, when determining an appeal, either confirm the determination of the HA or substitute his own determination for that of the HA.

(12) The Secretary of State shall notify the chemist in writing of his determination and shall in every case include with the notification a written statement of the reasons for the determination.

(13) At each of the premises at which a chemist provides pharmaceutical services he shall exhibit—

(a) a notice provided by the HA specifying the times at which the premises are open for the provision of drugs and appliances; and

(b) at times when the premises are not open, a notice, where practicable legible from outside the premises, [deleted by 1997/2451] specifying the addresses of other chemists included in the pharmaceutical list and the times at which drugs and appliances may be obtained from those addresses.

(14) An HA shall notify the chemist in writing of the names and addresses of other chemists included in the pharmaceutical list whose premises are in the neighbourhood and of the times at which they are required to provide pharmaceutical services.

(15) Where a chemist is prevented by illness or other reasonable cause from complying with his obligations under this paragraph, he shall, where practicable, make arrangements with one or more chemists whose premises are situated in the neighbourhood for the provision of pharmaceutical services during that time.

(16) A chemist may apply to an HA for a variation of the times at which, in accordance with a determination under this paragraph ('the earlier determination'), a pharmacist is required to be normally available, and sub-paragraphs (3) to (13) shall apply to the making and determination ('the subsequent determination') of an application under this sub-paragraph as if it were the first application by that chemist for the purposes of this paragraph.

(17) Where an application made under sub-paragraph (16) is approved, the earlier determination mentioned in sub-paragraph (16) shall cease to have effect and the subsequent determination mentioned in that sub-paragraph shall have effect instead—

(a) where the subsequent determination is made by an HA and no appeal is made, from the day falling 8 weeks after the date on which the chemist receives notification of that HA's determination; or

(b) where the subsequent determination is made on appeal, from the day falling 8 weeks after the date on which the chemist receives notification of the Secretary of State's determination.

(18) Where it appears to the HA, after consultation with or at the request of the Local Pharmaceutical Committee, that the times at which a pharmacist is available no longer meet the needs of persons in the neighbourhood for pharmaceutical services on working days between the hours of 09.00 and 17.30 (or 13.00 on an early closing day), it may review the terms of—

(a) any approval granted by the HA under sub-paragraph (7)(a) or (b) or by the Secretary of State under sub-paragraph (12); or

(b) any direction given under sub-paragraph (20)(a) by the HA or, on appeal, by the Secretary of State.

(19) On any review under sub-paragraph (18) the HA shall—

(a) give notice to the chemist of its proposed changes in the times at which the pharmacist is to be available; and

(b) allow him 30 days within which to make representations to the HA about its proposals.

(20) After considering any representations made in accordance with sub-paragraph (19)(b), the HA shall either—

(a) direct the chemist to revise the times at which the pharmacist is to be available in the manner specified in the direction; or

(b) confirm that the existing times of availability continue to meet the need for pharmaceutical services on working days between the hours of 09.00 and 17.30 (or 13.00 on an early closing day).

(21) The HA shall notify the chemist in writing of its determination under sub-paragraph (20), and where it gives a direction under head (a) of that sub-paragraph it shall include with the notification a statement in writing of the reasons for its determination and of the chemist's right of appeal under sub-paragraph (22).

(22) A chemist may, within 30 days of receiving notification under sub-paragraph (21), appeal in writing to the Secretary of State against a direction under sub-paragraph (20)(a).

(23) Sub-paragraphs (11) and (12) shall apply to any appeal made under sub-paragraph (22) but as though in sub-paragraph (12) any reference to a determination were a reference to a decision.

(24) A chemist in respect of whom a direction is given under sub-paragraph (20) shall revise the times of availability of the pharmacist so as to give effect to the direction –

(a) where the direction is given by the HA and no appeal is made, not later than 8 weeks after the date on which he receives notification under sub-paragraph (21); or

(b) where the direction is given or confirmed on appeal, not later than 8 weeks after the date on which he receives notification of the Secretary of State's decision.

(25) Where it appears to the HA, after consultation with the Local Pharmaceutical Committee, that the times at which a pharmacist is available –

(a) on working days before the hour of 09.00 or after the hour of 17.30 (or 13.00 on an early closing day); or

(b) on any Sunday, Good Friday, Christmas Day or bank holiday,

are not adequate to meet the needs of persons in the neighbourhood for pharmaceutical services at those times or on those days, the HA may (subject to sub-paragraphs (26) to (28)) direct the chemist to revise the times at which the pharmacist is to be available in the manner specified in the direction.

(26) No direction shall be given under sub-paragraph (25) unless a fee, allowance or other remuneration to be paid to any chemist so directed is included in the Drug Tariff or has been determined by the HA by virtue of regulation 18(1A) (as the case may be).

(26A) The requirements referred to in sub-paragraph (26) are that –

(a) the Health Authority must have offered to make such arrangements with the chemist; and

(b) the arrangements offered must have been such that under them a pharmacist would have been available as mentioned in sub-paragraph (26) at the revised times which the Health Authority proposes to require in its direction under sub-paragraph (25), but it is immaterial whether or not the chemist has accepted the offer of such arrangements.

(26B) If the Health Authority has not been directed (under section 41A(1)(a) or (b) of the Act) in the manner referred to in sub-paragraph (26) no direction shall be given under sub-paragraph (25) unless a fee, allowance or other remuneration to be paid to any chemist so directed is included in the Drug Tariff or has been determined by the Health Authority by virtue of regulation (1A) (as the case may be).

(27) Before giving any direction under sub-paragraph (25) the HA shall –

(a) give notice to the chemist of the revised times at which it proposes the pharmacist is to be available; and

(b) allow the chemist 30 days within which to make representations to the HA about its proposals,

and shall take any such representations into account.

(28) The HA shall notify the chemist in writing of a direction under sub-paragraph (25), and shall include with the notification a statement in writing of the reasons for its direction and of the chemist's right of appeal under sub-paragraph (29).

(29) A chemist may, within 30 days of receiving notification under sub-paragraph (28), appeal in writing to the Secretary of State against a direction under sub-paragraph (25).

(30) Sub-paragraphs (11) and (12) shall apply to any appeal made under sub-paragraph (29) but as though any reference to a determination—

(a) in sub-paragraph (11) were to a direction; and

(b) in sub-paragraph (12) were to a decision.

(31) A chemist in respect of whom a direction is given under sub-paragraph (25) shall revise the times of availability of the pharmacist so as to give effect to the direction—

(a) where the direction is given by the HA and no appeal is made, not later than 8 weeks after the date on which he receives notification under sub-paragraph (28); or

(b) where the direction is given or confirmed on appeal, not later than 8 weeks after the date on which he receives notification of the Secretary of State's decision.

5 Provision of drugs and fitting of appliances

(1) Drugs shall be provided either by or under the direct supervision of a pharmacist.

(1A) Where the pharmacist referred to in sub-paragraph (1) is employed by a chemist, the pharmacist must not be one—

(a) who, having been disqualified under 46(2)(b) of the Act (or under any corresponding provision in force in Scotland or Northern Ireland) from inclusion in the pharmaceutical list of the Health Authority (or, in Scotland, of a Health Board or, in Northern Ireland, of a Health and Social Services Board) is also the subject of a declaration under section 46(2)(c) of the Act (or any corresponding provision in force in Scotland or Northern Ireland) that he is not fit to be engaged in any capacity in the provision of pharmaceutical services; or

(b) who is suspended by direction of the Tribunal, other than in a case falling within section 49B(3) of the Act.

(2) Subject to paragraph 3(1), a chemist shall make all necessary arrangements—

(a) for measuring a person who presents a prescription for a truss or other appliance of a type requiring measurement and fitting by the chemist; and

(b) for fitting the appliance.

6 Particulars of chemists

A chemist shall give the HA, if it so requires, the name of any pharmacist employed by him for the provision of drugs for persons from whom he has accepted an order for the provision of pharmaceutical services under paragraph 3.

7 Charges for drugs

(1) Subject to regulations made under section 77 of the Act(**a**), all drugs, containers and appliances provided under these terms of service shall be provided free of charge.

(2) Where a chemist supplies a container in response to an order for drugs signed by a doctor under paragraph 43 of Schedule 2 to the Medical Regulations or supplies an oxygen container or oxygen equipment, other than equipment specified in the Drug Tariff as not returnable to the chemist, the container and equipment shall remain the property of the chemist.

(**a**) See SI 1989/419 as amended by SI 1991/1579.

8 Remuneration of chemists

(1A) A chemist who has undertaken to provide additional professional services within the meaning of regulation 16A shall, on request,

(a) make available to the Health Authority all records kept in accordance with regulation 16A(2)(c); and

(b) permit the HA or another person on its behalf at any reasonable time to inspect the premises from which those services are provided for the purpose of satisfying itself that those services are being provided in accordance with the undertaking.

(2) The HA shall make payments, calculated in the manner provided by the Drug Tariff or in accordance with any determination made by virtue of regulation 18(1A) (subject to any deduction required to be made by regulations made under section 77 of the Act) to chemists in respect of drugs and appliances, containers, medicines measures and dispensing fees.

(2A) The HA shall make such payments, if any, as are provided for by the Drug Tariff or by any determination made by virtue of regulation 18(1A) to chemists who provide additional professional services within the meaning of regulation 16A.

(3) Where a chemist so requires, the HA shall afford him reasonable facilities for examining all or any of the forms on which the drugs or appliances provided by him were ordered, together with particulars of the amounts calculated to be payable in respect of such drugs and appliances and the HA shall take into consideration any objections made by the chemist in relation to those amounts.

(4) Where so required by the Local Pharmaceutical Committee or any organisation which is, in the opinion of the Secretary of State, representative of the general body of chemists, the HA shall give the Local Pharmaceutical Committee or the organisation in question similar facilities for examining such forms and particulars relating to all or any of the chemists which it represents.

8A Professional standards

(1) A pharmacist whose name is on the pharmaceutical list shall provide pharmaceutical services and exercise any professional judgement in connection with the provision of such services in conformity with the standards generally accepted in the pharmaceutical profession.

(2) A chemist who employs a pharmacist in connection with the provision of pharmaceutical services shall secure that the pharmacist complies with the requirements set out in sub-paragraph (1).

10 Withdrawal from pharmaceutical list

(1) Subject to sub-paragraph (2), a chemist may at any time give notice in writing to the HA that he wishes to withdraw his name from the pharmaceutical list and his name shall be removed accordingly on the expiry of the period of three months from the date of such notice or of such shorter period as the HA may agree.

(2) Where representations are made to the Tribunal under section 46 of the Act (disqualification of practitioner) that the continued inclusion of a chemist in the pharmaceutical list would be prejudicial to the efficiency of pharmaceutical services, he shall not, except with the consent of the Secretary of State, be entitled to have his name removed from such a list pending the determination of the proceedings on those representations.

10A Complaints

(1) Subject to sub-paragraph (2), a chemist shall establish, and operate in accordance with this paragraph, a procedure (in this paragraph and in paragraph 10B referred to as a 'complaints procedure') to deal with any complaints made by or on behalf of any person to whom he has provided pharmaceutical services.

Rider A

(2) The complaints procedure to be established by a chemist may be such that it also deals with complaints made in relation to one or more other chemists.

(3) The complaints procedure to be established by a chemist who provides pharmaceutical services from more than one set of premises may be such that it relates to all those premises together.

(4) A complaints procedure shall apply to complaints made in relation to any matter reasonably connected with the chemist's provision of pharmaceutical services and within the responsibility or control of—

(a)   a chemist;

(b)   where the chemist is a body corporate, any of its directors or former directors;

(c)   a former partner of the chemist;

(d)   any pharmacist employed by the chemist;

(e)   any employee of the chemist other than one falling within sub-paragraph (d).

and in this paragraph and paragraph 10B, references to complaints are to complaints falling within this sub-paragraph.

(5) A complaint may be made on behalf of any person with his consent, or—

(a)   where he is under 16 years of age—

     (i)   by either parent, or in the absence of both parents, the guardian or other adult person who has care of the child, or

     (ii)   where he is in the care of an authority to whose care he has been committed under the provisions of the Children Act 1989(**a**) or in the care of a voluntary organisation, by that authority or voluntary organisation; or

(b)   where he is incapable of making a complaint, by a relative or other adult person who has an interest in his welfare.

(6) A complaint may be made as respects a person who has died by a relative or other adult person who had an interest in his welfare, or where he was as described in paragraph (a)(ii) of sub-paragraph (5), by the authority or voluntary organisation.

(7) A complaints procedure shall comply with the following requirements—

(a)   the chemist must specify a person (who need not be connected with the chemist and who, in the case of an individual, may be specified by his job title) to be responsible for receiving and investigating all complaints.

(b)   all complaints must be—

     (i)   recorded in writing;

     (ii)   acknowledged, either orally or in writing, within the period of three days (excluding Saturdays, Sundays, Christmas Day, Good Friday and bank holidays) beginning with the day on which the complaint was received by the person specified under paragraph (a), or where that is not possible as soon as reasonably practicable, and

     (iii)   properly investigated;

(c)   within the period of 10 days (excluding Saturdays, Sundays, Christmas Day, Good Friday and bank holidays) beginning with the day on which the complaint was received by the person specified under paragraph (a) or, where that is not possible as soon as reasonably practicable, the complainant must be given a written summary of the investigation and its conclusions;

(d)   where the investigation of the complaint requires consideration of any records relating to the person as respects whom the complaint is made, the person specified under paragraph (a) must inform him or the person acting on his behalf if the investigation will involve disclosure of information contained in those records to a person other than the chemist or a director, partner or employee of the chemist; and

---

(**a**)   1989 c. 41.

(e) the chemist must keep a record of all complaints and copies of all corresponsence relating to complaints, but such records must be kept separate from any records relating to the person by whom the complaint was made.

(8) At each of the premises at which the chemist provides pharmaceutical services he must provide information about the complaints procedure and give the name (or title) and address of the person specified under paragraph (7)(a); and where he provides supplemental services he must provide the same information to the person referred to in regulation 16(2)(a).

10B(1) A chemist must cooperate with any investigation of a complaint by the Health Authority in accordance with the procedures which it operates in accordance with directions given under section 17 of the Act, whether the investigation follows one under the chemist's complaints procedure or not.

(2) The cooperation requirted by sub-paragraph (1) includes —

(a) answering questions reasonably put to the chemist by the Health Authority;

(b) providing any information relating to the complaint reasonably required by the Health Authority; and

(c) attending any meeting to consider the complaint (if held at a reasonably accessible place and at a reasonable hour, and due notice has been given), if the chemist's presence at the meeting is reasonably required by the Health Authority.

The Medicines for Human Use (Marketing Authorisations Etc.) Regulations 1994, SI No. 3144

3 Marketing authorisations for relevant medicinal products

(1) Except in accordance with any exception or exemption set out in the relevant Community provisions and subject to paragraphs 1 and 3 of Schedule 1–

(a) no relevant medicinal product shall be placed on the market; and

(b) no such product shall be distributed by way of wholesale dealing,

unless a marketing authorisation in respect of that product has been granted in accordance with the relevant Community provisions by the licensing authority or the European Commission, and is for the time being in force in accordance with those provisions.

(2) Schedule 1 shall have effect for the purpose of making certain exceptions or exemptions from paragraph (1), and for imposing certain obligations in connection with such exceptions and exemptions.

4 Applications for the grant, renewal or variation of a United Kingdom marketing authorisation

(1) Every application for the grant, renewal or variation of a United Kingdom marketing authorisation for a relevant medicinal product shall be made in accordance with the relevant Community provisions, subject to any provision of Community law affecting parallel imports, and the applicant shall comply with so much of the relevant Community provisions as impose obligations on applicants as are applicable to the application or the consideration of it.

(2) Every application shall be made in writing, shall be signed by or on behalf of the applicant and shall, unless the licensing authority otherwise direct, be accompanied by any fee which may be payable in connection with that application.

(5) An application for the grant of a marketing authorisation shall include a statement indicating–

(a) whether the relevant medicinal product is one that should be available–

(i)   only on prescription;

(ii)   only from a pharmacy; or

(iii) on general sale; and

(b) what, if any, provisions of the authorisation are proposed concerning the method of sale or supply of the product (including, in particular, any proposed restrictions affecting the circumstances of the use or promotion of the product).

5 Consideration, and grant or refusal, of an application for, or for renewal or variation of, a United Kingdom marketing authorisation

(1) The licensing authority shall consider every application for the grant, renewal or variation by them of a marketing authorisation in accordance with the relevant Community provisions, and shall grant, renew or vary, or refuse to grant, renew or vary the authorisation in accordance with those provisions.

(2) The licensing authority shall publish in the Gazette notice of every authorisation granted by them.

(3) Schedule 2 shall have effect to regulate the procedure for receiving advice and representations before granting, renewing or varying, or refusing to grant, renew, or vary, a marketing authorisation.

(4) A marketing authorisation shall, unless previously renewed or revoked, be valid for the period (not exceeding five years) specified in it beginning with the date on which it is granted, but where an application for the renewal of such an authorisation is made in accordance with Article 10 of the 1965 Directive the marketing authorisation shall remain in force pending the decision of the licensing authority on that application.

6 Revocation, suspension or variation of a United Kingdom marketing authorisation or the suspension of the use or marketing of medicinal products

(1) The licensing authority may and, where appropriate shall, subject to and in accordance with the relevant Community provisions, revoke, suspend or vary a marketing authorisation for a relevant medicinal product.

(5) Where, under the preceding provisions of this regulation or the provisions of Council Regulation (EEC) No. 2309/93, the licensing authority or the European Commission revoke or suspend a marketing authorisation, or where the licensing authority suspend the use, supply or marketing of a product, or where the relevant Community provisions so permit or require, the licensing authority may and, where appropriate, shall give written notice to the person who is or, immediately before its revocation or suspension, was the holder of the authorisation, requiring him to take all reasonably practicable steps to—

(a) inform wholesalers, retailers, medical practitioners, patients and others who may be in possession of relevant products of the revocation or suspension, the reasons for it, and the action (if any) to be taken to restrict or prevent further use, supply or marketing;

(b) withdraw from the market in the United kingdom and recover possession of such products within the time and for the period specified in the notice.

7 Obligations of holders of marketing authorisations, and offences by holders of marketing authorisations and other persons

(1) Every holder of a United Kingdom marketing authorisation for a relevant medicinal product shall comply with all obligations which relate to him by virtue of the relevant Community provisions (apart from Regulation (EEC) No. 2309/93) including, in particular, obligations relating to providing or updating information, to making changes, to applying to vary the authorisation, to pharmacovigilance, and to labels and package leaflets.

(2) The holder of a marketing authorisation shall maintain a record of reports of which he is aware of suspected adverse reactions in accordance with the relevant Community provisions which shall be open to inspection by a person authorised by the licensing authority, who may take copies of the record and, if the licensing authority so directs, the authorisation holder shall furnish the licensing authority with a copy of any such reports of which he has a record or of which he is or subsequently becomes aware.

(3) The holder of a marketing authorisation shall keep such documents as will facilitate the withdrawal or recall from sale or supply of any relevant medical product to which the authorisation relates.

(4) Schedule 3 shall have effect to create certain criminal offences in connection with the obligations of applicants for, and holders of, marketing authorisations and other persons arising under the relevant Community provisions.

8 Control of retail sale or supply of relevant medicinal products

(1) Paragraphs (2) or (3) applies where a Community marketing authorisation for a relevant medicinal product is subject to any condition or restriction which attaches to the authorisation under Article 9.3(b) of Council Regulation (EEC) No. 2309/93.

(2) If the condition or restriction is to the effect that the product is to be sold or supplied only in accordance with a prescription given by a person who, in relation to the product, is an appropriate practitioner for the purposes of section 58 of the Act, the appropriate Ministers shall, subject to Article 3.4 of Council Directive 92/26/EEC (power to waive the application of the other provisions of that Article), give effect to the condition or restriction—

(a) by exercising their powers under section 58 or 60 of the Act; or

(b) where it appears to them that such an exercise would not be immediately practicable, by means of a written direction addressed to the holder of the authorisation.

(3) If the condition or restriction is not to that effect, the appropriate Ministers shall give effect to it—

(a) by the exercise of any other statutory power available to them for that purpose; or

(b) if there is no such power, by means of a written direction addressed to the holder of the authorisation.

(4) Except as provided by paragraph (2), the appropriate Ministers shall not exercise their powers under section 58(1) or, subject to paragraph (5), section 60 of the Act in relation to any relevant medicinal product for which a Community marketing authorisation has been granted.

(5) Paragraph (4) does not prevent the appropriate Ministers from exercising their powers under section 60 of the Act for the purposes mentioned in subsection (2) of that section.

SCHEDULE 1   Regulation 3(2)

EXEMPTIONS AND EXCEPTIONS FROM THE PROVISIONS OF REGULATION 3

1 Regulation 3(1) shall not apply to a relevant medicinal product supplied in response to a bona fide unsolicited order, formulated in accordance with the specification of a doctor or dentist and for use by his individual patients on his direct personal responsibility, but such supply shall be subject to the conditions specified in paragraph 2.

2 The conditions mentioned in paragraph 1 are that—

(a) the relevant medicinal product is supplied to a doctor or dentist or for use in a registered pharmacy, a hospital or a health centre under the supervision of a pharmacist, in accordance with paragraph 1;

(b) no advertisement or representation relating to the relevant medicinal product is issued with a view to it being seen generally by the public in the United Kingdom and that no advertisement relating to that product, by means of any catalogue, price list or circular letter is issued by, at the request or with the consent of, the person selling that product by retail or by way of wholesale dealing or supplying it in circumstances corresponding to retail sale, or the person who manufactures it, and that the sale or supply is in response to a bona fide unsolicited order;

(c) the manufacture or assembly of the relevant medicinal product is carried out under the supervision of such staff and such precautions are taken as are adequate to ensure that the product is of the character required by and meets the specifications of the doctor or dentist who requires it;

(d) written records as to the manufacture or assembly in accordance with sub-paragraph (c) are made and maintained and are available to the licensing authority or the enforcement authority on request by them or either of them;

(e) the relevant medicinal product is manufactured, assembled or imported by the holder of an authorisation referred to in Article 16 of Council Directive 75/319/EEC which relates specifically to the manufacture, assembly or import of relevant medicinal products to which paragraph 1 applies; and

(f) the relevant medicinal product is distributed by way of wholesale dealing by the holder of a wholesale dealer's licence.

3(1) Subject to the following sub-paragraphs, regulation 3(1) shall not apply to anything done —

(a) by a doctor or dentist which relates to a relevant medicinal product specially prepared by him, or to his order, for administration to one or more patients of his or, where that doctor or dentist is a member of a group of doctors or dentists working together to provide general medical or dental services, to one or more patients of any other doctor or dentist of that group, and consists of procuring the manufacture or assembly of a stock of the product with a view to administering the product to such patients; or

(b) in a registered pharmacy, a hospital or health centre and is done there by or under the supervision of a pharmacist, and consists of procuring the manufacture or assembly of a stock of relevant medicinal products with a view to dispensing them in accordance with paragraph 1.

(2) The exemption conferred by sub-paragraph (1) shall not apply to procuring the manufacture of relevant medicinal products unless those products are to be manufactured by the holder of a manufacturer's licence which relates specifically to the manufacture or assembly of relevant medicinal products to which paragraph 1 applies.

(3) The exemption conferred by sub-paragraph (1) shall not apply to anything done by a doctor or dentist in relation to a stock held by him of such relevant medicinal products in excess of a total of 5 litres of fluid and 2.5 kilograms of solids of all relevant medicinal products to which that sub-paragraph relates.

4(1) Regulation 3(1) shall not apply to the placing on the market by way of supplying of any relevant medicinal product to which this paragraph relates if the conditions of sub-paragraph (3) are satisfied.

(2) The relevant medicinal products to which this paragraph relates are relevant medicinal products which are for use by being administered to one or more human beings and which may be lawfully sold by retail or supplied in circumstances corresponding to retail sale, otherwise than in accordance with a prescription by a doctor or dentist.

(3) The conditions referred to in sub-paragraph (1) are —

(a) that the relevant medicinal product is sold or supplied to a person exclusively for use by him in the course of a business carried on by him for the purposes of administering it or causing it to be administered to one or more human beings otherwise than by selling it;

(b) that, if sold or supplied through the holder of a wholesale dealer's licence, the relevant medicinal product is sold or supplied to such a person, and for such use by him, as is described in head (a) above;

(c) that, where the manufacture or assembly of the relevant medicinal product is procured, it is procured by such a person, and for such use by him, as is described in head (a) above;

(d) that no advertisement or representation relating to the relevant medicinal product is issued with a view to it being seen generally by the public in the United Kingdom and that no advertisement relating to that product, by means of any catalogue, price list or circular letter, is issued by, at the request or with the consent of, the person selling that product by retail or by way of wholesale dealing or supplying it in circumstances corresponding to retail sale, or the person who manufactures it, and that the sale or supply is in response to a bona fide unsolicited order;

(e) that the relevant medicinal product is prepared by or under the supervision of a pharmacist; and

(f) that the relevant medicinal product is manufactured by the holder of a manufacturer's licence which relates specifically to the manufacture of relevant medicinal products to which paragraph 1 applies.

5(1) Regulations 3(1) shall not apply to a radiopharmaceutical for human use –

(a) which is prepared at the time at which it is intended to be administered; and

(b) which is prepared, in accordance with the manufacturer's instructions and by the person by whom it is to be administered, exclusively from a kit, generator or precursor (or from more than one of these) in respect of which a marketing authorisation is in force; and

(c) the administration of which is not or will not be a contravention of regulation 2 of the Medicines (Administration of Radioactive Substances) Regulations 1978.

(2) In this paragraph –

'generator' means any system incorporating a fixed parent radionuclide from which is produced a daughter radionuclide which is to be removed by elution or by any other method and is to be used in a radiopharmaceutical;

'kit' means any preparation to be reconstituted or combined with radionuclides in a final radiopharmaceutical, usually prior to its administration;

'precursor' means a radionuclide produced for the radio-labelling of another substance prior to its administration, other than a radionuclide which is incorporated in or produced from a generator or is included in a radiopharmaceutical;

'radiopharmaceutical' means any relevant medicinal product which when ready for use contains one or more radionuclides included for a medicinal purpose.

6 Any person who sells or supplies a relevant medicinal product in accordance with any of paragraphs 1 to 4 shall maintain, and keep for a period of at least 5 years, a record showing –

(a) the source from which that person obtained that product;

(b) the person to whom and the date on which the sale or supply was made;

(c) the quantity of each sale or supply;

(d) the batch number of the batch of that product from which the sale or supply was made; and

(e) details of any suspected adverse reaction to the product so sold or supplied of which he is aware.

7 A person required to maintain the records mentioned in paragraph 6 shall –

(a) notify the licensing authority of any suspected adverse reaction such as is mentioned in head (e) of that paragraph which is a serious adverse reaction; and

(b) make available for inspection at all reasonable times by the licensing authority the records mentioned in that paragraph.

OFFENCES, PENALTIES ETC.

Offences

1 Any person who, in breach of the relevant Community provisions or of these Regulations, places a relevant medicinal product on the market without holding a Community or United Kingdom marketing authorisation in respect of that product, or otherwise than in accordance with the terms of such an authorisation, shall be guilty of an offence.

2 Any person who, in the course of a business carried on by him, sells, supplies, manufactures or assembles, or procures the sale, supply, manufacture or assembly of, a relevant medicinal product, or who has in his possession a relevant medicinal product, knowing or having reasonable cause to believe that the product was or is intended to be placed on the market contrary to paragraph 1 shall be guilty of an offence.

3 Without prejudice to any other sanction which may be available for the enforcement of conditions attaching to marketing authorisations, any holder of a marketing authorisation for a relevant medicinal product who contravenes any condition of the authorisation shall be guilty of an offence.

4 Where the use, supply or marketing of a relevant medicinal product is suspended in accordance with regulation 6 or Council Regulation (EEC) No. 2309/93, any person who sells, supplies or markets, or procures the sale, supply or marketing of, that product knowing, or having reasonable cause to believe, that such use, supply or marketing is suspended, shall be guilty of an offence.

5 Any person who is or, immediately before its revocation or suspension, was the holder of a marketing authorisation who fails to comply with a notice given to him under regulation 6(5) (notice to take all reasonably practicable steps to publish information concerning revocation or suspension or to recover possession of products affected) shall be guilty of an offence.

6 Any holder of a marketing authorisation who fails promptly to —
  (a) update information concerning the product or any connected matter as required by Article 4 of the 1965 Directive or Article 6 of Council Regulation (EEC) No. 2309/93; or
  (b) take any steps reasonably necessary to take account of technical and scientific progress for the purposes of making any changes or amendments as required by Article 9a of the 1965 Directive or Article 15.1 of Council Regulation (EEC) No. 2309/93; or
  (c) introduce any changes or make any amendments that may be required in accordance with those Articles; or
  (d) provide information to the EMEA, the Commission or the licensing authority as required by Article 15.2 of Council Regulation (EEC) No. 2309/93; or
  (e) submit any application to the licensing authority or the Community to make any changes or variation as required by Article 9a of the 1965 Directive or Article 15.3 of Council Regulation (EEC) No. 2309/93,
shall be guilty of an offence.

7 Any person responsible for placing on the market a relevant medicinal product authorised by the Community or by the licensing authority who, at any time, does not have at his disposal an appropriately qualified person responsible for pharmacovigilance as required by Chapter 3 of Title II of Council Regulation (EEC) No. 2309/93 or Chapter Va of Council Directive 75/319/EEC shall be guilty or an offence.

8 Any person responsible for placing a relevant medicinal product on the market who fails to report to the licensing authority any suspected adverse reaction, or to submit to the licensing authority any records of suspected adverse reactions as required by Chapter 3 of Title II of Council Regulation (EEC) No. 2309/93 or Chapter Va of Council Directive 75/319/EEC, shall be guilty of an offence.

9 Any person responsible for placing a relevant medicinal product on the market who fails to make or maintain a detailed record of any suspected adverse reaction as required by Chapter 3 of Title II of council Regulation (EEC) No. 2309/93, or Chapter Va of Council Directive 75/319/EEC shall be guilty of an offence.

10 Any person who, while employed or engaged as an appropriately qualified person responsible for pharmacovigilance for the purposes of Chapter 3 of Title II of Council Regulation (EEC) No. 2309/93, or Chapter Va of Council Directive 75/319/EEC fails to —
  (a) establish or maintain a system for collecting and collating information about suspected adverse reactions;
  (b) prepare for the licensing authority a report on any such reactions; or
  (c) ensure that a request from the licensing authority for the provision of additional information necessary for the evaluation of the benefits and risks afforded by a relevant medicinal product is answered fully and promptly,
as required by any provision of any such Chapter, shall be guilty of an offence.

11 Any holder of a marketing authorisation who sells or supplies or procures the sale or supply of a relevant medicinal product to which the authorisation relates —
  (a) the labelling of which, or any package leaflet accompanying which, does not comply with; or
  (b) without a package leaflet required to be provided by virtue of,
the applicable requirements of Council directive 92/27/EEC or of Schedule 5 to these Regulations, shall be guilty of an offence.

12 Where, in relation to a relevant medicinal product —
  (a) the labelling of the product, or any package leaflet accompanying the product, does not comply with; or
  (b) the product is not accompanied by a package leaflet required to be provided by virtue of,
the applicable requirements of Council Directive 92/27/EEC or Schedule 5, any person, other than the holder of the marketing authorisation for that product, who in the course of a business carried on by him, sells or supplies or procures the sale or supply of that product knowing, or having reasonable cause to believe, that the labelling does not so comply or, as the case may be, that the product is not so accompanied, shall be guilty of an offence.

13 Any person who fails to keep any record required under paragraph 6 of Schedule 1, or to give notice or make it available for inspection as and when required under paragraph 7 of that Schedule, shall be guilty of an offence.

Penalties

14 Any person guilty of an offence under any of the preceding paragraphs shall be liable —
(a)   on summary conviction, to a fine not exceeding the statutory maximum;
(b)   on conviction on indictment, to a fine or to imprisonment for a term not exceeding two years or to both.

Miscellaneous

15(1) Where an offence is committed under any of paragraphs 8, 9 or 10 by a person mentioned in those paragraphs who is acting as the employee or agent of another person, the employer or principal of that person shall be guilty of the same offence.
(2) Where a Scottish partnership is guilty of an offence under these Regulations in respect of any act or default which is shown to have been committed with the consent or connivance of, or to be attributable to any neglect on the part of, a partner in th partnership, he, as well as the partnership, shall be guilty of that offence and shall be liable to be proceeded against and punished accordingly.

16 Where the holder of a marketing authorisation is charged with an offence under these Regulations in respect of anything which has been manufactured or assembled to his order by another person and had been so manufactured or assembled as not to comply with the provisions of that authorisation, it shall be a defence for him to prove —
(a)   that he had communicated the provisions relating to the authorisation to that other person; and
(b)   that he did not know, and could not by the exercise of reasonable care have known, that those provisions have not been complied with.

SCHEDULE 5   Regulation 11

LABELS

1 Interpretation
In this Schedule, unless the context otherwise requires —
'dispensed relevant medicinal product' means a relevant medicinal product prepared or dispensed in accordance with a prescription given by a practitioner;
'relevant medicinal product on a general sale list' means a relevant medicinal product of a description, or falling within a class, specified in an order under section 51 of the Act which is for the time being in force;
'requirements' includes restrictions;
'retail sale' has the same meaning as in section 131 of the Act; and
'supply in circumstances corresponding to retail sale' has the same meaning as in section 131 of the Act.

2 Introductory
The requirements of this Schedule supplement those of Council Directive 92/27/EEC relating to —
(a)   special warnings necessary for particular medicinal products;
(b)   the legal status for supply to the patient, in accordance with Council Directive 92/26/EEC;
(c)   identification and authenticity.

3 Dispensed relevant medicinal products

(1) Subject to the following provisions of this Schedule, where a relevant medicinal product is a dispensed relevant medicinal product the container of that product shall be labelled to show the following particulars —

  (a) where the relevant medicinal product is for use by being administered to a particular human being, the name of the person to whom the relevant medicinal product is to be administered;
  (b) the name and address of the person who sells or supplies the product;
  (c) the date on which the product is dispensed; and
  (d) where the relevant medicinal product has been prescribed by a practitioner, such of the following particulars as he may request —
   (i)   the name of the relevant medicinal product or its common name;
   (ii) directions for use of the relevant medicinal product; and
   (iii) precautions relating to the use of the relevant medicinal product,
   or where a pharmacist, in the exercise of his professional skill and judgment, is of the opinion that any of such particulars are inappropriate and has taken such steps as in all the circumstances are reasonably practicable to consult with the practitioner but has been unable to do so, particulars of the same kind as those requested by the practitioner as appear to the pharmacist to be appropriate.

(2) Where the container of a dispensed relevant medicinal product is enclosed in a package immediately enclosing that container the particulars set out in sub-paragraph (1) may be omitted from the container if that package is labelled to show such particulars.

(3) Where a number of containers or packages, or of containers and packages, of dispensed relevant medicinal products all of the same description are enclosed in a package, sub-paragraph (1)(d) shall be deemed to have been complied with if such of the particulars referred to in that sub-paragraph as would, apart from this sub-paragraph, be required to be shown on each container or package, or on each container and package so enclosed, are shown on either one or more containers or packages or such containers and packages as the case may be.

4 Delivery and storage

(1) Subject to the following provisions of this Schedule, where for the purposes of transport, delivery or storage a number of packages of relevant medicinal products all of the same description, not being relevant medicinal products to which paragraph 1 of Schedule 1 applies, are enclosed in a package, such package shall be labelled to show the following particulars —

  (a) any special requirements for the storage and handling of the product;
  (b) the expiry date of the product; and
  (c) the manufacturer's batch number.

(2) Sub-paragraph (1) does not apply to any package in the form of a packing case, crate or other covering used solely for the purposes of transport or delivery (but not storage) of containers and packages of relevant medicinal products each of which is labelled in accordance with the provisions of this Schedule.

5 Relevant medicinal products on a general sale list

(1) Subject to the following provisions of this Schedule, where a relevant medicinal product on a general sale list, not being a dispensed relevant medicinal product, is sold by retail, or supplied in circumstances corresponding to retail sale or by means of an automatic machine or is in the possession of any person for the purpose of such sale or supply, every container and every package immediately enclosing a container of such product, being a product described in any of the following sub-paragraphs, shall be labelled to show the words and particulars set out in such sub-paragraph or sub-paragraphs —

(a)   if the product contains aloxiprin, aspirin or paracetamol, the words 'If symptoms persist consult your doctor' and, except where the product is for external use only, the recommended dosage;

(b)   if the product contains aloxiprin, the words 'Contains an aspirin derivative';

(c)   If the product contains aspirin, except where the product is for external use only or where the name of the product includes the word 'aspirin' and appears on the container or package, the words 'Contains aspirin';

(d)   if the product contains paracetamol, except where the name of the product includes the word 'paracetamol' and appears on the container or package, the words 'Contains paracetamol';

(e)   if the product contains paracetamol, the words 'Do not exceed the stated dose';

(2) Where a container or package is required by this paragraph to show —

(a)   words set out in more than one of sub-paragraphs (b), (c) and (d) of sub-paragraph (1), there may be substituted for those words other words showing that the product contains more than one of the substances aloxiprin, aspirin and paracetamol and naming the substances so contained, except that in the case of aloxiprin the words 'aspirin derivative' shall appear and the word 'aloxiprin' need not appear;

(b)   words set out in one or more of those sub-paragraphs, such words shall appear in a prominent position and shall be within a rectangle within which there shall be no other matter of any kind, except that where words set out in more than one of the said sub-paragraphs appear on the container or package then any of them may together be within a rectangle within which there shall be no other matter of any kind.

(3) Where a container or package is required to be labelled to show the words 'Do not exceed the stated dose', such words shall appear adjacent to either the directions for use, where such directions appear on the container or package, or the recommended dosage, where such recommendation appears on the container or package.

(4) Where a container or package is required to be labelled to show the words 'Do not exceed the stated dose', such words shall not be required to be shown if, by virtue of paragraph 6, the words set out in head (a) of sub-paragraph (2) of that paragraph are required to be, and are, shown.

(5) Without prejudice to the operation of sub-paragraph (1), where a relevant medicinal product, not being a dispensed medicinal product, is —

(a)   sold by retail; or

(b)   supplied in circumstances corresponding to retail sale; or

(c)   in the possession of a person for the purpose of such sale or supply; or

(d)   sold by way of wholesale dealing,

then, if the product is a product referred to in regulation 8 of the Medicines (Sale or Supply) (Miscellaneous Provisions) Regulations 1980 which is not presented for sale in the manner described in relation to that product in that regulation, every container and every package immediately enclosing a container of that relevant medicinal product shall be labelled to show the capital letter 'P' within a rectangle within which there shall be no other matter of any kind.

6 Relevant medicinal products not on a general sale list

(1) Subject to the following provisions of this Schedule, where a relevant medicinal product to which any of the restrictions imposed by section 52 of the Act (sale or supply of medicinal products not on general sale list) apply is sold by retail, or supplied in circumstances corresponding to retail sale or is offered or exposed for sale by retail, every container and every package immediately enclosing a container of such a product —

(a)   shall be labelled in accordance with the provisions of paragraph 5 as if such provisions applied to such containers and packages as they apply to containers and packages of relevant medicinal products on a general sale list;

(b) shall, if the product is described in any head of sub-paragraph (2), be labelled to show the words and particulars set out in that head, except that where words set out in more than one of heads (a), (b) and (c) of that sub-paragraph appear on the container or package then the word 'Warning' need not appear more than once, and where the product is a dispensed relevant medicinal product then the words set out in those heads need not appear;

(c) shall, unless any of the provisions of paragraph 7 apply to such container or package or the product is a dispensed relevant medicinal product, be labelled to show the capital letter 'P' within a rectangle within which there shall be no other matter of any kind.

(2) The descriptions and words referred to in sub-paragraph (1) are—

(a) if the product would be subject to restrictions imposed under section 58 of the Act but for an exemption from any such restrictions conferred by an order made under that section by reason of the proportion or level in such product of any substance, except where the product is for external use only or contains any of the substances described in head (c) of this sub-paragraph the words 'Warning. Do not exceed the stated dose';

(b) if the product is for the treatment of asthma or other conditions associated with bronchial spasm or contains ephedrine or any of its salts, except where the product is for external use only, the words 'Warning. Asthmatics should consult their doctor before using this product';

(c) if the product contains an antihistamine or any of its salts or molecular compounds, except where the product is for external use only or where the marketing authorisation contains no warning relating to the sedating effect of the product in use, the words 'Warning. May cause drowsiness. If affected do not drive or operate machinery. Avoid alcoholic drink';

(d) if the product is embrocation, liniment, lotion, liquid antiseptic or other liquid preparation or gel and is for external use only, the words 'For external use only';

(e) if the product contains hexachlorophane, either the words 'Not to be used for babies' or a warning that the product is not to be administered, except on medical advice, to a child under two years.

(3) The requirement of sub-paragraph (1)(c) shall apply to every container and every package immediately enclosing a container of a relevant medicinal product which is sold by way of wholesale dealing and which is not a relevant medicinal product on a general sale list.

(4) Where a container or package is required by this paragraph to be labelled to show any of the words or particulars specified in heads (a) to (e) of sub-paragraph (2), such words or particulars shall be within a rectangle within which there shall be no other matter of any kind, except that where words or particulars set out in more than one head of that sub-paragraph appear on the container or package then any of them may be together within a rectangle within which there shall be no other matter of any kind.

7 Prescription only relevant medicinal products

Subject to the following provisions of this Schedule, every container and every package immediately enclosing a container of a relevant medicinal product which is subject to restrictions imposed under section 58(1) of the Act (relevant medicinal products on prescription only) shall, if the product is described in heads (d) or (e) of sub-paragraph (2) of paragraph 6, be labelled to show the words and particulars set out in that head and shall, except where the product is sold by retail or supplied in circumstances corresponding to retail sale or is the subject of an exemption, by virtue of the provisions of section 58(4)(a), from any of the restrictions imposed by section 58(2) of the Act, be labelled to show the letters 'POM' in capital letters within a rectangle within which there shall be no other matter of any kind.

8 Exemptions

Nothing in this Schedule shall require the labelling of —

(a) any package in the form of a transparent wrapping or cover to a container and package of a relevant medicinal product or any package the whole or part of which is transparent or open if the particulars shown on the labelled container enclosed in that package are clearly visible;

(b) any package in the form of a wrapping paper, paper bag or similar covering in which the container and package of a relevant medicinal product labelled in accordance with the provisions of this Schedule is placed when such relevant medicinal product is sold by retail or supplied in circumstances corresponding to retail sale; or

(c) any container or package immediately enclosing the container of a relevant medicinal product which is for export;

(d) any container which is —

(i) an ampoule or other container of not more than 10 millilitres nominal capacity which is immediately enclosed in a package which is labelled in accordance with those provisions of paragraphs 5 to 7 which apply to such package;

(ii) in the form of a wrapper consisting of paper, film, plastic material, metal foil or other sheet or strip material or in the form of a bubble, blister or other sealed unit consisting of such sheet or strip material, enclosing one or more dosage units of a relevant medicinal product and such container is immediately enclosed in a package which is labelled in accordance with those provisions of paragraphs 5 to 7 which apply to such package;

(iii) where the package immediately enclosing such a container as is described in head (ii) above is itself in the form of a bubble, blister or other sealed unit as is mentioned in that head and is part of a continuous series comprising a sheet or strip of like packages and is required to be labelled to show any of the words, particulars or letters referred to in paragraphs 5 to 7, such requirements shall be deemed to have been complied with if the said words, particulars or letters, as the case may be, are displayed at frequent intervals on the said sheet or strip of such packages.

The Code of Ethics of the Royal Pharmaceutical Society of Great Britain

Preface

The Code of Ethics has recently undergone substantial revision. The new code was finally adopted at the Society's annual general meeting in May 2001.

- Part 1 replaces the previous preface to the Code
- Part 2 replaces Principles Four and Five of the Code and Standard 7 of the Appendix to the Code
- The remaining Code and Appendix are now termed Part 3.

Part 1: pharmacists' ethics

The public places great trust in the knowledge, skills and professional judgment of pharmacists. This trust requires pharmacists to ensure and maintain, throughout their career, high standards of personal and professional conduct and performance, up-to-date knowledge and continuing competence relevant to their sphere of practice whether or not they work in direct contact with the public.

The Royal Pharmaceutical Society of Great Britain seeks to safeguard and promote the interests of the public and the profession by identifying the key responsibilities of a pharmacist.

Ethics has been described as the systematic study of moral choices; it concerns the values that lie behind them, the reasons people give for them and the language used to describe them. Ethical decision making is the process whereby one recognises that a problem needs to be overcome or a difficult choice made, identifies the possible courses of actions, chooses one, takes it and then accepts responsibility.

The exercise of professional judgment requires identification and evaluation of the risks and benefits associated with possible courses of action. On occasions there may not be a right or wrong answer. Different people may reach different decisions on a single set of circumstances and each may be justifiable.

Many of the issues pharmacists are called upon to resolve are unambiguous and the decision will be obvious. However, when faced with ethical dilemmas pharmacists are expected to use their professional judgment in deciding on the most appropriate course of action. They must be able to justify their decisions to their peers, and to any person or organisation which may be affected by their actions, including individual patients, the public, the National Health Service, their employers, and other health care professionals. Pharmacists may be accountable to any of these.

Disreputable behaviour or breach of a professional responsibility or requirement identified in the Code could form the basis of a complaint of professional misconduct. The Society's disciplinary committees, in considering whether or not action should follow, take into consideration the circumstances of an individual case and do not regard themselves as being limited to those matters which are mentioned in this document.

Key responsibilities of a pharmacist

Pharmacists understand the nature and effect of medicines and medicinal ingredients, and how they may be used to prevent and treat illness, relieve symptoms or assist in the diagnosis of disease. Pharmacists in professional practice use their knowledge for the wellbeing and safety of patients and the public.

- At all times pharmacists must act in the interests of patients and other members of the public, and seek to provide the best possible health care for the community in partnership with other health professions. Pharmacists must treat all those who seek their professional services with courtesy, respect and confidentiality. Pharmacists must respect patients' rights to participate in decisions about their care and must provide information in a way in which it can be understood.
- Pharmacists must ensure that their knowledge, skills and performance are of a high quality, up to date, evidence based and relevant to their field of practice.
- Pharmacists must ensure that they behave with integrity and probity, adhere to accepted standards of personal and professional conduct and do not engage in any behaviour or activity likely to bring the profession into disrepute or undermine public confidence in the profession.

Part 2: Standards of professional performance

A. Personal responsibilities

Pharmacists' prime concern, irrespective of their sphere of work, must be for the wellbeing and safety of patients and the public. Some roles pharmacists undertake attract specific professional responsibilities. For example, pharmacists who own a pharmacy, superintendent pharmacists, or pharmacist managers in hospitals and trusts must ensure that procedures designed to minimise risks are formulated and applied. Pharmacists providing professional services in any sphere of practice must ensure that their own work procedures are safe and effective.

The public and the profession are entitled to expect that pharmacists providing services will comply with the specific professional responsibilities associated with them and comply with any other accepted codes of practice and statutory requirements applicable to their sphere of practice.

A.1 Pharmacists providing professional services

Pharmacists assuming responsibility for any pharmacy function whether as an employee, locum, adviser or otherwise are professionally accountable for all decisions to supply a medicine or offer advice, and must ensure that:

(a) they only accept work where they have the requisite skills and fitness for the tasks to be performed. All pharmacists must establish sufficient information about the work to enable an assessment to be made;

(b) they undertake continuing professional development relevant to their professional duties;

(c) all activities they undertake are covered by professional indemnity arrangements;

(d) they do not work in conditions that do not enable them to comply with the key responsibilities of a pharmacist;

(e) the requisite facilities, equipment and materials are accessible to enable the provision of the service to professionally accepted standards;

(f) if any tasks are to be delegated they are delegated to persons competent to perform them, for example, any assistant who is given delegated authority to sell medicines under a protocol should have undertaken, or be undertaking, an accredited course relevant to their duties;

(g) they and other staff work within standard operating procedures where these exist;

(h) they agree terms and conditions and abide by them;

(i) they honour commitments to provide professional services unless this is impossible. If they are not able to honour a commitment the pharmacy owner or other responsible person must be informed at the earliest opportunity in order that alternative arrangements may be made;

(j) they take action to report to the prescriber and relevant authorities, suspected adverse drug reactions where this is likely to assist in the future treatment of the patient, or the future use of the medicine;

(k) before accepting employment pharmacists must disclose any factors which may affect their ability to provide services. Where pharmacists' religious beliefs or personal convictions prevent them from providing a service they must not condemn or criticise the patient and they or a member of staff must advise the patient of alternative sources for the service requested;

(l) if they become aware that a person has received pharmaceutical care of a standard less than the person had a right to expect they provide, if possible, an explanation of what happened, whether or not they are the person responsible;

(m) they report to the Society concerns that a pharmacist's professional competence or ability to practise may be impaired and put the public at risk.

A.2 *Pharmacists who own a pharmacy, superintendent pharmacists and pharmacist managers in hospitals and trusts or other fields of practice*

Before assuming the role of pharmacist owner, superintendent pharmacist or pharmacist manager in a hospital or trust pharmacists must be satisfied that they are able to comply with the responsibilities set out below. Pharmacist owners, superintendent pharmacists and pharmacist managers in hospitals and trusts or other fields of practice have a personal professional responsibility:

(a) to ensure the observance of all legal and professional requirements in relation to pharmaceutical aspects of the business. They are responsible for ensuring that a retrievable record of the pharmacist taking responsibility for the provision of each pharmacy service is maintained and that an identifiable pharmacist is accountable for all activities of non-pharmacists involved in the provision of pharmacy services;

(b) to ensure that all professional activities undertaken by them or under their control are covered by adequate professional indemnity arrangements;

(c) to satisfy themselves that the supplier, the source and the quality of any medicines or pharmaceutical ingredients are reputable. Medicines must normally be obtained from licensed wholesalers, the manufacturer or via a central purchasing or inter-branch transfer system. Records must be kept of the source of all medicines obtained by any other means and of measures taken to ensure the safety and efficacy of them. This standard is not intended to cover loans from professional colleagues;

(d) to ensure that all staff are informed of the professional activities they are expected to undertake. Clear instructions should be provided, designed to identify and minimise risks and reviewed regularly. Where possible standard operating procedures should be drafted;

(e) not to seek to impose conditions on pharmacists which may adversely affect their ability to comply with their professional and legal duties;

(f) to ensure that adequate support staff and information about the pharmacy are provided to enable all pharmacists, including temporary staff and locums, to perform their duties effectively;

(g) to satisfy themselves that pharmacists employed or engaged by them are aware of the need to undertake continuing professional development relevant to their professional duties;

(h) to ensure that pharmacists and other staff employed by them or under their management have the requisite knowledge, skills and fitness to perform work delegated to them and comply with work instructions;

(i) to ensure that pharmacists and other staff employed by them are sufficiently competent in English. Competency in other languages common to the area is desirable;

(j) to ensure that working conditions, facilities, equipment and materials enable the provision of services to professionally accepted standards;

(k) to have procedures to deal with incidents where there is a threat to the health of a patient or the public and review practices in the light of incidents;

(l) to ensure that effective measures are in place for protecting the confidentiality of person identifiable data;

(m) to ensure that an effective complaint handling procedure exists, whereby all complaints are dealt with promptly, constructively and honestly;

(n) to report to the Society concerns that a pharmacist's professional competence or ability to practise may be impaired and put the public at risk;

(o) to notify the Society in writing of any changes in the ownership of registered pharmacy premises, or superintendent pharmacist of a body corporate.

A.3 Preregistration tutors and pharmacists supervising preregistration trainees

Preregistration tutors and preregistration managers must ensure that section XX of the Society's Byelaws, relating to preregistration training, is complied with.

Tutors and preregistration managers must ensure that:

(a) preregistration trainees they assess understand and comply with the key responsibilities of a pharmacist and are competent. The public may be put at risk if a tutor or manager confirms the competence of a trainee who has not attained the required standard;

(b) preregistration trainees receive wide-ranging experience of professional practice;

(c) preregistration training meets the needs of the trainee;

(d) preregistration trainees are properly supervised, in particular in relation to their responsibilities for services to the public;

(e) the progress of preregistration trainees is reviewed regularly, with honest and constructive feedback;

(f) preregistration trainees are encouraged to self-appraise their performance;

(g) reports of trainees' performance provided to the Society are honest and objective;

(h) they reflect on work processes and outcomes, evaluate their own performance and take action to develop their expertise and knowledge.

B. Professional competence

The public, the profession and the NHS expect pharmacists to develop their professional performance to provide a high level of care to patients.

(a) Pharmacists must continually review the skills and knowledge required for their field of practice, identifying those skills or knowledge most in need of development or improvement and audit their performance as part of the review.

(b) Pharmacists must, each year, undertake a minimum of 30 hours' continuing education structured to meet their personal needs, and be able to provide evidence of such.

(c) Pharmacists must be ready and able to provide information and advice about any medicine supplied by them or under their authority.

(d) Pharmacists giving advice to prescribers, patients and others must be able to demonstrate competence and knowledge of medicines within the relevant therapeutic class.

(e) Pharmacists must be alert to potential adverse drug reactions and drug interactions and respond accordingly.

C. Confidentiality

The public expects pharmacists and their staff to respect and protect confidentiality. This duty extends to any information relating to an individual which pharmacists or their staff acquire in the course of their professional activities. Confidential information includes personal details and medication, both prescribed and non-prescribed.

Pharmacists must ensure that:

(a) the confidentiality of information acquired in the course of their professional activities is respected and protected, and is disclosed only with the consent of the individual other than in the circumstances defined below in (b).

(b) information is disclosed without the patient's consent only in the following circumstances:

(i) where the patient's parent, guardian or carer has consented to the disclosure and the patient's apparent age or health makes them incapable of consent;

(ii) Pharmacists should be aware that information about services provided to adolescents should not normally be disclosed to their parents.

(iii) where disclosure of the information is to a person or body empowered by statute to require such a disclosure;

(iv) where disclosure is directed by a coroner, judge or other presiding officer of a court, Crown Prosecution Office in England and Wales and Procurator Fiscal in Scotland;

(v) to a police officer or NHS Fraud Investigation Officer who provides in writing confirmation that disclosure is necessary to assist in the prevention, detection or prosecution of serious crime;

(c) where necessary to prevent serious injury or damage to the health of the patient, a third party or to public health;

(d) they do not disclose information relating to the prescribing practices of identifiable prescribers or their practices, other than for the necessary purposes of the NHS or other health care provider, unless the prescriber has given his written informed consent to the disclosure;

(e) access to confidential information within the pharmacy is restricted to those who require that information and who are themselves subject to an obligation of confidentiality;

(f) the requirements of data protection legislation for data collection and use are complied with;

(g) confidential information is effectively protected against improper disclosure when it is disposed of, stored, transmitted or received;

(h) pharmacy computer and manual systems which include patient specific information incorporate access control systems to minimise the risk of unauthorised or unnecessary access to the data. Pharmacy computer systems which include patient specific information and which are linked to the internet or other networks must incorporate measures such as data encryption to eliminate the risk of unauthorised access to confidential data.

Part 3: Service specifications

The application of the key professional responsibilities described in Part 1 to the following activities indicates that the provision of these services should incorporate the following professional requirements. Pharmacists should build upon these requirements when developing professional services to enable the public to receive services that reflect the best possible pharmaceutical practice. These service specifications must be read in conjunction with each other to ensure that in providing a service account is taken of all relevant professional requirements.

When providing any professional service pharmacists should ensure that the tenets of clinical governance are followed:
that an identifiable pharmacist is accountable for all activities undertaken;

- that they and staff providing services are suitably trained and competent to perform the tasks required;
- that any necessary equipment and suitable facilities are available for the provision of the service and that these are maintained in good order;
- that risk assessment and management procedures have been identified and are followed;
- that adequate records are maintained to enable the service to be monitored.

The following service specifications cover a range of services; some are core services which will be provided by the majority of pharmacies, others are additional professional services which pharmacists may wish to be involved in.

1. Publicity, promotion and information

It is in the public interest for pharmacies to provide information about their opening hours and services available. Any information or publicity material regarding pharmacy services must be accurate and honest. The public and the profession would not expect any products or services advertised or otherwise promoted, to be injurious to health when properly and responsibly used.

(a) All information and publicity for goods and services must be legal, decent and truthful; be presented and distributed in a manner so as not to bring the profession into disrepute; and not abuse the trust or exploit the lack of knowledge of the public.

(b) Information and promotional material relating to professional services must be compatible with the role of pharmacists as skilled and informed advisers about medicines, common ailments, general health care and well being. It should be presented so as to allow the recipient to decide independently whether or not to use a service and should not disparage the professional services of other pharmacies or pharmacists.

(c) Pharmacists must not make any unsolicited approach, for promotional purposes, directly to a member of the public by way of a telephone call, e-mail, or visit made without prior appointment.

(d) Pharmacists must ensure that promotions (materials and campaigns) for medicines aimed at the public:

(i) emphasise the special nature of medicines;

(ii) do not make any medicinal claim not capable of substantiation;

(iii) are consistent with the summary of product characteristics approved by the Medicines Control Agency as part of the licensing procedures;

(iv) do not promote a medicine by way of endorsement by a pharmacist, or comparison with other products. A pharmacist may recommend a product in response to a request for advice from an individual patient;

(v) do not promote inappropriate or excessive consumption or use of medicines or their misuse, injudicious or unsafe use which may be injurious to health.

(d) Pharmacists may advertise the prices at which they sell medicines and price discounts. Promotions for pharmacy medicines which seek to persuade consumers to obtain medicines that are not wanted or quantities substantially in excess of those wanted are considered to be professionally unacceptable. (At present almost all proprietary medicines are subject to resale price maintenance (RPM) controls imposed by contract as permitted by legislation, and price discounting of these medicines could result in legal action being taken to secure compliance with the contractual provisions. This provision of the Code of Ethics does not override or affect RPM; it reflects the provisions of new competition law.)

2. Stock

The public and the profession are entitled to expect all stock to be obtained from a reputable source and be of high quality and fit for the intended purpose.

(a) Pharmacists must not purchase or supply any medicines, food supplement or health care related product where they have reason to doubt its quality or safety.

(b) Pharmacists must report to the Royal Pharmaceutical Society, the Medicines Control Agency, Veterinary Medicines Directorate or the marketing authorisation holder any instance where they suspect that they have been offered or have been supplied with counterfeit or defective medicines. Such medicines must be isolated from other pharmacy stock and withheld from sale or supply.

(c) Pharmacy stock must be stored under suitable conditions appropriate to the nature and stability of the product concerned. Particular attention must be paid to protection from contamination, sunlight, atmospheric moisture and adverse temperatures. During storage medicines must be retained in the manufacturer's original packaging. Pharmacists must exercise their knowledge of stability of materials to segregate for disposal any substances that are likely to have deteriorated, or have been in stock for unduly long periods or have reached their expiry dates.

(d) All stocks of medicines in the pharmacy must have batch and expiry details. Medicines may only be removed from blister or foil packs at the time of dispensing to assist an individual patient.

(e) Medicines returned to a pharmacy from a patient's home, a nursing or residential home must not be supplied to any other patient.

(f) Pharmacists must not purchase for sale on registered pharmacy premises, any product which may be injurious to public health or bring the profession into disrepute. This includes tobacco products other than nicotine replacement therapies, alcohol and products intended to mask signs of alcohol or drug consumption.

3. Pharmacy premises and facilities

The profession expects all parts of pharmacy premises to be kept clean and orderly to reflect the professional health care image of pharmacy, and to facilitate a safe system of work. The public is entitled to expect that any part of premises from which professional services are provided is readily identifiable and well maintained. The public and the profession expect a pharmacy offering professional services to have the resources to ensure competent provision of the service. These requirements apply to both registered retail pharmacy premises and hospital pharmacies.

(a) Premises must be safe for the public and people working there. All statutory requirements must be complied with, e.g. health and safety, occupier's liability, disability discrimination legislation, etc., and high standards of hygiene must be ensured.

(b) A designated area reserved for pharmacy services should be easily identifiable and arranged to enable services to be provided efficiently. Arrangements for the sale of pharmacy medicines must ensure that the sale is made by a pharmacist or a person acting under the supervision of a pharmacist. Pharmacy medicines must not be accessible to the public by self-selection.

(c) The size and organisation of the dispensary must reflect the volume and work flow, and facilitate effective communication and supervision.

(d) Refrigerators used for pharmaceutical stock must be capable of storing products between 2C and 8C. They must be equipped with a maximum/minimum thermometer which is checked on each day the pharmacy is open and the maximum and minimum temperatures recorded. Appropriate action must be taken to rectify any identified deficiency.

(e) Arrangements must be made for the regular collection and safe disposal of pharmaceutical waste and other refuse.

4. Supply of prescribed medicines

4.1 Dispensing procedures in community pharmacies and for hospital outpatients

The public is entitled to expect the service to be accurate, accessible and reasonably prompt, and the medicines to be of appropriate quality, with a sufficiently long expiry date to cover the course of treatment, and to be suitably packaged and labelled for the intended recipient. The profession expects pharmacists to seek to maintain adequate stock holdings.

(a) Dispensing must be under the supervision of a pharmacist, who must be available to intervene and advise.

(b) Every prescription must be professionally assessed by a pharmacist to determine its suitability for the patient. Pharmacists must ensure that the patient receives sufficient information and advice to enable the safe and effective use of the medicine.

(c) Pharmacists must implement procedures to minimise the risks of dispensing errors or contamination of medicines, incorporating checks to reduce special risks associated with particular products.

(d) Where a product is ordered on a prescription a pharmacist must supply a product with a marketing authorisation, where such a product exists and is available, in preference to an unlicensed medicine or food supplement.

(e) Except in an emergency, pharmacists must not substitute any other product for a specifically named product without the approval of the patient or carer and the prescriber, or a hospital drug and therapeutics committee.

(f) All solid dose and all oral and external liquid preparations must be dispensed in reclosable child resistant containers unless:

(i) the medicine is in an original pack or patient pack such as to make this inadvisable;

(ii) the patient has difficulty in opening a child resistant container;

(iii) a specific request is made that the product shall not be dispensed in a child resistant container; or

(iv) no suitable child resistant container exists for a particular liquid preparation;

(v) the patient has been assessed as requiring a compliance aid.

(g) Labelling of dispensed products must be clear and legible and include the details required by the labelling regulations under the Medicines Act and where appropriate any cautionary and advisory labelling recommended by the current British National Formulary.

(h) Where it is not possible to dispense a prescription in its entirety, the patient, their carer or representative, should be informed at the outset and be given the opportunity to take the prescription to another pharmacy. A legible note detailing the name and quantity of the medication outstanding must be provided and a record kept in the pharmacy. Wherever possible the patient, their carer or representative, must be informed when the balance will be available for collection.

(i) Dispensed medicines should normally be supplied directly to the patient or their carer in the pharmacy, where there is an opportunity for face-to-face contact, and the pharmacist has access to records and references which enable him to provide the best pharmaceutical service. Service Specification 8 must be complied with whenever dispensed medicines are not to be handed over in the pharmacy direct to the patient, their carer or representative.

4.2 Medicines for hospital inpatients

Patients, hospital staff and management teams are entitled to expect pharmacists involved in the supply of medicines to ensure that the systems in place are adequate to assure the safe and accurate supply and usage of medicines.

This service specification applies to all supplies of medicines for hospital in-patients whether supplied as ward stocks or on an individual named patient basis.

(a) Pharmacists must adopt procedures to support appropriate use of medicines and minimise the risks of dispensing errors or contamination of medicines, incorporating checks to reduce special risks associated with particular products.

(b) Medication must be clearly and legibly labelled.

(c) Sufficient information must be provided to ensure that all medicines supplied to in-patients are likely to be used safely, effectively and appropriately. Patient information leaflets must be available to the ward.

(d) Medicines brought in to hospital by patients remain the property of the patient; they must not be supplied to anyone else.

(e) All medicines returned from a ward or hospital department must be examined under the direction of a pharmacist, to assess their suitability for being returned into stock. Date expired medicines must be destroyed.

5. Patient medication records

The public is entitled to expect the best available pharmaceutical care from pharmacies. In order to provide that care, pharmacists and their staff need timely and accurate information to be held on pharmacy computer systems or in manual records.

Patients are entitled to expect that any information stored about them will be pertinent, accurate and up to date, stored securely and treated as confidential and used only for the purpose for which it is was obtained.

Pharmacists must be aware that individual patients have a right, under data protection legislation, to inspect records held about them provided that suitable notice is given.

The pharmacy patient medication record system must:

(a) be notified to the Data Protection Commissioner;

(b) incorporate access control mechanisms to minimise the risk of unauthorised or unnecessary access to patient specific data;

(c) have the facility to identify drug interactions and be able to highlight those which are potentially hazardous;

(d) provide for the collection, storage and display of patient medication records containing the following as a minimum:

(i) sufficient information about the patient to allow accurate identification;

(ii) the identity of the patient's GP;

(iii) prescription details (quantity supplied, directions, date of dispensing, any balance owed).

6. Repeat medication services

A repeat medication service is a service operated in co-operation with local prescribers, in which pharmacists will provide professional support to assist in the rational, safe, effective and economic use of medicines.

(a) The pharmacy must operate a patient medication record (PMR) system, notified to the Data Protection Commissioner, and ensure that an audit trail exists to identify each request and supply so as to enable the service to be monitored.

(b) The request for the service must come from the patient or their carer and be recorded in writing. Pharmacists may not act as the carer for this purpose.

(c) Unless this information is already available from the prescription form, pharmacists must establish with the prescriber the period for which repeat prescriptions will be issued. Pharmacists must be alert to the possibility of the patient needing earlier review. On dispensing the final repeat the pharmacist must remind the patient or their carer, preferably in writing, of the need to visit the prescriber.

(d) Pharmacists may institute a patient reminder system but may not request a repeat prescription from a surgery before obtaining the patient or carer's consent.

(e) At the time of each request the pharmacist must establish which items the patient or their carer considers are required and ensure that unnecessary supplies are not made. At this stage pharmacists must also use their professional judgment to decide whether concordance or other problems encountered by the patient may require early reference to the prescriber.

(f) Records of all interventions should be kept in order to be able to deal with any queries that may arise and to advise the prescriber.

7. Prescription collection services

Prescription collection services encompass any scheme whereby a pharmacy receives prescriptions other than directly from the patient, their carer or representative.

(a) Prescriptions must be collected by individuals acting in accordance with directions given by the pharmacist.

(b) Pharmacists must ensure that the procedures for the collection of prescriptions safeguard patient confidentiality and the security of prescriptions.

(c) The request for the ongoing service must come from the patient or carer and the pharmacy must ensure that a procedure for recording the initial request, preferably consisting of written authorisation, exists.

(d) All requests to the doctor for repeat prescriptions must be initiated by the patient or carer and be made directly to the surgery unless the pharmacy is offering a repeat medication service in compliance with Service Specification 6.

(e) On receipt of prescriptions pharmacists must ensure that the pharmacy is authorised to receive and dispense them. Any prescriptions received for which the pharmacy does not have the patient's or their carer's consent must be returned to the surgery for collection by the patient or carer or be directed to the pharmacy authorised to receive the prescription.

8. Delivery services

A delivery service is one where medicines are handed over to a patient or their carer other than on the registered pharmacy premises. The provisions detailed in this service specification also apply to rural collection points. On each occasion a service is requested pharmacists must use their professional judgment to assess whether direct face-to-face contact with the patient or their carer is necessary.

In addition to complying with all other professional requirements relating to the sale or supply of medicines pharmacists are responsible for ensuring that the delivery mechanisms used:

(a) are safe and that the medicines will be delivered promptly to the intended recipient with instructions for use. Unless alternative delivery arrangements have been made, medicines must only be handed over to the patient or their carer and before doing so the delivery person must confirm with the patient or their carer that the name and address of the patient is correct;

(b) cater for any special storage requirements of the product;

(c) enable a verifiable audit trail to be kept identifying the initial request for the service and each delivery and attempted delivery so that the service can be monitored. Wherever possible a signature should be obtained indicating safe delivery of the medicines.

9. On-line pharmacy services

The public is entitled to expect the same high quality pharmaceutical care irrespective of whether the service is provided on-line or face-to-face on pharmacy premises. At all times pharmacists must act in the best interests of the patient and seek to provide the best possible health care.

Pharmacy websites must clearly display the name of the owner of the business and the address of the pharmacy at which the business is conducted.

In addition to complying with all other professional requirements relating to the sale or supply of medicines pharmacists must ensure compliance with the following:

(a) Security and confidentiality

(i) Pharmacists must ensure that the confidentiality and integrity of all patient information is protected. All patient data transmissions must be encrypted to prevent the possibility of access by the internet service provider or any other unauthorised party;

(ii) National Health Service patient data must comply with security standards and other requirements determined by the NHS Executive;

(b) Request for supply of medicines

(i) In all cases where a pharmacy medicine is requested or recommended, pharmacists must ensure that sufficient information is available to enable a professional assessment of the request and that they have an opportunity to provide appropriate counselling or advice. Advice must be available to all prospective purchasers of general sale list medicines and vitamin and mineral supplements;

(ii) Pharmacists providing on-line pharmacy services must advise patients to consult a convenient pharmacy whenever a request for a medicine or the symptoms described indicate that the patient's interests would be better served by a face-to-face consultation;

(c) Information and advice

(i) All information related to specific products must comply with the marketing authorisation, the patient information leaflet and the Medicines (Advertising) Regulations;

(ii) Information relating to medicines must include all relevant details of contra-indications and side-effects;

(iii) Non-patient specific health care advice, such as that relating to the treatment of symptoms or specific conditions, first aid, travel precautions, etc, provided on pharmacy web sites must be of a high professional standard and the pharmacist assuming professional responsibility for the provision of that advice must be identified;

(iv) Product recommendations may only be given in respect of individual patients and a record must be kept of the pharmacist assuming professional responsibility for the recommendation;

(v) Before a patient receives a pharmacy or prescription only medicine pharmacists must ensure that the patient receives sufficient information to enable the safe and effective use of the medicine. Procedures for dealing with requests for supplies of medicines and/ or delivery arrangements must ensure that this occurs;

(d) Record keeping

(i) The pharmacy must maintain information about supplies of medicines sufficient to guard against risks of abuse or misuse;

(ii) Records must be kept to identify the pharmacist authorising every supply of a P or POM medicine following an e-mail request to purchase.

10. Sales of pharmacy medicines

The public is entitled to expect that medicines purchased over the counter will be safe, effective and appropriate for the condition to be treated and the intended recipient. The following requirements apply to pharmacy medicines intended for human use and pharmacy only veterinary medicines.

All staff whose work regularly includes the sale of pharmacy medicines must be competent and instructed to refer customers to the pharmacist where appropriate. Pharmacists responsible for the provision of professional services in a pharmacy must ensure that the following standards are observed in the sale of pharmacy medicines.

(a) Pharmacists or assistants asked for advice on treatment must obtain sufficient information to allow an assessment to be made that self-medication is appropriate, and to enable a suitable product or products to be recommended. Advice on the use of products must be provided.

(b) Pharmacists must ensure that when a product is requested by name the procedures for sales of medicines provide for professional advice and intervention whenever this can assist in the safe and effective use of pharmacy medicines. Pharmacists or assistants must provide any advice relevant to the product and the intended consumer.

(c) Pharmacists must be personally involved whenever this is necessary to provide an acceptable standard of pharmaceutical care. Assistants must be trained to know when the pharmacist should be consulted.

(d) Procedures must ensure that the particular care needed is provided when supplying products for children, the elderly and other special groups or individuals or where the product is for animal use.

(e) Pharmacists must ensure that they are involved in the decision to supply any medicine, which requires their intervention. Such medicines may include those that have recently become available without prescription, that may be subject to abuse or misuse, or where the marketing authorisation for non-prescription use is restricted to only selected conditions. Pharmacists and their staff must be aware of the abuse potential of certain OTC products and should not supply where there are reasonable grounds for suspecting misuse.

11. The supply of emergency hormonal contraception as a pharmacy medicine

Pharmacists in personal control of a pharmacy must ensure that the following standards are observed in the supply of emergency hormonal contraception as a pharmacy medicine. As with all medicines pharmacists must have sufficient knowledge of the product to enable them to make an informed decision when requests are made.

(a) Pharmacists must deal with the request personally and decide whether to supply the product or make a referral to an appropriate health care professional.

(b) Pharmacists must ensure that all necessary advice and information is provided to enable the patient to assess whether to use the product.

(c) Requests for emergency hormonal contraception must be handled sensitively with due regard being given to the patient's right to privacy.

(d) Only in exceptional circumstances should pharmacists supply the product to a person other than the patient.

(e) Pharmacists should whenever possible take reasonable measures to inform patients of regular methods of contraception, disease prevention and sources of help.

12. Complementary therapies and medicines

The public trusts pharmacists to offer informed advice on treatments and medicines, and the profession expects pharmacists to ensure that they are competent in any area in which such advice is given.

Pharmacists providing homoeopathic or herbal medicines or other complementary therapies have a professional responsibility:

(a) to ensure that stocks of homoeopathic or herbal medicines or other complementary therapies are obtained from a reputable source of supply;

(b) not to recommend any remedy where they have any reason to doubt its safety or quality;

(c) only to offer advice on homoeopathic or herbal medicines or other complementary therapies or medicines if they have undertaken suitable training or have specialised knowledge.

13. Health care information and advice

Pharmacists are encouraged to contribute to the promotion of healthy lifestyles. By increasing public awareness of health promotion issues and participating in disease prevention strategies pharmacists can work actively towards improving the nation's health.

The public and other health care professions are entitled to expect pharmacists and their staff to be able to provide up to date, accurate and reliable advice and information on a wide range of health care issues. Pharmacists and staff providing information and advice on health related issues must:

(a) have an adequate level of current knowledge and information about relevant subjects;

(b) ensure that all advice is independent and not compromised by commercial considerations;

(c) seek appropriate and sufficient information from the enquirer to enable them to provide informed advice;

(d) continually review their knowledge and keep up to date regarding new products and new policies for health promotion;

(e) be aware of local and major national and topical health promotion initiatives;

(f) work in partnership with patients and other health care professionals in seeking to promote healthy lifestyles and respect patients' rights to be involved in decisions about their health.

14. Diagnostic testing and health screening

Pharmacists working in primary care are well placed to provide diagnostic testing and health screening services to the public, who would expect any such service to be safe and accurate.

Pharmacists providing diagnostic testing or health screening services must:

(a) ensure that before providing a service all staff have completed any training required to ensure competency with the equipment and procedures to be used and in the interpretation of results. They must be aware of the limits of the tests provided. The pharmacy must have a designated area, not in the dispensary, with suitable facilities to perform the tests and provide counselling;

(b) institute and operate an appropriate quality assurance programme in order to ensure the reliability of the results produced;

(c) ensure that equipment is maintained in good order to ensure that performance is unimpaired;

(d) keep up to date with developments in the field and ensure that they are aware of current advice or local guidance on when to refer patients to their general medical practitioner;

(e) before undertaking a test provide an explanation to the patient of the procedure to be adopted and obtain the patient's consent;

(f) communicate test results to the patient in a manner in which they can be understood. Patients should be fully informed about the significance of the results and must be provided with any necessary counselling and available information;

(g) ensure that adequate documentation is maintained to enable the service to be audited.

15. Emergencies

Increasingly the public looks to pharmacists in community practice for help and assistance, sometimes in emergencies.

(a) Pharmacists must consider using their rights to make emergency supplies of medicines whenever a patient has an urgent need for a medicine. They must consider the medical consequences, if any, of not supplying.

(b) Where pharmacists are not able to make an emergency supply of a medicine they should do everything possible to advise the patient how to obtain essential medical care.

(c) Pharmacists must assist persons in need of emergency first aid or medical treatment whether by administering first aid within their competence or by summoning assistance and/or the emergency services. The Society's booklet, "Emergency first aid: guidance for pharmacists", provides guidance on action in life-threatening situations.

16. Collection and disposal of pharmaceutical waste

These services include the collection and disposal of unwanted medicines returned to the pharmacy by patients and other members of the public, or from wards, clinics or other departments in a hospital, and the disposal of obsolete pharmacy stock.

(a) Within the hospital sector pharmacists must ensure that a standard operating procedure dealing with waste management, including pharmaceutical waste, is in place.

(b) Pharmacists must ensure that a contract has been made with an authorised carrier for the collection and disposal of pharmaceutical waste at regular intervals or on demand.

(c) All pharmaceutical waste must be segregated from pharmacy stock and promptly transferred to disposal containers.

(d) Pharmacists must ensure that consignment notes and any other requisite documentation are completed and copies kept to comply with legal requirements.

17. Advisory services to nursing and residential homes

This service specification applies to any service intended to facilitate the safe, effective, and appropriate usage of medicines, dressings and appliances, their storage, stock control or disposal, and the associated record keeping in nursing and residential homes and hospices. Pharmacists providing advisory services must ensure that:

(a) they have undertaken adequate training relevant to the services being provided;

(b) they visit the home regularly by appointment. All staff visiting the home should carry identification;

(c) they have contact, regularly and as frequently as needed, with medical and nursing personnel responsible for the care and medical treatment of residents;

(d) they undertake professional assessments to ensure appropriate usage of medicines in the home;

(e) they assess and advise on procedures to ensure safe and accurate administration of medicines;

(f) all necessary supplementary information, e.g. patient information leaflets, is available at the home;

(g) they advise on the safe disposal of unwanted medicines supplied by the pharmacy and of other pharmaceutical and clinical waste, in compliance with legal requirements;

(h) adequate records are maintained to enable them to deal with any queries that may arise and to enable audit of the service;

(i) where they do not supply the medicines to the home they liaise with the pharmacy that does.

18. Domiciliary oxygen services

Domiciliary oxygen services comprise the supply of oxygen and associated equipment to a patient's home and the provision of advice on the use of oxygen in the home.

(a) The pharmacy must operate a patient medication record system, notified to the Data Protection Commissioner.

(b) The pharmacy must have the facilities, as laid down in statute, for the safe storage of oxygen cylinders and oxygen concentrators and display the required statutory warning signs.

(c) Personnel involved in the provision of domiciliary oxygen services must be suitably trained to undertake the tasks required of them and should carry identification.

(d) All patients receiving domiciliary oxygen for the first time must be visited by the pharmacist or a suitably trained and competent member of staff to instruct the patient or their carer on the use of oxygen in the home.

(e) Pharmacists must ensure that all necessary safety information is provided to the patient or their carer.

(f) Sets must be serviced regularly in accordance with the manufacturer's recommendations.

(g) Pharmacists must maintain adequate records of supplies and advice given to enable the regular audit of the service.

19. Services to drug misusers

Services to drug misusers include the dispensing and/or supervision of patient self-administration of methadone and other products dispensed on instalment prescriptions.

(a) The pharmacy must operate a patient medication record system, notified to the Data Protection Commissioner.

(b) Pharmacists must liaise with health care professionals and others involved in the care of the patient having due regard for the patient's confidentiality.

(c) If pharmacists anticipate or experience problems of unacceptable behaviour by a patient they should enter into an agreement with the patient for the future provision of the service. This should detail the services that the pharmacist will provide and also outline the pharmacist's expectations of the patient, the reasons why and any action to be taken if the patient's conduct becomes unacceptable. Pharmacists may decline to provide a service to a patient whose conduct is unacceptable.

(d) The pharmacy must not deviate from the instructions given on the prescription. Sugar- and/or colour-free products have a greater potential for abuse than syrup based and coloured products and must not be dispensed unless specifically prescribed.

(e) Patients must be treated with respect and courtesy and where self-administration occurs due regard must be given to the provision of a quiet area in order to provide some privacy for both the patient and other members of the public.

(f) Only in exceptional circumstances should pharmacists supply clean injecting equipment for drug misusers if the pharmacy has no arrangements for taking back contaminated equipment. Purchasers of injecting equipment should be advised of the availability of disposal facilities at the pharmacy and should always be encouraged to dispose of used syringes and needles safely.

20. Needle and syringe exchange schemes

Needle and syringe exchange schemes involve the provision of clean syringes and needles and the collection of contaminated equipment used by substance and drug misusers.

(a) Pharmacists must be aware of local facilities for drug misusers and have established contacts with other health care professionals involved in the care of drug misusers.

(b) All staff who may be involved in the service must be instructed on procedures to be followed to minimise risks.

(c) Supplies of syringes and needles must be made by pharmacists or trained staff.

(d) Individuals must be encouraged to return used contaminated equipment in approved disposal containers, but a supply of clean equipment must not be refused if they omit to do so.

(e) Used equipment must be disposed of, preferably by the individual, into a properly designed sharps container available in the pharmacy.

(f) Suitable arrangements must be made for the disposal of full sharps containers.

21. Extemporaneous preparation/compounding

This service specification is not intended to cover the reconstitution of dry powders with water or other diluents.

The public is entitled to expect that products extemporaneously prepared in a pharmacy will be prepared accurately, suitable for use and meet the accepted standards for quality assurance.

Pharmacists wishing to be involved in extemporaneous preparation must ensure that they, and any other staff involved, are competent to undertake the tasks to be performed and that the requisite facilities and equipment are available.

(a) A product should only be extemporaneously prepared when there is no product with a marketing authorisation available and where the pharmacist is able to prepare the product in compliance with accepted standards.

(b) Equipment must be maintained in good order to ensure that performance is unimpaired.

(c) Pharmacists must be satisfied as to the safety and appropriateness of the formula for the product.

(d) Ingredients must be of sourced from recognised pharmaceutical manufacturers and be of a quality accpeted for use in the preparation and manufacture of pharmaceutical products. All calculations and, where possible, measurements should be checked. Pharmacists must pay particular attention to substances which may be hazardous and require special handling techniques.

(e) The product must be labelled with the necessary particulars, including any special requirements for the safe handling or storage of the product, and an expiry date.

(f) Records must be kept for a minimum of two years but if possible for five years. The records must include the formula, the ingredients and the quantities used, their source, batch number and expiry date. Where the preparation is dispensed in response to a prescription the records must also include the patient's and prescription details and the date of dispensing. A record must be kept of personnel involved including the identity of the pharmacist taking overall responsibility.

22. *Aseptic dispensing services from non-licensed units*

Aseptic dispensing includes manipulations such as reconstitution, dilution and transfer of a sterile preparation avoiding microbiological contamination and maintaining a physicochemical stability, under the supervision of a pharmacist.

(a) The preparation of products intended for administration to humans must be in accordance with the principles of good manufacturing practice throughout the process. This is encompassed in the documents "Quality assurance of aseptic preparation services" and "Aseptic dispensing for NHS patients" and any subsequent revisions.

(b) The decision to prepare a product aseptically should be made in the context of the clinical needs of the patient. The pharmacist must ensure that the product complies with the standards to be expected for that product.

(c) Personnel involved in aseptic dispensing must be suitably trained to enable them to work safely and competently.

(d) The facilities and the service as a whole must be regularly audited and faults and deficiencies once identified must be promptly rectified.

23. *Patient group directions*

Pharmacists involved in writing and/or approving patient group directions are accountable for their content and must therefore ensure that:

(a) they only approve directions which comply with legal requirements;

(b) the staff training specified will enable safe operation of the patient group direction;

(c) the appropriate people have been involved in the drafting and approval of the patient group direction;

(d) they have up-to-date knowledge relating to the clinical situation covered by the patient group direction, the medicine and its use for the indications specified in the patient group direction;

(e) they are familiar with their role and responsibilities and the government advice set out in relevant guidance. (HSC 2000/026 (England only), WHC: (2000) 116 (Wales only) or HDL (2001) 7 (Scotland only).)

Pharmacists involved in the supply and/or administration of a prescription only medicine under a patient group direction must:

(f) ensure that they have up-to-date knowledge relating to the clinical situation covered by the patient group direction, the medicine and its use for the indications specified;

(g) ensure that they have undertaken any training required for operation of the patient group direction;

(h) be satisfied that the patient group direction is legally valid and that it has been approved by the relevant health authority or other NHS body;

(i) ensure that when supplies are made the agreed protocol is followed and that the information specified in the patient group direction is recorded. These records must include the identity of the pharmacist assuming responsibility for each supply.

Index